The Complete
Aromatherapy Tutor

*A structured course to achieve
professional expertise*

Joanna Hoare

with Sarah Wilson

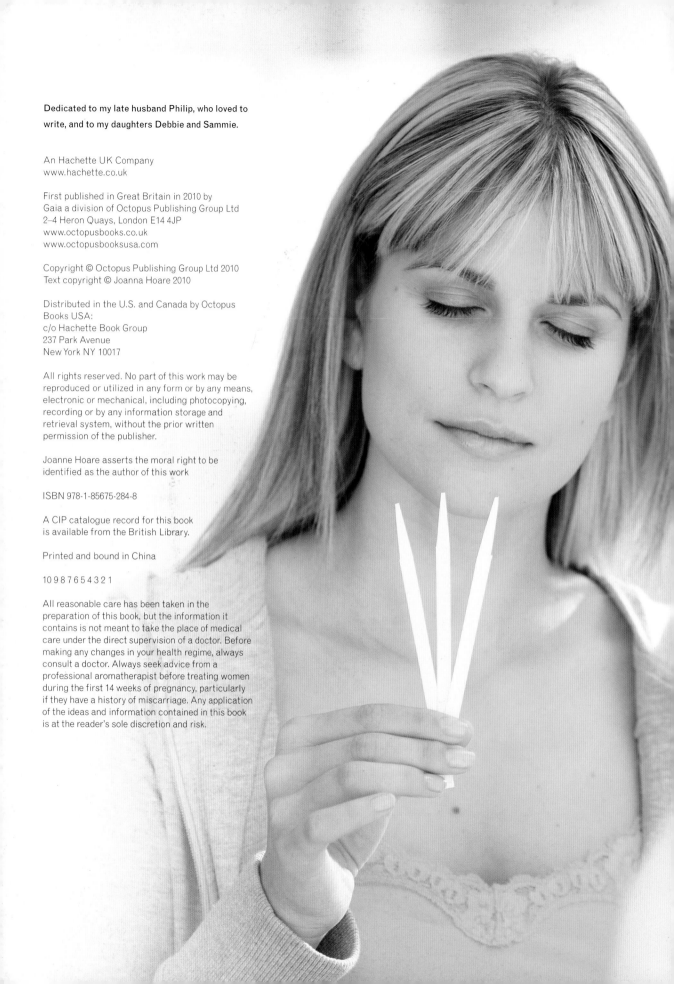

Dedicated to my late husband Philip, who loved to
write, and to my daughters Debbie and Sammie.

An Hachette UK Company
www.hachette.co.uk

First published in Great Britain in 2010 by
Gaia a division of Octopus Publishing Group Ltd
2–4 Heron Quays, London E14 4JP
www.octopusbooks.co.uk
www.octopusbooksusa.com

Distributed in the U.S. and Canada by Octopus
Books USA:
c/o Hachette Book Group
237 Park Avenue
New York NY 10017

ISBN 978-1-85675-284-8

A CIP catalogue record for this book
is available from the British Library.

Printed and bound in China

10 9 8 7 6 5 4 3 2 1

All reasonable care has been taken in the
preparation of this book, but the information it
contains is not meant to take the place of medical
care under the direct supervision of a doctor. Before
making any changes in your health regime, always
consult a doctor. Always seek advice from a
professional aromatherapist before treating women
during the first 14 weeks of pregnancy, particularly
if they have a history of miscarriage. Any application
of the ideas and information contained in this book
is at the reader's sole discretion and risk.

The Complete
Aromatherapy
Tutor

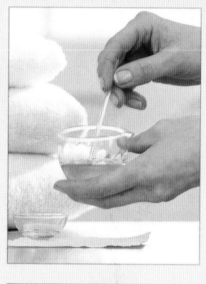 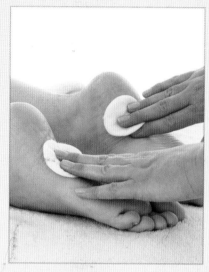 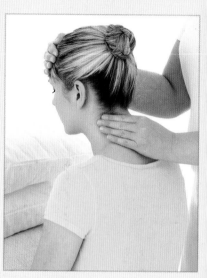

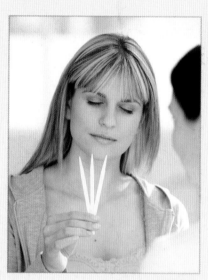 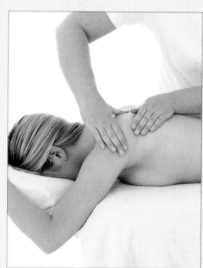 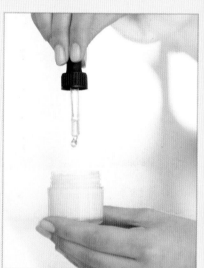

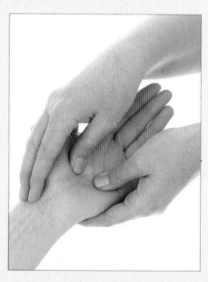 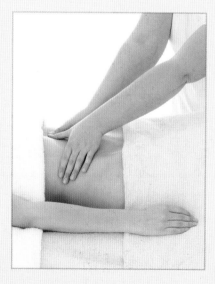 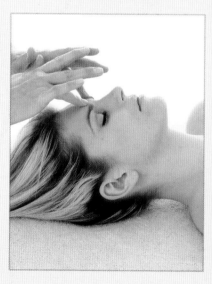

Contents

Introduction 6

How to use this book 7

1 The origins of aromatherapy 8

2 The science of essential oils 18

3 Choosing and using essential oils 36

4 Directory of essential oils 56

5 Aromatherapy massage 110

6 Body systems 158

7 Aromatherapy for special conditions 212

8 How to become a successful aromatherapist 240

Glossary 250

Index 252

Acknowledgements 256

Introduction

Plant oils have long been recognized for their healing properties. They have been used continually throughout Europe and the Far East for thousands of years.

In the West, there is evidence that the Ancient Egyptians extracted oils from plants and the Greeks and Romans used them both for hygiene and for medicinal purposes. In the East, essential oils are used in incense that is burned in temples, as they have been for centuries.

I have been an International Federation of Aromatherapists (IFA) member, examiner and principal tutor since the IFA first started their examinations at the Royal Masonic Hospital in the 1980s. Having been involved in aromatherapy for over 30 years I have seen complementary medicine, especially aromatherapy, progress from being regarded as superficial to now being accepted as one of the most popular alternative therapies.

Practitioners trained today learn that aromatherapy is a gentle holistic therapy that draws its healing powers from the plant world, helping to re-establish harmony and revitalize the malfunctioning parts of the body. The oils that are used have the ability to balance the mind, body and emotions and to make people look and feel good.

Nowadays, aromatherapy uses essentials oils for a therapeutic effect but advanced clinical aromatherapy uses the essential oils for the relief of pain, insomnia, infection and depression. Research has clearly shown that smell has a profound physiological effect and essential oils working on the nervous system, which is the most easily disturbed of the bodily systems in the modern world, help to relax or uplift the mind. I have seen this particularly in my volunteer work with cancer patients over the past ten years.

This book is a comprehensive reference for all aspects of aromatherapy and its ability to heal. I hope you enjoy it.

Joanna Hoare

The International Federation or Aromatherapists is the longest-established governing body for Professional Aromatherapy in the world. The Federation is an international organisation with training schools and members worldwide and has been at the forefront of developments within the aromatherapy profession, pioneering the use of aromatherapy in hospitals, hospices, special care units and general practice.

For more information, see the IFA website
www.ifaroma.org

How to use this book

This is a book for anyone interested in learning about or working with aromatherapy, whether you are training to become a practitioner or you are already a practising therapist.

This book gives you a complete view of aromatherapy, providing you with a thorough foundation, including an understanding of how aromatheray works and a knowledge of how to use it.

Reading through the book, you will learn about the origins of aromatherapy and about the key figures in its history and development.

The basic botanical and chemical principles behind aromatherapy are then explained in detail, before a chapter on how to choose essential oils for each client and how to blend them with carrier oils for massage.

A comprehensive directory of essential oils follows, which includes information on where each oil is from, the properties of the plant from which it is extracted, the method used to extract it and lists of complementary oils and most common uses.

A chapter on massage takes you step by step through sequences for the whole body, using photographs of a professional aromatherapist and focusing on the position of the hands and fingers. The next chapter explains basic anatomy system by system, detailing the workings of the body and how aromatherapy can be used to treat each organ or system.

Finally, there are chapters containing information on which oils can be used for specific illnesses and health conditions and on how to set up your own practice.

LEARNING STEP BY STEP

The aromatherapy massage routines are broken down into a series of steps, each one accompanied by a photograph showing you exactly how to move your hands to treat the part of the body in question. This example shows the different pieces of information that you can expect to encounter in each step-by-step massage sequence.

Photographs of an aromatherapist show you exactly how to perform each movement.

The introduction tells you exactly which part of the body you'll be working on, what position the client should be in and what the aim of the sequence is, whether it be to drain lymph, calm the nerves or release tension.

Step-by-step instructions guide you through the specific technique used, explaining the motions your hands and fingers should make and the pressure you should use.

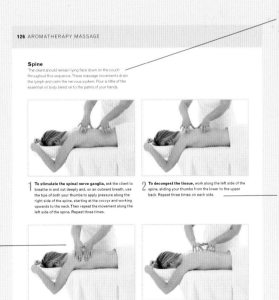

126 AROMATHERAPY MASSAGE

Spine
The client should remain lying face down on the couch throughout this sequence. These massage movements drain the lymph and calm the nervous system. Pour a little of the essential oil body blend on to the palms of your hands.

1 **To stimulate the spinal nerve ganglia,** ask the client to breathe in and out deeply and, on an outward breath, use the tips of both your thumbs to apply pressure along the right side of the spine, starting at the coccyx and working upwards to the neck. Then repeat the movement along the left side of the spine. Repeat three times.

2 **To decongest the tissue,** work along the left side of the spine, sliding your thumbs from the lower to the upper back. Repeat three times on each side.

3 Use 'butterfly' movements, catching up the skin between both forefingers. Work from the sacrum towards the head. Then work from the spine out towards the lateral side of the body in three movements. Repeat on the other side, again working from the spine out to the sides and from the sacrum towards the head.

4 Liberate the lymph: apply pressure with the fingertips along the erectus spinus muscle. Flow fingers downwards laterally. Move hands up to repeat pressure and sliding movement at mid-spine and then the top of spine.

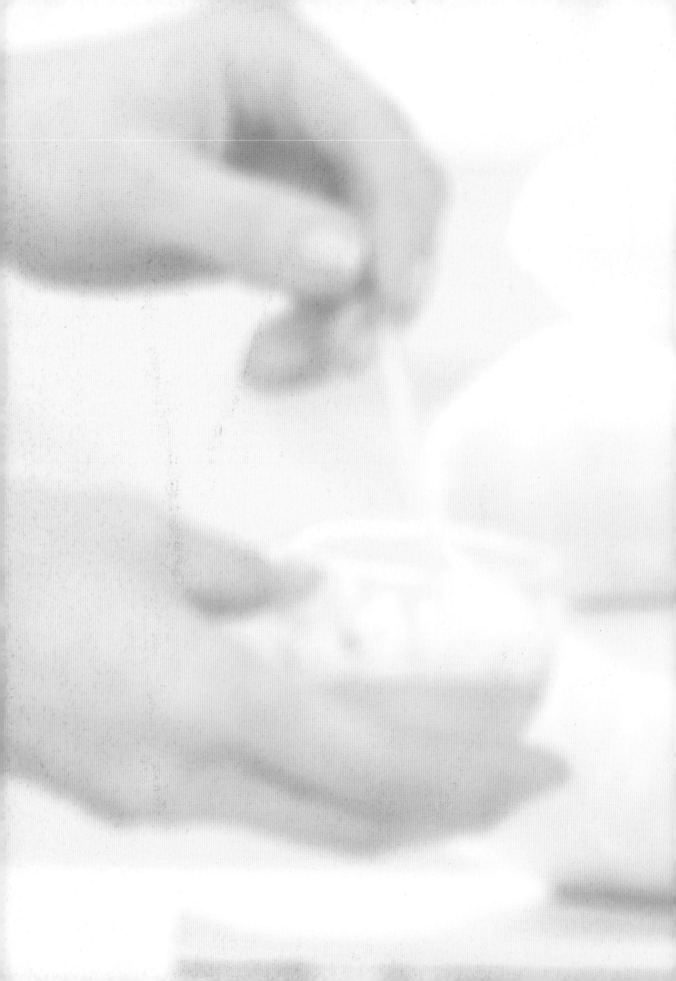

The origins of aromatherapy

Modern aromatherapy dates back to the 1930s and the work of the French chemist René-Maurice Gattefossé, who experimented with essential oils and realized their great healing potential. It is from these early beginnings, and from the pioneering work carried out in the last century, that aromatherapy developed into the widely recognized form of treatment that it is today. The use of essences from aromatic plants, however, pre-dates Gattefossé by millennia.

History and background 10

Aromatherapy today 14

Aromatherapy as a healing art 16

History and background

Aromatic extracts from plants have been used therapeutically for thousands of years and their use can be traced back to all the major early civilizations.

The ancient world

Since the earliest ages of mankind, aromatic fumigations have been used in daily rituals and during religious ceremonies as an expression and a reminder of an all-pervasive sacredness. Fragrance has been seen as a manifestation of divinity on Earth, a connection between human beings and the gods, medium and mediator, emanation of matter and manifestation of spirit.

India, where essential oils have been used for thousands of years, is probably the only place in the world where this tradition was never lost. Indian temples were built almost entirely of sandalwood to ensure that they had an aromatic atmosphere and, with a history of over ten thousand years, ayurvedic medicine is the oldest form of medical practice. The oldest surviving medical book, *Pen Tsao*, is a Chinese herbal by Chen Nang, and is dated at around 2800 BC. It contains information on over a hundred plants. As well as for medicines, the Chinese used aromatic herbs and burned aromatic woods and incense to show respect to their gods.

The Egyptians

The origins of aromatic medicine in Europe and the Western world can be traced back more than six thousand years, to the Egypt of the pharoahs. The Egyptians used a method known as infusion to extract the oils from aromatic plants, and incense was probably one of the earliest ways of using aromatics. The Egyptians took personal hygiene seriously, and the earliest recorded recipe for a body deodorant was found in the Ebers Papyrus of 1500 BC. They were practiced in massage, using fragrant massage oils after bathing, and were renowned for their skincare and cosmetics. The Egyptians were also experts at embalming, using essential oils with strong antiseptic properties so that the body tissue would be well preserved for thousands of years. The famous perfume kyphi was made by the Egyptians, but it was more than a perfume because it was also an antiseptic, a balsamic and a tranquillizer.

Egyptians practices influenced the whole of the Middle East and the Mediterranean basin. The Babylonians mixed perfume with mortar when building their temples, an art that was handed down to the Arabs, who built their mosques in the same way. King Solomon's famous temple in Jerusalem, competed in about 960 BC, was built of cedarwood and stone.

Phoenician merchants exported rich unguents and aromatic wines around the Mediterranean and the Arabian peninsula, and brought back precious cinnamon, frankincense, ginger and myrrh from their voyages to the Orient. Frankincense and myrrh were two of the Wise Men's offerings to the newborn baby Jesus.

The classical world

The ancient Greeks used aromatic substances in their bath-houses, and aromatic oils were extensively used for health. Importantly, the Greeks wrote down much of their medical knowledge, which was passed down the centuries. Hippocrates used and wrote about a great number of plant medicines, making observations that are still relevant to aromatherapy. Theophrastus wrote the first treatise on scent, which was called *Concerning Odours*. He took an inventory of all the Greek and imported aromatics and discussed ways in which they could be used. Pedanius Dioscorides wrote his book about herbal medicine, *De Materia Medica*, in the first century AD, but it remained the Western world's standard medical reference for at least twelve hundred years after his death. Much of our present medical knowledge of medicinal herbs originates from Dioscorides.

The Romans acquired much of their medical knowledge from the Greeks and went on to improve and increase the use of aromatics in hygiene, medicine and cosmetics. Galen (AD c.130–200), physician to several Roman emperors, contributed a great deal to the history of pharmacology.

The Middle Ages

During this period in Europe, neither bodies nor clothes were washed with great frequency, and aromatic herbs were strewn on the floors to help mask the smell. Glovemakers would impregnate their wares with

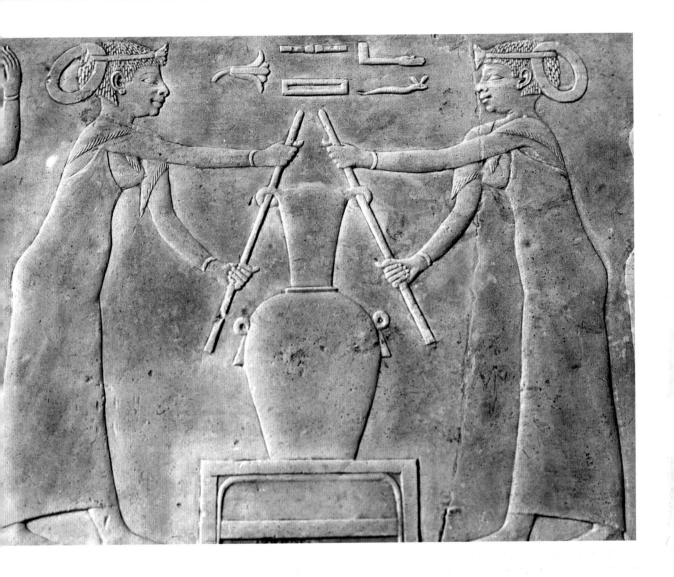

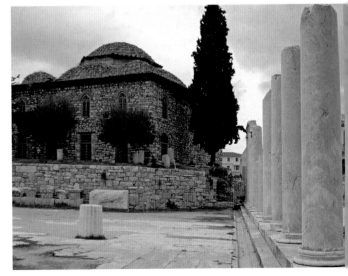

Egyptian serving women pressing flowers in a 'ling' to make medicinal oils and perfume. The ancient Egyptians extracted oils from aromatic plants for use in incense, deoderants, massage and embalming.

Ruins of the Bath House of the Four Winds (in foreground). The ancient Greeks and Romans used aromatic oils in bath houses, for hygiene purposes, and eventually used them in medicines and in cosmetics.

aromatic oils and it is recorded that these and other uses of aromatic substances were used to help survive plague epidemics. Pomanders – oranges stuck with cloves, or little bouquets of aromatic herbs – were carried to ward off infection, particularly the plague. Doctors often wore a 'nose-bag' for the same reason. It becomes clear that plant extracts were being used successfully for a variety of internal and external problems. In 1559, Conrad Gesner wrote that essential oils have the power to 'conserve all strengths, and to prolong life'.

On the other side of the world, the Aztecs were well known for their plant remedies and the conquistadors brought back knowledge of more medicinal plants and aromatic oils. Native North Americans also used aromatic oils and produced their own herbal remedies.

Parascelus, a physician, surgeon and alchemist in the 16th century, was the first to achieve and record the dissociation of active chemical agents in plants – something regularly performed today in modern pharmaceutical procedure. In the 17th century Nicholas Culpepper, a botanist, herbalist and physician, wrote his famous book *Complete Herbal*, from which people still quote today.

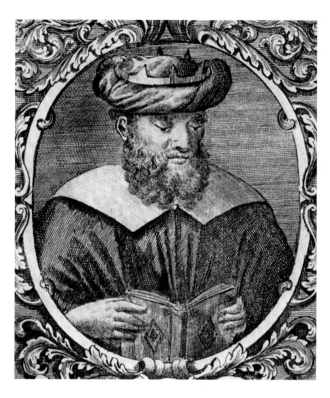

Avicenna was a late 10th- and early 11th-century Persian physician whose improvements to distillation equipment enabled him to be the first to produce a pure essential oil. He had a particular interest in rose essence.

AVICENNA

Avicenna was one of the most famous Arab physicians during a time when Arabic medicine was the most advanced in the Western world. He was born in AD 980 in Bukhara, Persia. He was responsible for improving the then very simple distillation equipment, simply by extending the length of the cooling pipe and forming it into a coil, allowing the steam to cool more quickly and efficiently, and refining the process so that a pure essential oil could be obtained for the first time. It would seem that his first successful distillation was *Rosa centifolia* from rose petals.

He wrote over a hundred books, one of which was on the beneficial effects of rose essence. Avicenna's two most famous books were *The Book of Healing*, which dealt with the natural sciences, psychology, astronomy and music, plus purely medical matters, and the *Canon of Medicine*, in which he summarized the medical knowledge of his Greek, Roman and Arab antecedents, adding his own findings to this summary. In the *Canon* he lists no fewer than 760 drugs.

The pioneers of aromatherapy

Aromatherapy as we know it today owes much to the pioneering work of French and Italian scientists during the 19th and 20th centuries.

Tuberculosis was once a very common disease in France, and it was noticed that workers in the processing of flowers and herbs stayed free of respiratory diseases. This led to the first recorded laboratory test, in 1887, on the antibacterial effects of essential oils, as it was these that were thought to be responsible for the good health of the workers. This began the earliest scientific research into essential oils and their effect on micro-organisms, carried out in France by Chamberland and validated by Cadac and Meunier. It showed that essential oils killed micro-organisms of glandular and yellow fever.

Dr René-Maurice Gattefossé, who is believed to have coined the term *aromathérapie,* was a chemist. His contribution to aromatherapeutic history is that, in 1910, he severely burnt his hands while conducting an experiment in his laboratory that resulted in an explosion. As a reflex action he immersed his hand in a nearby container that contained lavender essential oil. Gattefossé found that the pain in his hands lessened and the healing process was more pronounced from this inadvertent application of the lavender.

Between 1920 and 1930 Italian scientists conducted experiments dealing with the psychological effects of essential oils. Dr Renato Cayola and Dr Giovanni Garri discussed the effects of essential oils on the nervous system, blood pressure, breathing rate and pulse rate, both scientists having studied their stimulating and calming effects. They also observed the bacteria-destroying capabilities of essential oils.

The French army surgeon Dr Jean Valnet used essential oils as antiseptics to treat wounds and severe burns during the Indochina war of 1948–59. After the war he went on to treat patients using essential oils in his capacity as a doctor. He then began to treat patients in psychiatric hospitals with essential oils and other plant products, with great success. In 1964 he wrote *The Practice of Aromatherapy*.

Professor Paoli Rovesti conducted research on the psychological effects of essential oils on patients suffering from depression and hysteria. In 1975 he led an archeological expedition to Pakistan in order to investigate finds connected with the use of beauty products by the Indus Valley civilization five thousand years ago. In the museum of Taxilla, a town at the bottom of the Himalayas, he found a perfectly preserved distillation apparatus or still, made of terracotta. Scientific dating of this equipment placed it at 4000 BC.

Around the same time, the biochemist Marguerite Maury was researching the use of essential oils for therapeutic and cosmetic purposes. She used massage as the basis for her medical/cosmetic therapy and made a study of the way in which the aromatic essences work on the physical body, the mind and also on the skin. Her natural skincare knowledge seems to be largely based on ancient Indian and Chinese information.

The current trend in aromatherapy has much of its origins in Marguerite Maury's work. The late Micheline Arcier met Marguerite Maury at a beauty therapy conference in 1959. This led to Micheline Arcier's lifelong devotion to aromatherapy, training with both Marguerite Maury and Dr Jean Valnet.

Micheline Arcier was one of the first training establishments accredited to the well-established International Federation of Aromatherapists, which was formed in 1985 as the leading body for aromatherapy in the UK and elsewhere in the world. It has successfully laid down standards of practice as well as promoting aromatherapy to the medical profession and public alike.

MARGUERITE MAURY

Marguerite Maury (1895–1968) is known as the mother of modern aromatherapy practice. She was a pioneer of her time, starting her research in the 1940s and continuing right up until her death. Her book *Le Capital Jeunesse*, which was first published in 1961 and translated into English, as *The Secret of Life and Youth*, by Daniele Ryman in 1964, is a valuable resource for aromatherapists today. Maury worked tirelessly and discovered the value of the active zone of aromatic particles, paying particular notice to their effects through skin absorption and inhalation.

She tried to prove and demonstrate through her research the effects of essential oils and lectured all over Europe, opening aromatherapy clinics in Paris, Switzerland and England. She won international prizes in 1962 and 1967 for her research in essential oils and cosmetology. Her work lives on in modern aromatherapy and the aromatherapy profession will be eternally grateful for her outstanding contribution.

Nicholas Culpeper catalogued hundreds of medicinal herbs and in 1653 published his findings in his *Complete Herbal*, which had a profound impact on medicine.

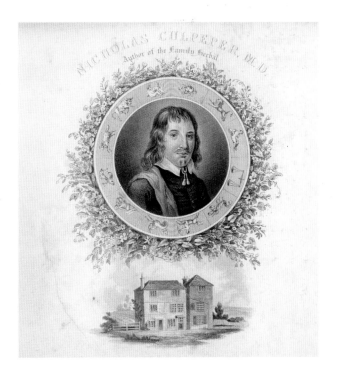

Aromatherapy today

As the medical profession has become more interested in alternative remedies, increasing evidence has emerged that aromatherapy works. As a result, the benefits are now widely recognized and aromatherapy is being taken more seriously.

Research studies

Research and clinical studies in laboratories throughout the world show the positive effects of aromatherapy. Much of this research is concerned with the antiseptic and antibiotic powers of essential oils and their allopathic (disease-countering) properties.

When applied topically, some essential oils, including tea tree, have antibacterial and antiseptic properties. There is a strong case for the use of essential oils in hospitals. As they are antiseptic, they can help prevent the spread of airborne infection, a problem in many hospitals. Tea tree oil has been studied for treating a variety of infections, and has been indicated as being as effective as antibiotics at killing off the MRSA superbug.

Since the early 1980s, researchers at Warwick University in the UK have been studying olfaction and the influence of essential oils when inhaled. Essential oils can be effective physiologically, where they work on the actual physical condition, but also psychologically, where they work via the sense of smell and the effect it has on the mind. There are many studies that demonstrate how essential oils can positively affect mood and the sense of well-being, creating either stimulating or relaxing effects: rosemary, for example, works as a stimulant, and lavender as a relaxant. Other studies have shown the beneficial effects of specific oils: peppermint oil, for example, can help keep your digestive system healthy.

Research is also being carried out in the field of coronary care, care of the elderly and sleep disorders. When applied to the skin or inhaled, essential oils are absorbed into the bloodstream and metabolized in the body. Aromatherapy may help calm agitation and improve the quality of life for those with Alzheimer's disease or other dementia, according to research in the *British Medical Journal*. It suggested that the therapy could help ease the behavioural problems common in people with dementia and help people suffering from cancer to feel more positive. There is a strong connection between touch and massage and a sense of well-being, and this is one of the guiding principles of aromatherapy.

Aromatherapy's role in complementary medicine

Aromatherapy is based on holistic principles, treating the whole person rather than a set of symptoms. ('Holistic' stems from the Greek term *holos*, meaning 'whole' or 'entire'.) It is a very humane process, based on touch, communication and dealing with people, instead of reaching automatically for the prescription pad. Therapists will establish a complete picture of an individual's case by asking detailed information about lifestyle, diet, exercise, medical history and general health. The idea is that if people are involved in their own healthcare and the advice makes sense to them, then the outcome is likely to be much better. The emphasis is on strengthening the body's immune system, and looking at the root cause of the problem and how it can be addressed.

The essential oils used in aromatherapy are chosen to improve physical and emotional well-being. Essential oils extracted from plants possess distinctive therapeutic properties, which can be utilized to improve health and prevent disease. Essential oils can be used alongside other treatments as part of an integrated approach to health problems. Some of the popular oils used in aromatherapy today include lavender (soothing, calming), rosemary (stimulating) and tea tree (antiseptic). Aromatherapy is also popular in beauty treatments, where essential oils are used in skin and bodycare products and massages to enhance the skin's condition.

Aromatherapy is compatible with all other natural therapies, with the possible exception of homeopathy. It is thought that some essential oils negate the healing powers of homeopathic remedies. However, most practitioners prefer to stick to one therapy at a time. If, for example, a patient is going to an acupuncturist and an aromatherapist at the same time, neither is going to know how much effect their particular treatment is having.

As soon as an odour molecule enters the nose it can positively affect mood, thereby improving emotional well-being, whether through stimulation or relaxation.

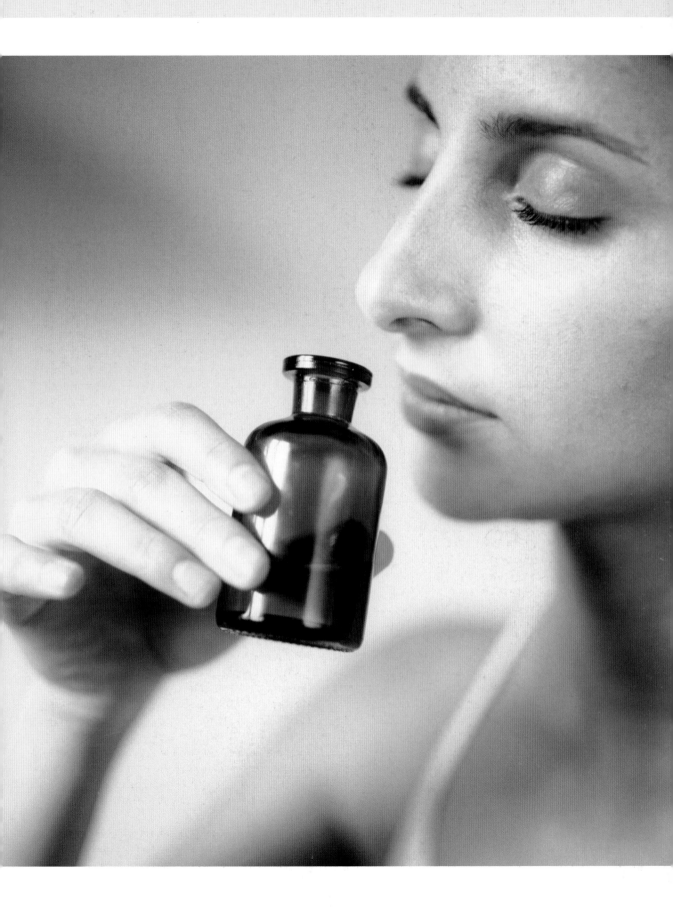

Aromatherapy as a healing art

While essential oils should not replace conventional medicine, they can play a prominent role in maintaining general health and mental well-being.

The benefits of aromatherapy

Aromatherapy is beneficial in many ways. It can provide a boost when you need to be alert or promote calmness during tense and stressful situations. People of all ages can benefit from aromatherapeutic treatment, either to get them well or to give them a general lift. The psychological benefits of aromatherapy are undisputed.

Aromatherapy is also effective as preventive medicine, having the power to boost the immune system and counteract the negative effects of stress. Life often puts great pressures on our bodies and minds: long hours at a computer screen, over-processed food, poor air quality, poor posture, lack of sleep and pressures of time and money all take their toll. Stress and sickness often go hand in hand – the term 'integral biology' is often used to describe the way in which physical, environmental and social factors interact and affect our general health and well-being.

Studies show that those therapies thought to be most beneficial are those that include massage and relaxation techniques. Indeed, one of the reasons aromatherapy is so popular today is that it is a relaxing, hands-on therapy that has wonderful benefits in terms of boosting well-being and relieving the tensions and worries that so often accompany a stressful lifestyle.

Aromatherapy is regularly used to help the physical ills and discomforts that can be brought on or exacerbated by everyday life. Peppermint and eucalyptus oils may reduce pain associated with headaches, according to researchers in Germany. They found that applying the oils with a sponge to the forehead and temples reduced the pain in over 50 per cent of cases. Essential oils, either inhaled or massaged into the skin, can help to maintain focus and energy levels throughout a long working day or when battling exhaustion or jet lag. They have been shown to be effective in increasing attention and memory, and in helping overcome ADHD (attention deficit hyperactive disorder). Researchers in America are working on a study to see if some smells can help weight loss.

Essential oils can also help with a wide range of common physical disorders, ranging from asthma to menopausal and menstrual problems, and including minor aches and pains, skin disorders such as acne and eczema, and infections such as cystitis and bronchitis. Aromatherapists do not tend to treat the more serious ailments such as epilepsy, cancer or meningitis, although aromatherapy can be of great assistance to patients in

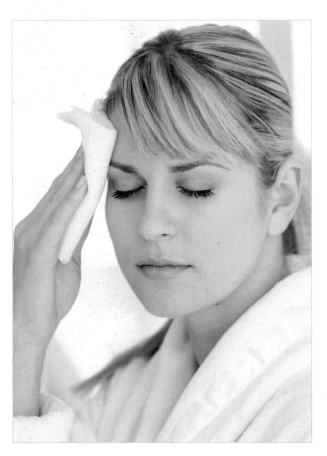

Help to reduce the pain of a headache by holding a cloth soaked in a cooling blend of essential oils to the forehead or temples.

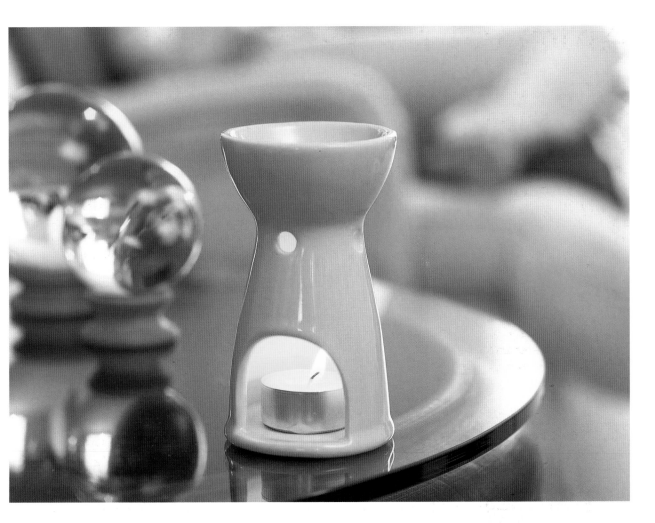

Filling a room with the aroma of essential oils can help with a wide range of physical and emotional problems, from improving headaches and increasing attention and memory, to simply relaxing you after a long day.

complementing medical treatment as long as the practitioner has the cooperation of a doctor. Chapter Seven covers how aromatherapy can help.

Most essential oils are sold in bottles that dispense the oils by the drop and these should not be used undiluted on the skin. An exception to this rule is when there is a small burn or sting. Then, a small amount of lavender (*Lavandula angustifolia*) or tea tree (*Melaleuca alternifolia*) may be used. The frequency of treatment depends very much on the skin area covered and the absorbtion of the blended essential oil. The reaction to the application of essential oils applied to different individuals varies enormously and must be taken into account.

THE HOLISTIC APPROACH TO HEALTH

In *The Secret of Life and Youth*, Marguerite Maury points out that aromatherapy treatments alone are not enough to give us health, youth and happiness. They should be supported by a healthy, balanced lifestyle. This includes eating a healthy, balanced diet that is rich in seasonal foods, not over-indulging in food or alcoholic drinks, getting plenty of regular sleep, balancing the emotions, and trying to lead a stress-free existence in which you are not constantly rushing around. Some of these things may be difficult to achieve but there is no doubt that clients will be grateful for any advice that can help to make them happier and that will support treatments in restoring vitality.

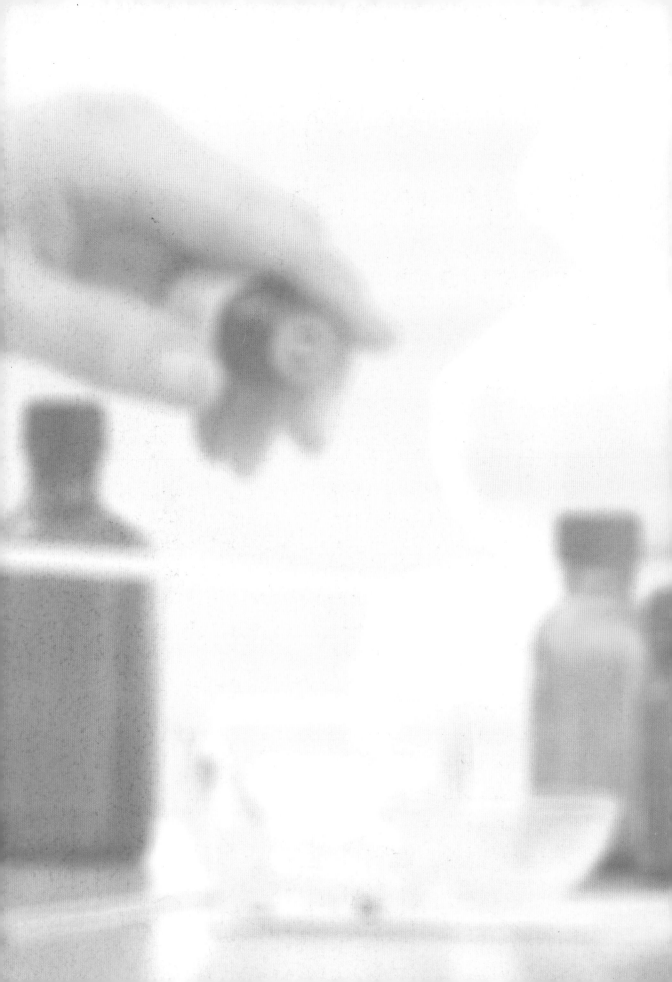

The science of essential oils

With the growing scientific interest in aromatherapy, and the increasing numbers of research projects and scientific papers being published, it is essential for aromatherapists to have a good grounding in the science behind the art. This includes the basic chemical make-up of essential oils, the life cycles of plants and how their conditions of growth affect the oils they produce. It is also important to understand something of the mechanisms involved in our perception of smells and the ways in which essential oils are absorbed by the skin, knowledge that is invaluable when it comes to choosing the appropriate oils for treatment.

Chemistry basics 20

Plant anatomy and metabolism 24

Plant classification 27

Plant aromatics 29

The sense of smell 32

Absorption through the skin 34

Chemistry basics

The essential oils used in aromatherapy have been described as a cocktail of chemicals. The chemistry relevant to essential oils is related to the types of molecules that form them, so understanding structure means looking at them at the atomic and molecular level.

Atoms

Atoms are the basic components of all substances in the physical world; they form the smallest unit of an element that can exist in a stable form. An element is a substance consisting of chemically identical atoms. As an example of the size of an atom, an ordinary aluminium bottle top is composed of about 3,500 million million million atoms of the element aluminium. Each element is designated by a one- or two-letter abbreviation. The most important elements in aromatherapy are carbon (C), oxygen (O), hydrogen (H), nitrogen (N) and sulphur (S).

Although atoms are the smallest unit, they are themselves made up of several parts. They consist of a nucleus, which contains protons and neutrons, and one or more electrons that orbit the nucleus in a series of layers or 'shells'. Protons have a positive electrical charge (+), neutrons have no electrical charge (0) and electrons have a negative electrical charge (-).

Atoms strive for stability, which happens when there is a balance of positive protons and negative electrons that produces a total electrical charge of zero. An atom of helium, with two electrons and two protons, is innately stable, but most atoms are not and therefore look to bond with other atoms to share electrons and achieve stability and make up their full complement of electrons (see box).

Hydrogen (H), the most common atom in the Universe, has the simplest possible structure. It has one proton (+) in its nucleus and one orbiting electron (-). Therefore it has one empty space in its single outer shell.

Helium (He) has two protons (+) and two neutrons (0) in its nucleus and two orbiting electrons (-). There are no empty spaces in its outer shell so this atom is stable.

Carbon (C) has six protons (+) and six neutrons (0) in its nucleus and six orbiting electrons (-): two in the first shell and four in the second shell. Therefore it has four empty spaces in its outer shell.

Oxygen (O) has eight protons (+) and eight neutrons (0) in its nucleus and eight orbiting electrons (-): two in the first shell and six in the second shell. Therefore it has two empty spaces in its outer shell.

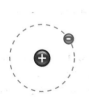

Hydrogen (H)

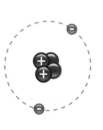

Helium (He)

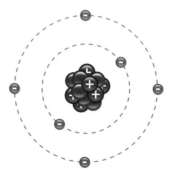

Carbon (C)

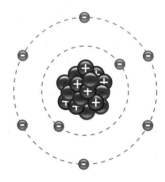

Oxygen (O)

Molecules

Atoms can bond with other atoms of the same type – long chains of carbon atoms bonded together are the basis of life on Earth – but most seem to prefer diversity. When atoms of two or more different elements bond together to form a single substance they form molecules. A molecule of water, for example, is a bond of two atoms of hydrogen and one atom of oxygen (H_2O). A molecule is a compound, in that it is comprised of more than one element, but it is not the same as a mixture: it cannot be separated and retain its identity.

The properties of a molecule depend on the nature, number and spatial arrangement of the atoms of the elements of which it is composed. The larger the molecule the lower its volatility, or ability to evaporate. The molecules of essential oils are mostly small, and so essential oils are inclined to be volatile, which means they evaporate quickly.

The chemical composition of essential oils

Almost all molecules found in essential oils are composed of carbon, hydrogen and oxygen. As atoms attach themselves to each other and bond they form molecular chains that branch off into forms that can become extremely complex. The two formations that occur most often in the molecules of essential oils are isoprene units, which consist of a branched chain of five carbon compounds, and aromatic rings. Aromatic rings can be formed by as few as three carbon atoms, but five or six is more common. The term was coined due to the sweet smell of many of the compounds formed in this way.

The chemistry of an essential oil is usually determined by two factors:

- the chemical nature of the essences synthesized by the plant, which depends both on its species and the conditions under which it is grown (see page 31).
- the extraction process. For example, the process of steam distillation extracts only the volatile and water-insoluble constituents of a plant. See Chapter Three for the different extraction processes.

There are two main classes of compounds in essential oils:

- terpenes, which consist only of carbon and hydrogen
- oxygenated compounds, which include oxygen as well as carbon and hydrogen. These are classified according to their functional groups (see page 22).

THE STRUCTURE OF ATOMS

Orbiting electrons arrange themselves in layers or shells around the nucleus. The innermost shell can contain a maximum of two electrons and, and once an atom has its full complement, electrons begin to congregate in the second shell, which can contain up to eight electrons, then in the third shell, which can accommodate a further 18 electrons, and so on.

Atoms aim to have a full outer shell of electrons. They achieve this by bonding with other atoms to effectively lose, gain or share electrons. If, in bonding, one atom loses an electron to another so they can both achieve their full complement, and this results in one of the atoms becoming positive and the other negative, they are said to have formed an ionic bond. If the atoms share electrons in order to reach their full complement they have formed a covalent bond.

Terpenes

The terpenes are a large and very important family of aromatic unsaturated hydrocarbons. (They are called unsaturated because they contain less than the maximum number of hydrogen atoms.) Their names can be recognized by the common suffix: -ene.

The molecules of terpenes consist of two or more isoprene units, and are classified according to their size:

- monoterpenes have two isoprene units and contain 10 carbon atoms (C^{10})
- sesquiterpenes have three isoprene units and contain 15 carbon atoms (C^{15})
- diterpenes have four isoprene units and contain 20 carbon atoms (C^{20}).

Terpenes occur in the chemical make-up of most essential oils (tea tree is approximately 30 per cent terpenes). Most commonly these are monoterpenes, whose high volatility and low odour means that they do not contribute greatly. Sesquiterpenes and diterpenes occur less frequently but are noted for their strong odour. Caryophyllene, for example, is a sesquiterpene that contributes to the distinctive fragrances of oils as diverse as ylang ylang, lavender and Atlas cedarwood.

Functional groups

An essential oil derives its particular fragrance and therapeutic properties from how its component atoms of hydrogen, carbon and oxygen combine in different oxygenated compounds. These fall into a number of groups, known as functional groups, which share certain characteristics. A single oil may contain dozens of different compounds from some or all of the groups, each contributing to its individual character.

Aldehydes

The suffix -al in the constituent of an essential oil indicates the presence of an aldehyde. The citrus-like fragrance of lemongrass is a very familiar and recognizable fragrance, and the aldehydes responsible for this are citral and citronellal. The latter is also found in *Eucalyptus citriadora*.

Therapeutic properties
- Local anti-inflammatory, with a direct and indirect action on the inflammation.
- Calming and soothing, directly affecting the central nervous system.
- Rubefacient, increasing localized blood flow.
- Stimulating action on the exocrine glands of the digestive tract.
- Aerial antiseptic, slowing the spread of airborne infections.
- Antifungal, having strong antiseptic properties.

Ketones

The suffix **-one** indicates a ketone, for example, verbenone (found in rosemary) and thujone (found in thuja, wormwood and sage). Ketones are hydrophilic or water-loving compounds, which means that they may also be found in hydrosols after the steam distillation of plant materials (see page 40).

Therapeutic properties
- Healing and regenerative effect on damaged skin, promoting tissue formation.
- A mucolytic action and, when in action with other chemical groups, has been found to be effective for mucopurulent conditions of the respiratory and reproductive systems.
- Essential oils with high amounts of ketones are useful for rapid reabsorption in the treatment of extensive bruising following severe injuries.

- Essential oils containing high amounts of ketones have a stimulating effect on the central nervous system, but may have a neurotoxic effect after prolonged use.

Alcohols

The suffix -ol indicates a member of an alcohol group, for example, linalol (in petitgrain and thyme) and geraniol (in rose, rose geranium and palmarosa). These essential oils also have substantial proportions of monoterpene alcohols.

Therapeutic properties
- Anti-infection – antiseptic, bactericidal and antiviral.
- Diuretic – causes increased production of urine.
- Immunostimulant – helping the immune system.
- Heart-toning – working on the circulatory system.

Acids

Organic compounds of this type are rarely found in significant quantity in essential oils. The most common examples are benzoic acid, which is found in benzoin, and geranic acid, found in geranium. Acids have a low volatility. However, when an acid is combined with an alcohol is produces an ester, which is a major aromatic compound.

Esters

These molecules are found in an essential oil as a result of the addition of an alcohol to an acid. An easy way of recognizing an ester is by the suffix -yl on the name of the alcohol, and -ate on that of the acid, for example, the addition of acetic acid to linalol produces the ester linalyl acetate. Esters are usually very fruity and fragrant. Those present in essential oils are highly volatile, that is, they evaporate quickly when exposed to the air. The highest level of esters are produced on the full bloom of the flower.

Therapeutic properties
- Sedative – directly calming the central nervous system.
- Antispasmodic – some esters are powerful

spasmolytics. (The antispasmodic properties of Roman chamomile are largely influenced by its ester content.)

- Antifungal – some esters are active against the fungus *Candida*; for example, linalyl acetate found in high concentrations in lavender, clary sage and petitgrain. Geranium contains esters that give it considerable antifungal properties.

Phenols

As phenols share some but not all of the properties of alcohols, they share the same suffix -ol, for example, thymol and carvacrol, which may cause some confusion. Phenols are some of the most beneficial molecules for anti-infectious use. An example is thymol, found in thyme, and eugenol, found in basil.

Therapeutic properties

- Bactericidal, fungicidal, viricidal and parasiticidal.
- Highly stimulating and have a marked anti-asthmatic effect due to their dilating action on the bronchi.
- Strong antispasmodic effect on smooth muscle.
- Immunostimulant.

Oxides

As oxides are usually derived from alcohols, they keep the name of the alcohol with the addition of 'oxide'; for example, linalool oxide. A common example of an oxide found in essential oils is cineole, commonly known as 1,8 cineole, the main constituent of eucalyptus.

Therapeutic properties

- Strong expectorant – oxides stimulate the mucous glands of the respiratory tract.

Lactones and coumarins

Lactones are known by their common names, as the chemical names are too lengthy. These names tend to end with -in; for example, helenalin in arnica, but can also end with -one; for example, umbelliferone, found in umbelliferous plants such as carrot and angelica. Lactones have an enhanced ketonic action (see boxes) that is shown by their strong mucolytic action. Coumarins are derived from lactones and their names similarly tend to end with -in or -one.

Therapeutic properties

- Lactones stimulate the liver.
- Coumarins have a special affinity with the central nervous system. They are:
  - anti-convulsive, calming and sedative
  - anti-coagulant
  - sudorific – acting on the nervous system to encourage perspiration.

IMPORTANT INFORMATION ABOUT LACTONES AND COUMARINS

If used incorrectly, essential oils containing a high percentage of lactones or coumarins are potentially neurotoxic. They may burn the skin and are also known to cause skin allergies. Fortunately, they only exist in small amounts in most essential oils.

Coumarins and their related **furocoumarins** may produce photosensitivity and should not be administered before sunbathing or sunlamp treatments. **Bergaptene**, the furocoumarin contained in bergamot is well known for its UV-sensitizing effect. It is thought to affect the DNA in the cells responsible for the production of the skin pigment melanin. A lack of melanin means that the skin is no longer protected from UV rays, which can cause burning or even skin cancer.

CAUTIONS

The application of large quantities of aldehydes to the skin may have an irritant or sensitizing effect.

Use essential oils with high amounts of ketones with care.

Ethers are also identified by the suffix '-ol' but in aromatherapy the only ether of importance is anethol, which is found in high levels in aniseed oil. The oil is predominantly spasmolytic and carminative and used as an aid to digestion.

Phenols may cause a fever-like reaction (hyperthermia). All phenolic compounds may produce slight liver toxicity, which becomes noticeable when they are used in high doses for extended periods of time.

The presence of cineole in *Eucalyptus globulus* means it should not be used on young babies because it is too strong and closes the air sacs.

Plant anatomy and metabolism

Every aromatherapist should have a basic understanding of the anatomy of plants and their life cycle, in order to appreciate how a plant's formation and growth influence the style, quality and therapeutic power of the oil it produces.

Cells and tissues

Plants are composed of different types of cells. Like animal cells, these basically consist of a cell membrane that encloses the cytoplasm and a nucleus, together with distinct structures known as organelles, which have various functions in the cell (see page 160 for the structure of a human cell). However, unlike animal cells, plant cells are surrounded by a rigid cellulose cell wall, which prevents moisture escaping from the cell.

An organelle of particular importance is the chloroplast, which is found mainly in the cells of the leaves. Chloroplasts contain the green pigment chlorophyll (from the Greek words *chloros*, meaning 'green' and *phyllon*, meaning 'leaf'), which capture the energy of sunlight and play an essential role in photosynthesis (see page 26).

The cells are arranged into tissues, which can be described according to their functions:

- packing tissue (or parenchyma), which is a soft tissue with large spaces between the cells; this sometimes secretes oils or resins of interest to aromatherapists
- supporting tissues, which are fibrous/woody and help to support the plant and transport water and nutrients
- glandular tissue, which contains various structures that produce gum, mucilage, resins, oils and so on.

The root system

A plant's root system serves two functions and is typically formed of two types of root. A series of large branching roots or a single long deep root (taproot) anchors the plant in the soil, and a mass of finer, fibrous roots are responsible for absorbing minerals, nutrients and water that are then transported to the leaves to be converted into nutrition for the plant (see page 26). Roots also provide a means of storing nutrients, and some plants develop notably swollen storage depots (tubers): potatoes are a common example.

In addition to the true root system, many plants develop structures that can be mistaken for roots because they develop at or below ground level:

- Rhizomes are modified stems, with a series of swollen nodes, which grow just beneath the soil surface, e.g. ginger (*Zingiber officinale*).
- Bulbs are modified buds used as storage organs, e.g. members of the onion family (*Allium* spp.)
- Corms are swollen stems used for storage, e.g. crocus (*Crocus* spp.) and water chestnut (*Eleocharis dulcis*)

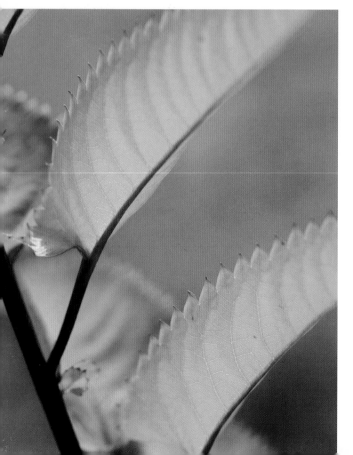

The size, shape and structure of leaves vary according to the method used by a particular plant to process chlorophyll, transport and store food and water, and to defend itself. Chlorophyll is vital in processing sunlight for photosynthesis.

Flower section This shows the male and female parts that are involved in fertilization and reproduction.

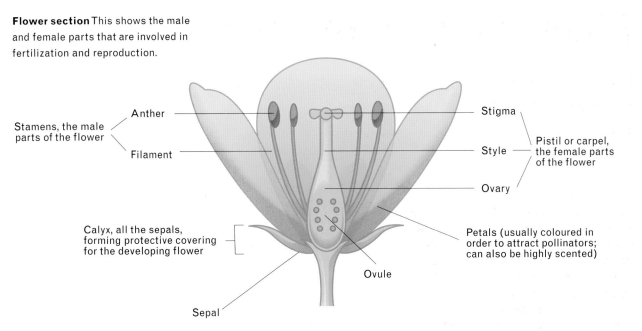

Stamens, the male parts of the flower

Anther

Filament

Stigma

Style

Pistil or carpel, the female parts of the flower

Ovary

Calyx, all the sepals, forming protective covering for the developing flower

Petals (usually coloured in order to attract pollinators; can also be highly scented)

Ovule

Sepal

The shoot system

The part of the plant that is above the ground is known as the shoot system. This consists of the supporting stems, stalks or trunk and branches, the leaves and, in the case of the majority of plants, the flowers.

Stems or trunks

These provide structural support for the plant and provide the means by which water, minerals and storage substances (such as glucose) move around the plant through specialized tissues, called xylem and phloem, which are continuous throughout the root, stems and leaves. In some herbaceous plants, the stems as well as the leaves and flowers are aromatic.

Leaves

Leaves are a plant's organs of respiration and transpiration, carrying out gaseous exchange in a similar way to the human lungs (see Photosynthesis and transpiration, page 26). Their structure, shape, size and texture varies enormously according to their particular adaptations for photosynthesis, water metabolism, food storage and defence. Many leaves are aromatic.

Flowers, fruits and seeds

Although there are exceptions, most plants reproduce sexually, by pollination, and the role of the flower is to attract pollinators. How they do this depends on the pollinator they wish to attract, which is why some flowers have brightly coloured petals or alluring markings or (if they need night-time pollinators) petals of a luminous whiteness. Smell is another strong attractant (see Plant aromatics, page 29).

Bracts are colourful modified leaves that protect the flower of some plants.
Perianth describes the petals and calyx together, especially if they cannot be distinguished from each other.
In some species, the male and female parts are formed on different flowers or even on different plants.

Once pollinated the role of the flower is over. The petals will drop (some may remain for some time but change colour to indicate that pollination has taken place); scent will fade. This explains the importance of timing when harvesting flowers for making essential oils.

The seeds that will produce the next generation of plants can take a multitude of forms, from tiny grains that are wind-blown to new locations to nuts in a hard protective casing or stones surrounded by a fleshy fruit. A number of seeds provide essential oils for aromatherapy, including avocado, black pepper and apricot kernel.

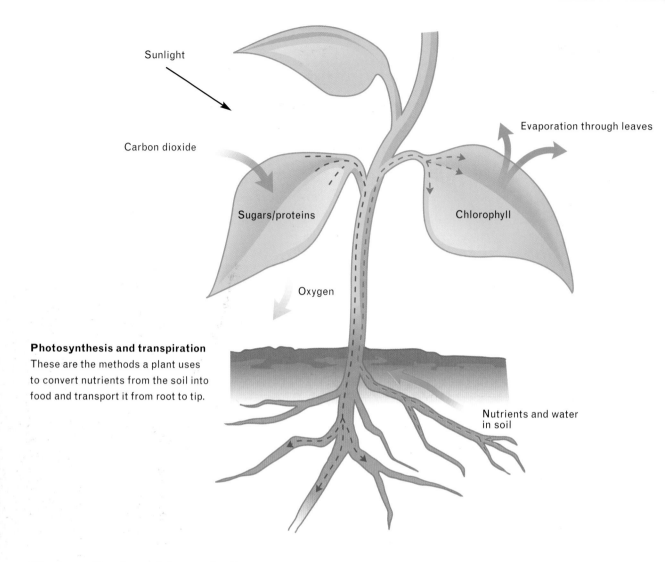

Sunlight

Carbon dioxide

Evaporation through leaves

Sugars/proteins

Chlorophyll

Oxygen

Photosynthesis and transpiration
These are the methods a plant uses
to convert nutrients from the soil into
food and transport it from root to tip.

Nutrients and water
in soil

Photosynthesis and transpiration

Unlike animals, which obtain their energy from the foods
that they eat, green plants can make their own food by
metabolizing basic elements in a series of physical and
chemical processes.

Photosynthesis is a chemical reaction that occurs
naturally in the leaves of green plants when they are
exposed to light. It converts the basic nutrients the
plant has absorbed through its roots into the starches,
sugars and proteins it needs to flourish.

Photosynthesis can only take place if the following
factors are present:

- a supply of energy in the form of sunlight
- water
- carbon dioxide, which diffuses naturally into the leaf
  tissue from the surrounding air
- chlorophyll, the green pigment in the chloroplasts.

In the presence of sunlight, which is captured by the
chlorophyll, the carbon dioxide reacts with the water
to form a carbohydrate (such as the sugar glucose) and
oxygen. The plant then breaks down the sugar in order
to obtain the energy for growth and reproduction, and
releases the oxygen into the atmosphere.

It is the evaporation through the leaves that creates
the suction that pulls water and the nutrients it bears in
through the roots and right up through the plant's entire
height. This process is known as transpiration. The
cellular structure of the plant then permits a return flow
of the photosynthesized nutrients throughout the plant in
a process called translocation.

Only during the 20th century has a scientific
understanding developed of the way plants are able
to trap sunlight and convert it to chemical energy,
although even now some of the steps in the process
are still not understood.

Plant classification

Plant identification is very important in aromatherapy – for example, the lavender oil extracted from *Lavandula angustifolia* will not be the same as that extracted from *Lavandula latifolia*. In addition, a knowledge of the family to which a plant belongs can guide you in the choice of oils and an understanding of how they work.

How plants are classified

Plant are classified according to shared features that reflect their natural and evolutionary relationships with other plants, based on the accumulated research and interpretation of structure and development by generations of botanists. They are usually based on features such as:

- the structure, number and position of the leaves on the stem
- the shape and positioning of the flowers and the numbers of their component parts (petals, stamens, etc.)
- the structure of the fruit.

Using these criteria, the plant kingdom breaks down into a series of ever more specific groupings, according to the number of features that each group has in common.

The basic unit is the **species**, abbreviated as sp. (singular) and spp. (plural). Individual plants of the same species share a common ancestry, are nearly identical in structure and behaviour, and are relatively stable in nature.

Closely related species that have features in common are grouped together in the same **genus** (plural genera), Genera that have features in common are grouped together as a **family**. Families are grouped within a **class** and classes within an **order**. The three levels of classification that are of most interest to aromatherapists are family, genus and species.

Plants in the same family tend to produce their essential oils in particular parts. For example species in the Lamiaceae and Myrtaceae families produce their essential oils mostly in the leaves, the Rosaceae family mostly in the flowers, and species of the Rutaceae family (which covers all the citrus plants) produce them in the flowers, fruits and leaves.

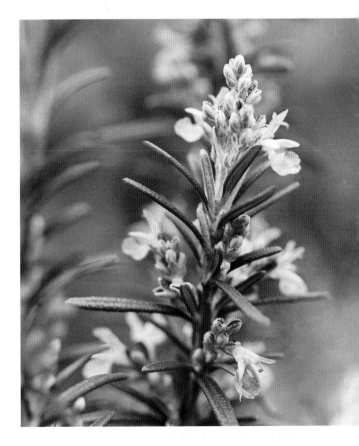

The large Lamiaceae family This family includes many herbal plants that yield useful essential oils. Despite the variety of shapes and styles, they have a number of features in common, including the arrangement of their leaves and their seedheads (four 'nutlets' inclosed by the calyx). A particular distinguishing feature is the flower. It has four or five petals, the larger bottom petal forming a lip (the former family name was Labiatae or 'lipped'). The flowers usually occur in dense clusters or whorls near the junction of the leaf and stem; and usually have four (rarely five) stamens.

Nomenclature

The binomial system of plant naming, devised by Linnaeus, enables us to identify every plant species precisely. Each species is given a botanical name in Latin consisting of two parts:

- The **generic name**, which identifies the genus (like a surname, or family name, e.g. Smith)
- The **specific name**, which identifies the species (like a given name, e.g. Roger).

For example, the damask rose is *Rosa damascena*: *Rosa* is the genus name and *damascena* is the species name. It is a convention that these names should always be in italics, and the generic name, but not the specific name should always start with a capital letter. Family names are also capitalized but not italicized.

The species name can often provide a useful clue about the plant – *damascena* indicates that this was a rose originating from Damascus (or at least that area of the Near East). A specific name may relate to, among other characteristics, who first identified the plant, where it originated or its growth habit. Recognizing indicators

such as *rubra* (red) or *officinalis* (used for medicinal or culinary purposes) can help you become familiar with these botanical names.

Plant species can further divide into several categories. These differences may not always be apparent to a non-botanist, but they can influence the type and quality of the oil a plant produces.

Subspecies (subsp. or subspp.) are a distinct subdivision of a species that has developed differently, often due to geographical isolation. Their names are written as, e.g. *Lavandula stoechas* subsp. *lusitanica*. Lesser distinctions within a species may be labelled **variety** (var.) or **forma** (f.), written as, e.g. *Lavandula stoechas* var. *rosea*, *Lavandula stoechas* f. *leuchantha*. Human hybridization of plants has produced many cultivars, distinguished as, e.g.: *Lavandula stoechas* 'Kew Red'. See also Chemotypes, page 31.

The geographical location is also useful in identifying chemotypes. Basil oil from the Comoro Islands is the methyl chavicol chemotype whereas Australian Basil has a much sweeter linalol chemotype odour and this latter chemotype would be more sedating and relaxing whereas the former would be useful for alertness – often said to give a 'whiff of oxygen' to a tired brain.

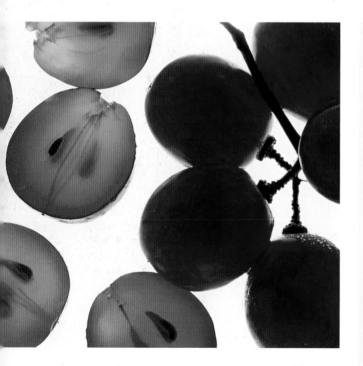

The binomial system of plant naming sees each plant given two Latin names – one which identifies its genus and one which identifies its species. Thus grapeseed is known as *Vitis* (meaning vine) *vinifera* (meaning wine-bearing).

EARLY CLASSIFICATION SYSTEMS

Taxonomy – the naming of plants and animals and their classification into groups (or *taxa*) – is one of the oldest branches of the science. Several systems of classification have been proposed over the centuries. In ancient Greece, for example, Pliny used size and shape to establish three primary groupings: herbs, shrubs and trees. In the Middle Ages, plants were grouped according to their use into: medicinal, edible and poisonous. Many common names describing how specific plants were used are still current, such as lungwort (*Pulmonaria* spp.) for lung diseases.

In the 18th century, the great Swedish botanist Carolus Linnaeus established a classification based on the number of stamens. His system has been superseded as science has refined how we see plants' relationships to each other, but his binomial system of nomenclature (see above), which replaced the clumsy and confusing naming systems that preceded it, is still the standard today.

Plant aromatics

The aromatic substances that plants produce are part of their means of survival. The nature of this aroma varies from family to family, from species to species and even within different parts of the same plant.

Why do plants produce aromatic substances?

Plants are thought to produce aromatic substances – volatile, essential or ethereal oils – for two reasons: as a defence, to deter animals from eating them, or as an attraction, to ensure pollination or seed dispersal. Plants may adopt one or both of these strategies. The western azalea (*Rhododendron occidentale*), for example, has skunk-scented leaves to deter browsers and sweetly perfumed flowers to attract pollinators.

Defence – aromas in leaves

The leaves of many plants are covered with tiny cells containing aromatic oils. Many of these oils belong to a family of chemical compounds known as terpenes (see page 21). These oils not only make the leaves unappetizing or nauseating to animals searching for food, but they also evaporate readily on hot days, cooling the surface of the leaves. In addition, some terpenes are thought to inhibit the growth of neighbouring plants and seeds when carried into the soil on water droplets.

Attraction – aromas in flowers

The fragrance, colour and shape of flowers, either alone or in combination, serve to attract pollinators. Some flowers produce a fragrance that is only perceptible at short range, sometimes only when the pollinator has already landed on the flower; other fragrances attract pollinators from much greater distances.

The nature of a flower's fragrance varies according to the type of pollinator that it wishes to attract. Fragrances to attract bees and butterflies are typically pleasantly sweet, while flowers such as the night-blooming jasmine (*Cestrum nocturnum*), which need to attract night-time moths, are heavier and cloying. Not all odours designed to attract are pleasant: some plants exude a smell like rotting meat, to attract fly pollinators. It is interesting to note the animal/human communication – for instance, evaporating molecules may irritate the mouth of a grazing animal or they may repel certain insects. On the other

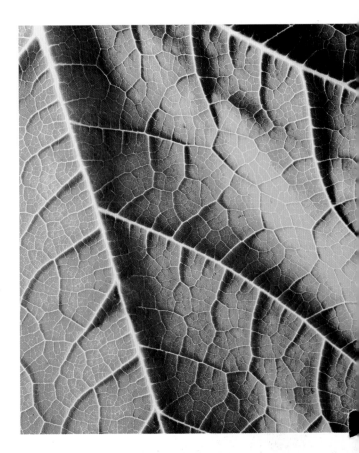

The surface of an aromatic leaf is covered with cells containing aromatic oils. If you crush an aromatic leaf, such as a peppermint leaf, between your fingers, the cells release the oils and you get a wonderful burst of aroma.

hand we know that bees are particularly attracted to mints and lemon balm.

The strength of a plant's aromatic oils is also related to how and where it is grown: some tropical aromatic plants prefer the heat and sun to give off their heady perfumes whereas in a more temperate climate the plant odours are more subtle (see *Terroir*, page 31).

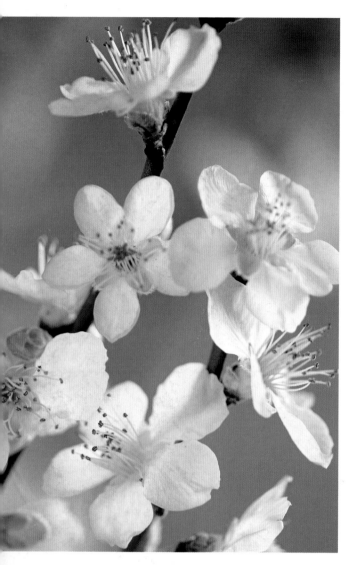

Sweet almond blossom *(Prunus dulcis var. amygdalis)* is the source of a commonly used carrier oil which is obtained from the kernels of the plant by cold pressing.

Oil-producing structures

Different plant cells produce different types of oil. This explains the differences in the chemical composition of the volatile oils produced in the leaf, the stem and the flower of a plant. The fragrant essences of flowers are usually secreted by epidermal cells in the petals, whereas the production of oil by other parts of plants usually involve oil-secreting hairs.

The surfaces of many plants are pubescent, meaning that they are covered with hairs (or trichomes). These hairs may occur over the entire surface of the plant or just certain parts, such as the leaves or the calyx of the flower, and may be fine or coarse. Those that are designed to secrete oil contain specialized secretory tissues, which develop from a single epidermal cell with a large nucleus and dense cytoplasm (see Cells, page 24).

Secretory hairs can either be **capitate** (have one or two head cells) or **peltate**, having as many as ten head cells. In the peltate hairs, the walls of the head cells separate from the outer cuticle, forming a space and causing expansion of the cuticle. It is in these spaces that the oil is stored.

Oil-storage structures

Oils are stored in various structures in plants, and the capacity of a plant varies according to its species, age and the age of its individual secretory cells.

Glandular cells, hairs and scales

These are single- or multi-celled protuberances, or 'pockets' on the surface of the plant's epidermis. Plants that store oils in this manner include thyme (*Thymus vulgaris*), sweet marjoram (*Origanum marjorana*), rosemary (*Rosmarinus officinalis*) and other members of the Lamiaceae family.

Oil cells and resin cells

Plants that devote special cells (still living in some cases) to storing oil or resin include members of the laurel family (Lauraceae), such as cinnamon (*Cinnamomum zeylanicum*) and ravensara (*Ravensara aromatica*).

Oil or resin canals

Some plants have developed tubular canals or ducts, formed by the expansion of the spaces between neighbouring glandular cells. These can be found in the seeds of umbellifers (Apiaceae) such as sweet fennel (*Foeniculum vulgare*) and coriander (*Coriandrum sativum*). Conifers also have resin canals from which large quantities of resin can be extracted. Some resins are collected by 'tapping', which involves piercing the bark of the tree and collecting the resin as it oozes out.

Oil reservoirs

These are formed when the walls of the secretory cells break down, creating a small sac which acts as an oil reservoir. (This is called secondary cavity formation and the reservoir is known as a lysigenous reservoir.) Members of the citrus family are particularly noted for their oil reservoirs.

Terroir and chemotypes

The French word *terroir*, often used in the wine industry, summarizes the effects of the growing conditions on a plant and therefore on the essential oil it yields. These conditions include:

- soil – the type of soil and its depth, texture, fertility and drainage, which can vary widely according to geographical situation
- location – altitude, sunny or shaded, sheltered or exposed, flat or sloping
- weather – the amount of rainfall and the time of year it falls can directly affect the size of flowers and seeds and the concentration of chemicals in the plant. Wind can also affect growth. Year-to-year variations on the same site can also be significant.

Samples of oil from otherwise identical plants grown in different regions or under different conditions are likely to have a different mixture of chemical compounds. This difference is described as a chemotype. Each essential oil is characterized by its chemotype. It may help to think of this as a 'recipe' for the oil that explains the mixture of compounds that it contains. For example, there are three main chemotypes of rosemary (*Rosmarinus officinalis*), respectively containing: camphor-borneol, 1,8 cineole and verbenone (see Functional groups, page 22). The chemotypes of such plants are often written as, e.g.(*Rosmarinus officinalis*) ct. borneol.

Just as *terroir* is a determining factor in the type of wine produced by the grapes on a vine, the type and quality of the soil and its exposure to the elements have an effect on plants from which essential oils are produced.

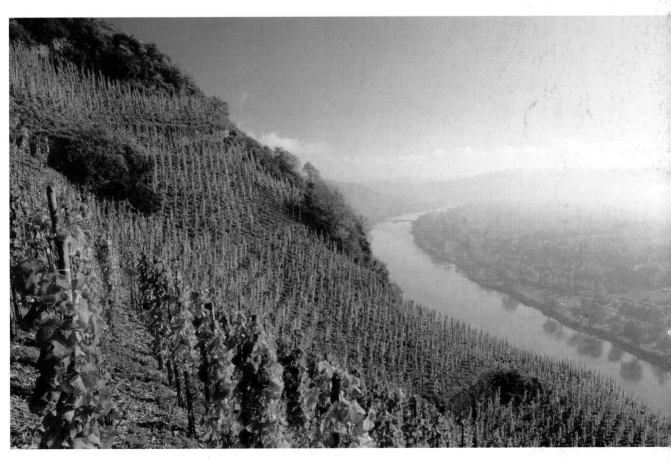

The sense of smell

The sense of smell or olfaction plays a very important role in aromatherapy. The human sense of smell is both primitive and sophisticated, and makes a fundamental contribution to our health and sense of well-being. Searching for the mechanism that triggers our sense of smell and the feelings it evokes is like a fascinating journey to the centre of the brain.

The physiology of olfaction

In order for a substance to be smelled it must be volatile, so that the molecules can enter the nostrils. The substance must be water-soluble, so that it can dissolve in the mucus in the nasal passages and thus make contact with the olfactory cells the mucus contains. It must also be fat-soluble, since the plasma membranes of the olfactory fibres are largely fatty.

As air is drawn through the nose, it is warmed and any odiferous molecules, like those of essential oils, dissolve in the mucus, which covers the lining of the nasal cavity. Located at the top and on both sides of the inner nasal cavity, approximately at eye level, is the olfactory bulb. This is little more than 1 cm (½ in) in diameter and is covered with a mucous membrane. This membrane, called the olfactory epithelium, is lined on both sides with a special tissue, consisting of about 10 million olfactory cells covered with a thin layer of mucus.

The cells of the olfactory membrane are nerve cells: this is the only place in the human body where the central nervous system is exposed and in direct contact with the environment. These nerve cells are replaced every 28 days. Each individual nerve cell bears a bundle of six to eight tiny hairs (or cilia), which are equipped with receptor cells. The structure of odour molecules is such that they fit, like pieces of a jigsaw, into a specific position on the receptor cells. Scientists have been studying for a long time how precisely odour molecules stimulate these tiny bundles of cilia before being carried to the brain by nerve cells in the form of electrical impulses.

The hairs attached to the nerve cells – up to 80 million of them – are capable of carrying a vast amount of information, more than any other known human analytical process. With every breath we take, we receive minute pieces of information about our environment. Our sense of smell has been highly tuned since birth, so it has a huge effect on us throughout life.

How we perceive smells

The sense of smell acts mainly on a subconscious level. It can be divided into two categories: primary (or instinctive) and secondary (learned by experience).

Primary sense of smell

This is part of our survival kit. A baby quickly learns to recognize the scent of its mother, and this forms part of the bonding process. The sense of smell means we can identify odours that are related to food or danger. At puberty we are subconsciously attracted to potential sexual partners by hormonal odours called pheromones.

Secondary sense of smell

From the moment we are born, our sense of smell grows and develops as we become increasingly aware of different odours, recognizing and associating them with pleasant or unpleasant experiences. The link between smell and emotions and memory is vital. This range of perceptions varies from person to person. In perfumery, the most important creator of a beautiful perfume is known as 'the nose' and can identify up to three thousand different scents. It can take up to 20 years to develop this skill.

Olfaction and aromatherapy

The acts of hearing and seeing require an energy stimulus in the form of sound or light. The sense of smell, on the other hand, simply requires the presence of an odour molecule, which is registered in the brain when air is exhaled or inhaled. Sharp, pungent odours, such of those of vinegar and ammonia, are carried by a particular set of nerve cells that respond to stimulation by these molecules, but fragrant substances pass on to the limbic system (like many other stimuli) without being registered by the cerebral cortex. They reach the innermost control centres in our brain, the place where information about

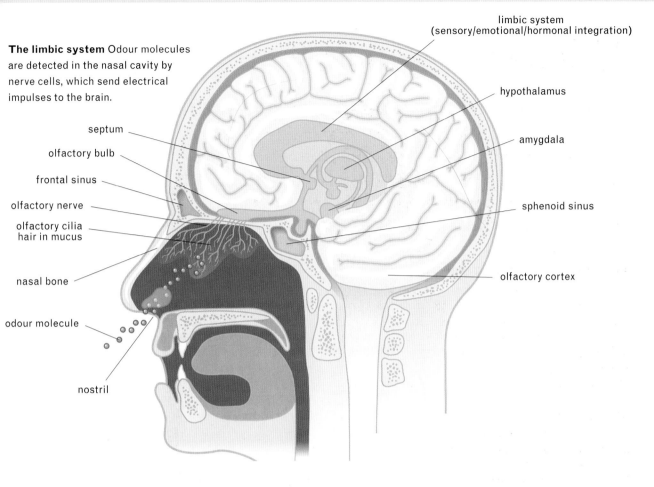

The limbic system Odour molecules are detected in the nasal cavity by nerve cells, which send electrical impulses to the brain.

limbic system
(sensory/emotional/hormonal integration)

hypothalamus

amygdala

sphenoid sinus

olfactory cortex

septum

olfactory bulb

frontal sinus

olfactory nerve

olfactory cilia
hair in mucus

nasal bone

odour molecule

nostril

THE LIMBIC SYSTEM

In terms of evolution, the limbic system (once actually called the olfactory brain) is one of the oldest parts of the brain. Its main components (the amygdala, thalamus, hypothalamus, pituitary and pineal glands, and hippocampus) are variously associated with the emotions, particularly pleasure, pain, anger, fear, sorrow and sexual feelings, as well as memory (both long-term and short-term), behavioural patterns, learning and mental activity. Some of these also play a role in regulating the body's responses to stimuli. The direct link between the olfactory receptor cells and the limbic area of the brain explains why smells can produce an emotional response and revive a past memory (scent memories persist for longer than visual memories). This is why certain odours can conjure up memories of past occasions.

odours is stored. In other words, our subconscious receives and responds to an odour before we are consciously aware of it.

This direct interaction with the nervous system and the brain is what gives essential oils so much of their therapeutic power, especially in the way they can affect mental activity and the emotions, which are controlled by the limbic system.

In part because of its complex relationship with memory and the emotions, our perception of individual fragrances is quite subjective, and the next chapter (in particular pages 50–55) looks in more detail at how odours can be analysed and the importance of creating pleasant as well as effective blends. Aromatherapists are not expected to become expert 'noses', but they must learn to educate their noses.

Aromas through the ages have been used to promote a sense of well-being and, if used correctly, they can be a powerful tool that can help us reconnect with nature. If the odour of an essential oil conjours up some pleasant associations, the psychological effect can help to balance the body and mind.

Absorption through the skin

The skin is the body's largest organ, and its ability to absorb essential oils provides the aromatherapist with the second principal way in which to introduce their therapeutic qualities into the body. The skin is also described as the body's integumentary system.

The skin's permeability

Skin accounts for approximately 12 per cent of our total body mass and one of its main functions is to protect against foreign substances entering the body. The skin, therefore, allows very little to penetrate it. Indeed, until 50 years or so ago it was assumed that the skin was completely impermeable. However, this is not entirely true. Microscopic substances (up to about twice the size of the average essential oil molecule) can be absorbed into the body, especially if, like essential oils, they are fat-soluble.

The first and principal barrier to absorption is the epidermis. This is breached by hair follicles and gland openings, and hydrophilic (water-attracting) molecules will find their way through the epidermis via the skin's sweat glands, while lipophilic (fat-attractive) molecules will enter via the sebaceous glands. (The structure of the skin and its various layers are described in detail in Chapter 6, see page 164.)

The skin The molecules of essential oils are small enough to be absorbed into the skin through hair follicles, sweat and sebaceous glands.

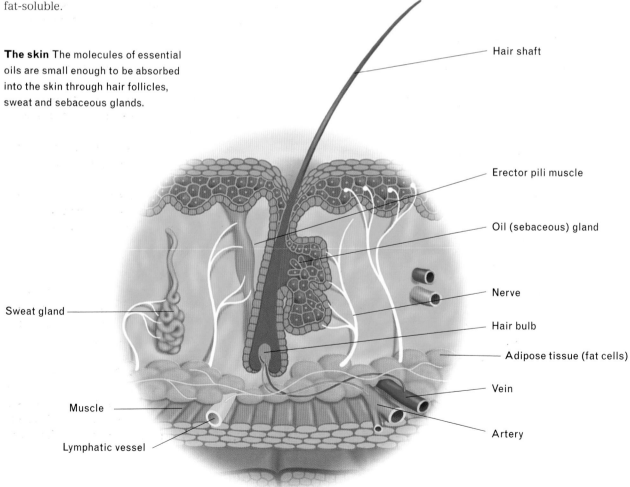

Hair shaft

Erector pili muscle

Oil (sebaceous) gland

Nerve

Hair bulb

Adipose tissue (fat cells)

Vein

Artery

Sweat gland

Muscle

Lymphatic vessel

The epidermis varies in thickness, being thickest on the soles of the feet and the palms of the hands and thinnest on the eyelids. Its permeability also varies: the skin on the legs, for example, is less permeable than the forehead or the inside of the wrists.

Below the surface

The epidermis has no supply of blood vessels, but once the essential oils have passed through to the dermis below they encounter the myriad blood vessels and lymph network that form a dense network at this level. They can then enter the blood and lymph circulatory systems and move swiftly around the body.

Absorption via the skin rather than via the digestive system gives the added advantage of entering the bloodstream directly, rather than passing first through the liver, which may filter part of their content. Additionally, because essential oils are fat-soluble, they are able to cross the blood–brain barrier and thereby enter the brain.

Rates of absorption

Several factors influence the rate at which essential oils can penetrate the epidermis. Skin that, through age or sun damage, is very dehydrated absorbs oils less easily, as its own reservoir cells of natural oils have diminished. Gender also makes a difference: a woman's additional subcutaneous fat layer means that her absorption of fat-soluble chemicals is generally higher than a man's.

The main variable of help to aromatherapists is temperature. Skin that is perspiring heavily inhibits absorption, because sweat glands cannot allow

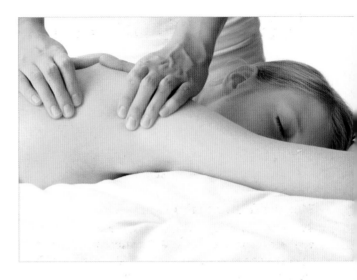

Aromatherapy massage is a relaxing treatment which encourages essential oils to penetrate the skin through the sweat and sebaceous glands.

substances to pass in through them while they are exuding moisture. Warm skin, on the other hand, is receptive, because:

- the warmth of the skin lowers the viscosity of the oil, facilitating its absorption
- warmth causes the blood vessels in the dermis to dilate, making it easier for the essential oils to enter the bloodstream
- the increased rate of blood flow near the skin's surface speeds the distribution of oils around the body.

As the rate of absorption increases to a greater extent if the skin is damaged or broken, it is very important to avoid these areas, thus preventing skin sensitization and skin irritation.

Methods of application

All the points above emphasize the advantages of an aromatherapy massage as a pleasant and effective means of encouraging absorption. A frequently used alternative method is a compress, to treat only a particular part of the body.

Essential oils are volatile, some highly so, and will evaporate quickly if allowed to do so. For this reason, it is always advisable to cover up those parts of a client's body that are not actually being massaged. The techniques of aromatherapy massage are explained in full in Chapter 5 (see page 110).

AN AROMATHERAPEUTIC BATH

Adding essential oils to bathwater is often recommended as a home treatment (see page 150). The number of drops advised for a bathful of water (only 6–8, and then diluted in a carrier oil) may seem too few to be effective, but super-hydrated skin absorbs the oils extremely effectively, and the warmth and relaxation of a bath are conducive to further encouraging the oils to penetrate the skin. There is also the added bonus of inhalation as the oils evaporate into the air around.

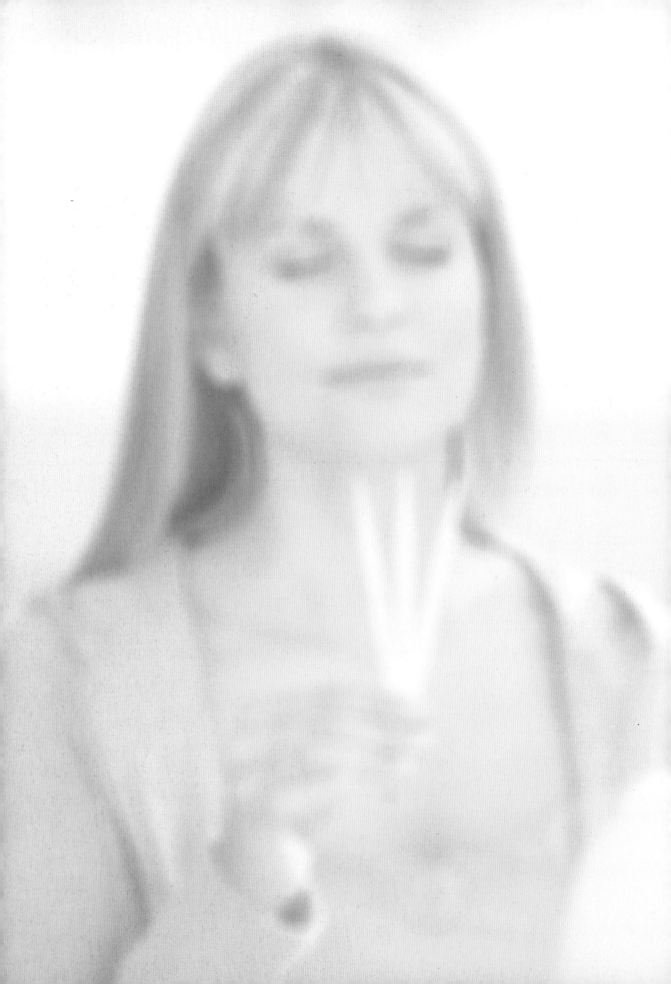

Choosing and using essential oils

Essential oils are extracted from an enormous range of plants using a variety of methods. Understanding both the time-consuming traditional methods and newer systems involving expensive equipment explains why pure, unadulterated essential oils are so prized and, in some cases, so costly. Once extracted, essential oils have the power to relieve, relax, stimulate and heal, but to realize their potential an aromatherapist needs to learn the art of blending them successfully.

Sources of essential oils 38

Distillation 40

Other methods of extraction 42

Buying essential oils 45

Carrier oils 46

Blending essential oils 50

Sources of essential oils

Essential oils form only the tiniest part of a plant's make-up. Different amounts of oil are produced by different species of plants, and by different parts of a plant, which is why some oils are more difficult to extract than others.

What is an essential oil?

Essential oils are sometimes referred to as essences but this is not strictly speaking correct. An essence is a substance produced by a plant in specialized secretory cells, which are found in the leaves, flowers, bark or roots, or in the fruit pulp or peel, usually near the surface. The essences are stored either in these cells or in special storage cells. An essence only becomes an essential oil after distillation. Only in a few cases, for example, citrus essential oils, is the essence itself used (see page 44).

PROPERTIES OF ESSENTIAL OILS

- Essential oils are usually liquids, although some (such as benzoin and rose otto) are semi-solids.
- Despite their name, they are usually non-greasy.
- They are volatile, evaporating in air to various degrees, and flammable. Consequently, they should always be stored in a cool place and kept away from naked flames.
- They are soluble in oil and alcohol, although they only form a suspension in water.
- They are aromatic, which is important in treatment.
- They are very powerful when undiluted, so they are usually diluted with a carrier oil or fat, or alcohol.

Most plants yield only one type of oil, and from a specific part of the plant. For example, basil (*Ocimum basilicum*) and pine (*Pinus sylvestris*) produce their essences in the leaves, while the carrot (*Daucus carota*) produces its essences in the seeds. The bitter orange (*Citrus aurantium* var. *amara*), on the other hand, produces three different oils, which are extracted by three different methods.

Methods of extraction

Once harvested, the plant material has to be processed in order to extract the plant essences. There are several different methods, most very labour-intensive. The processes of distillation and alternative methods are described on the next pages.

End products and by-products

The different methods of extraction described on the following pages vary in their suitability for certain plants, and some also produce by-products also used in aromatherapy or perfumery.

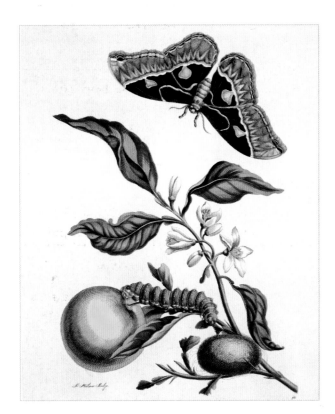

Bitter orange (*Citrus aurantium*) is the only plant that produces three different oils: bitter orange from the fruit, petitgrain from the leaves and neroli from the flowers.

Advantages and disadvantages of principal extraction methods

Extraction method	Advantages	Disadvantages
Distillation	An economical method of extracting large quantities of oils with simple apparatus	Involves high temperatures, which may affect the structure of the oils
Solvent extraction	Involves only low temperatures so is less damaging to the constituents of the oil	May contain solvent residues
Carbon dioxide extraction	Involves only low temperatures so is less damaging to the constituents of the oil	Very expensive because of the high-pressure equipment needed
Hydrocarbon extraction/ phytonic process	Fast and accurate	Expensive
Maceration	N/A	Slow and labour-intensive (now rarely used)
Enfleurage	Involves only low temperatures so is less damaging to the constituents of the oil	Very time-consuming and labour-intensive
Expression	Expressed oil is not subjected to heat	This process can only be used for citrus oils

Aromatic substances derived from plant materials

Distillation		Expression	Enfleurage	Solvent extraction		Maceration	
▼	▼	▼	▼		▼	Alcohol	Oil
essential oils	hydrosols	essences (citrus oils)	pomades	extracts	resinoids	▼	▼
			▼ ▼	▼	▼	tinctures	essential oils
			soap enfleurage absolutes (by alcohol extraction)	concretes	essential oils (by distillation)		
				▼			
				absolutes			

Distillation

Distillation is a centuries-old technique, traditionally carried out by small-scale artisan distillers. It follows the same principles as the distillation of spirits such as brandy or whisky.

Preparation

Flowers and leaves generally need very little preparation prior to distillation, although they sometimes need to be cut or grated in order to break down the walls of the plant cells and allow the volatile oil to escape. Likewise, hard fruits, seeds and bark may be reduced to small pieces or powder (a process called comminution) before distillation in order to expose their oil cells to the boiling water. Some leaves, such as patchouli (*Pogostemon cablin*), are left to ferment for a brief period in order to break down the cell walls.

Distillation involves heating a liquid or solid to a temperature at which it vaporizes, passing it through the plant material and then cooling the vapour, now containing the essences to be extracted, until it condenses back into a liquid or solid. Two main types of distillation are used in the production of an essential oil: water distillation and steam distillation.

Water distillation

The plant material is placed in the distillation vessel, together with a sufficient quantity of water, and the still head clamped into position. As it is heated the water boils, softening the plant material and releasing the essential oils from the oil glands. The oils vaporize, and the vapour (with the odour molecules) is carried up and into the condenser in the current of steam produced by the boiling water. In the condenser, the steam and essential oil vapour condense into their respective liquids, which then collect in the receiver.

Because the essential oil is less dense than the water, it separate outs, forming a layer on the surface of the condensed water. The oils are then drawn off and, if necessary, treated with anhydrous sodium sulphate to remove any residual water. The oil is then filtered and put into suitable containers for storage and transportation.

Steam distillation

This is a similar process, using the same principles, but steam from a separate boiler is injected into the distillation vessel and passed through the plant material. The pressure of the steam is greater than that of the atmosphere, so that its temperature is above the normal boiling point of 100°C (212°F). Volatile constituents that are insoluble in water are driven off in the steam, which, when cooled in the condenser, collect in the receiving vessel, as for water distillation.

Steam distillation extracts the essential oils more quickly than water distillation, minimizing the damage to the compounds in the oils. It is also good for the extraction of volatile compounds from the terpene family (see page 21).

There are also processes that are variations on these two main methods. Steam and water distillation is a hybrid between the two, as steam is generated in a separate apparatus and then passed through the still, which is filled with plant material and water.

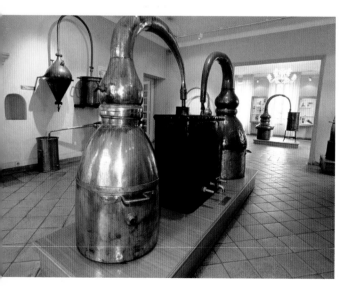

Early copper stills were very decorative and can be seen at the Parfumerie Museum in Grasse, a town in France that has had a perfume industry since the end of the 18th century.

Most essential oils are produced by distillation, the principles of which involve heating the relevant part of the plant, which releases the oil as a vapour, which is then condensed into the essential oil and water in the receiving tank.

Warmed outflow

Cooling condenser

Vaporized water and essential oils

Oil-yielding plant material

Cold water inflow

Cooled vapour and essential oil

Steam or heated water

Essential oil

Flower water (hydrosol)

Hydrodiffusion is a variation of direct steam distillation, the main difference being that the steam is introduced at the top of the still rather than at the base. Condensation of the oil/steam mixture occurs inside the still, directly below a perforated tray that supports the plant matter being processed. The advantages of this method are a lower consumption of steam, a shorter processing time and an increased yield of oil.

Redistillation (rectification)

Any essential oil containing non-volatile matter may be purified by redistillation, either in steam or by vacuum extraction. Redistillation is known as rectification and the products are known as rectified oils. Essential oils can be redistilled at different temperatures – a process known as fractional distillation – in order to obtain certain constituents and exclude others. Fractional distillation is similar to normal distillation, but the essential oil is collected in batches during the course of the redistillation instead of being continuously collected. These batches are called fractions. The fractional distillation of ylang ylang (*Canaga odorata*), for example, yields ylang ylang extra and ylang ylang No. 1, No. 2 and No. 3. The fractions of camphor (*Cinnamomun camphora*) are known as white, yellow and brown (the brown fraction is considered to be a hazardous essential oil and is not used by aromatherapists).

Cohobation is another type of distillation process mainly used for the extraction of Rose otto, redistilling the rose water and reeturning it to the original distillate.

HYDROSOLS

A hydrosol (also known as a hydrolat or floral water) is the water that is left after the essential oil has been removed from a distillate. It can only be produced during the distillation process and can be described as a 100 per cent non-alcoholic distillate. Hydrosols are not perfumed sprays, nor are they water to which droplets of essential oil have been added. They cannot be manufactured synthetically in the laboratory. Examples include rosewater and lavender water.

In his book *Medical Aromatherapy*, Dr Kurt Schnaubelt comments that aromatic hydrosols contain water-soluble, volatile components of a plant that often give them a fragrance similar to that of the essential oil but not as strong. Their composition also differs, being richer in water-compatible components and free of substances such as terpenes. This makes aromatic hydrosols highly tolerable, anti-inflammatory and antiseptic.

The use of hydrosols is now becoming more popular in aromatherapy. Some are used as toners or, in the case of tea tree (*Melaleuca alternifolia*) hydrosol, as an antiseptic foot-wipe before an aromatherapy massage.

Other methods of extraction

The other principal methods of extraction usually involve washing or immersing the plant material in a gas or solvent that absorbs the plant material's essential oils, sometimes along with other substances.

Solvent extraction

This is a very gentle process compared with distillation because it has less effect on the arrangement of the compounds in the essential oils. It is used for plants whose essential oils would be degraded by distillation, which applies when the plant material:

* cannot be heated, e.g. jasmine (*Jasminum officinale*)
* contains low concentrations of oil, e.g. rose (*Rosa centifolia*)
* contains resinous material, e.g. benzoin (*Styrax benzoin*).

Solvent-extracted oils have a richer fragrance, but non-volatile constituents, such as waxes and plant dyes, are extracted along with the essential oils.

The aromatic material is put in a closed vessel containing an organic solvent (acetone, benzene, propanone or hexane) which 'dissolves out' the oil, natural waxes, resinous material, chlorophyll and other pigments. The plant residue is repeatedly washed with the solvent to maximize the yield. The resulting solution is known as an **extract**.

The solvent is then removed by placing the extract in a still at a reduced pressure, which lowers the boiling point of the solvent so that only gentle heat is required to drive off the solvent, but not the essential oil, from the extract.

When cooled, the concentrated extract solidifies to a waxy consistency known as a **concrete**, which consists of up to 50 per cent odourless wax. The wax is removed by washing the concrete with alcohol, into which the essential oils dissolve. The alcohol mixture is then chilled and filtered, and the alcohol removed by vacuum extraction. The final residue is called an **absolute** (see box).

If the residue from the initial extraction is resinous, it is known as a **resinoid**. Benzoin (*Styrax benzoin*), myrrh (*Commiphora myrrha*) and frankincense (*Boswellia carteri*) are all resinoids. If they contain sufficiently volatile aromatic constituents, many resinoids will yield essential oils when distilled. Like concretes, resinoids are employed in perfumery as fixatives to prolong the effect of the fragrance. They are always base notes.

Carbon dioxide extraction

Supercritical (or hypercritical) carbon dioxide extraction is a relatively new method. It uses carbon dioxide at very high pressure to dissolve essential oils from a wide range of plant material. It has several advantages:

* The essential oil is not affected by heat
* The extraction is almost instantaneous (it takes just a few minutes) and is complete
* Because the solvent is virtually inert, there are no chemical reactions between the solvent and the aromatic substances.

By comparison, steam distillation takes up to 48 hours, it always leaves some residues of essential oils behind and many substances are oxidized in the process. The whole process takes place in a closed chamber, which means

ABSOLUTES

The main absolutes of interest to aromatherapists are the absolutes of rose (*Rosa damascena* or *R. centifolia*), jasmine (*Jasminum officinale* or *J. grandiflorum*) and neroli (orange blossom; *Citrus aurantium*). Absolutes have extremely high perfuming and therapeutic powers, and they generally need to be used in lower concentrations. They are normally coloured and are usually thicker and more viscous than essential oils, Rose absolute, for example, may solidify in the bottle at room temperature but quickly becomes liquid again when warmed in the hand.

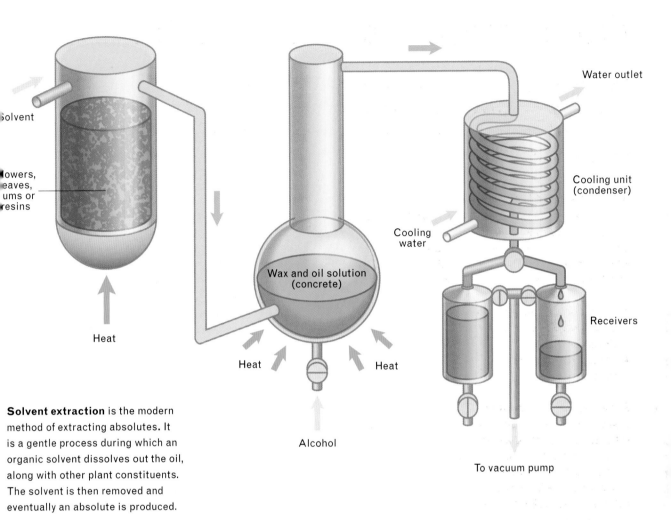

Solvent

Flowers,
leaves,
gums or
resins

Heat

Wax and oil solution
(concrete)

Heat

Heat

Cooling
water

Alcohol

Water outlet

Cooling unit
(condenser)

Receivers

To vacuum pump

Solvent extraction is the modern method of extracting absolutes. It is a gentle process during which an organic solvent dissolves out the oil, along with other plant constituents. The solvent is then removed and eventually an absolute is produced.

that even the most volatile and fragile fractions of the fragrance can be collected. Although the equipment is large and extremely expensive there are several processing plants around the world, all producing oils of excellent quality.

Hydrocarbon extraction

This method uses a hydrocarbon solvent, such as petroleum ether or hexane, to extract resinoids from naturally resinous materials such as balsams, resins, oleoresins and oleo gum resins, such as frankincense and myrrh. Resinoids can be viscous liquids, semi-solid or solid, and non-crystalline in character.

The phytonic process

This is a new, highly efficient and economical method of solvent extraction that uses environmentally friendly solvents, below room temperature and in a sealed

apparatus, to extract essential oils (phytols) from plants. This method ensures that the very delicate and heat-sensitive constituents of the essential oil are neither lost nor altered during extraction.

Maceration

To macerate in alcohol, the plant material (suitably broken down) is mixed with alcohol of an appropriate strength, then placed in a closed vessel and stirred occasionally until all the alcohol-soluble substances have passed from the plant into the alcohol. Then alcohol is then filtered and adjusted to correct the odour strength and allowed to mature (like wine) until its bouquet is perfectly smooth and representative of the best features of its natural source. This is called a **tincture**.

Macerating in oil involves placing the plant material in hot oil, which absorbs the plant's aromatic essence. New plant material repeatedly places the old until the oil is

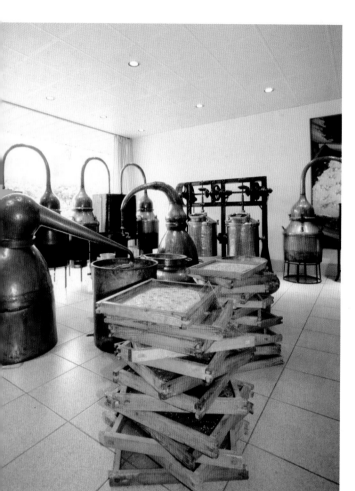

In the traditional method of enfleurage, freshly picked delicate flowers are spread on layers of fat and stacked in tiers. Over the course of many days the petals are renewed until the fat can absorb no more oil.

aromatic fat is known as a **pomade** and resembles a cream perfume. The oil is extracted from the pomade by diluting it in alcohol and then evaporating the alcohol. The remaining fat is used commercially to make soap. This laborious and expensive process has now been largely replaced by solvent extraction.

Expression

Expression is used solely for plants of the citrus family and, strictly speaking, produces an essence rather than an essential oil. It is similar to the process of cold-pressing used in the extraction of extra virgin olive oil from olives.

We are all familiar with the spray of oil that is released when scoring or zesting the skin of an orange or lemon. This happens because the oil in the citrus fruit is contained in little sacs just under the surface of the rind.

Manual expression involves cutting the fruits in half, removing the pulp and soaking the skins in warm water to soften them. They are then inverted around a sponge. This ruptures the oil cells and releases the oil, which is absorbed by the sponge. When saturated, the sponges are squeezed and the oil is collected into a vessel and then decanted.

This process has been largely superseded by mechanical methods. Whole fruits are fed from a hopper into a rotating drum containing rows of spikes that strips them of their outer peel, which is then pressed to extract the essence. The essence is rapidly separated from the other material, but there is a greater chance of enzyme action affecting the quality of the oil. The process (known as scarification) is usually carried out in a factory that produces fruit juice in order to maximize profits by using all parts of the fruits.

Expression is especially good for obtaining top notes (see page 50), such as bergamot (*Citrus bergamia*) and lemon (*Citrus limon*), which are very volatile.

Choice of extraction method

Different essential oils are created through a variety of extraction processes. The choice of extraction depends on the nature of the raw plant material and, although 90 per cent of essential oils used by aromatherapists are obtained by distillation, there are other plants too delicate to go through this process, such as Jasmine and Violet. Also resinous plants such as Benzoin must undergo solvent extraction and some citrus fruits must undergo expression.

perfumed. It was the traditional method of extracting the fragrance from rose petals in Persia, and the French perfumery house of Fragonard in Grasse still uses this type of maceration (followed by filtration to extract the essential oils).

Enfleurage

This traditional method of extracting the finest quality essential oils from delicate flowers such as violet, rose and jasmine is now almost obsolete, although Parfumerie Fragonard still obtains its essential oils in this way.

Sheets of glass in a wooden frame, called a chassis, are coated with a thin layer of fat, usually purified lard or beef fat. Freshly picked petals are spread by hand on the frames, which are stacked in tiers. As the fat absorbs the essence from the petals, faded petals are replaced by fresh ones. This is repeated until the fat can no longer absorb any more oil, a process that can take many days (three weeks in the case of jasmine). The resulting

Buying essential oils

The therapeutic properties of an essential oil depend on its chemical composition. In order to ensure that the oils you are using are pure and will have the desired effect, it is important to buy reputable brands and be alert to the sale of adulterated oils.

Why buy high-quality oils?

High-quality essential oils are often very expensive. This is a reflection of a number of factors:

- the time and effort involved in producing the plants
- the time and effort involved in harvesting the plants – which depend largely on the parts of the plant that are used and their oil content
- the costs of production – the extraction processes are often carried out on a fairly small scale and are time-consuming and labour-intensive, as well as requiring specialized equipment.

By buying high-quality essential oils, you can be sure that they contain the correct constituents in the correct proportions and that they will have the desired therapeutic properties. Synthetic and diluted oils are less predictable and less likely to be therapeutically effective.

In pure oils, there are hundreds of chemical constituents that interact when they are mixed together, enhancing their individual properties in a process known as synergy (see page 50). This process does not occur if synthetic oils are used.

Adulteration

Because pure oils are so expensive to produce, cheaper oils are now finding their way on to the market but these are generally of inferior quality due to adulteration. The main methods of adulterating essential oils are:

- adding a cheaper oil or diluting with alcohol or other spirit base
- adding a synthetic product
- substitution with a cheaper essential oil.

Practices such as adding cheaper lavandin to lavender oil, or adding cornmint oil (*Mentha arvensis*) to peppermint oil are, unfortunately, widespread. Of greater concern is the use of substitute products or 'nature-identical' synthetics: cassia oil has been found to contain synthetic cinnamic aldehyde, and 'red thyme oil' may be wholly synthetic. If the oil is not what you believe it to be, its effectiveness, and even safety, can be compromised.

Essential oils are used for many other purposes than aromatherapy, including food flavouring and in certain industrial processes. The International Standards Organization (ISO) and the Association Française de Normalisation (AFNOR) have set standards for essential oils in industrial terms, but the quality of oils used in aromatherapy can be difficult to ascertain, although most forms of adulteration can be revealed through gas chromatograph analysis. This underlines how important it is to buy from a reputable supplier that carries out its own quality-control testing.

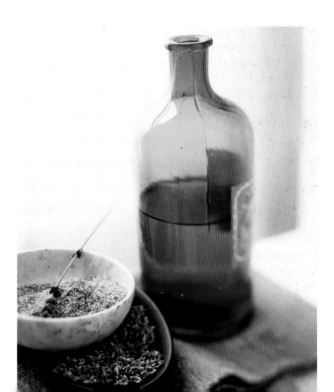

The time and effort that goes into producing good-quality essential oils means they can seem expensive. It is important to be aware that cheaper, adulterated oils are on the market and that these will not be as effective as the pricier, pure oils.

Carrier oils

Essential oils are too concentrated to be applied directly to the skin, so they are first blended with a lighter oil in order to dilute them and make them easier to apply. These lighter oils are known as carrier oils. The carrier oils used in aromatherapy are extracted from vegetable matter, nuts or seeds.

Types of carrier oils

Carrier oils are fixed, that is, they do not evaporate and have little or no smell. They are usually produced by cold-pressing (see page 44). Although a certain amount of heating and cooling is involved, temperatures do not usually exceed 60°C (140°F) so the characteristics of the oil remain largely unchanged. There are three main types of carrier oils:

- **Basic fixed oils**, such almond, grapeseed and peach kernel. These oils are pale, not too viscous and have very little smell. They can be used on the body and the face with or without the addition of essential oils.
- **Specialist fixed oils**, such as avocado, jojoba and wheatgerm. These are usually darker, more viscous and heavier. They are generally used in small amounts, blended with lighter carrier oils.
- **Macerated oils**, such as calendula and carrot. They are best described as plant extracts and, because of the way they are produced (see box), have additional therapeutic properties. They are particularly good for the skin, and may be added in small amounts to a blend or applied to the skin on their own.

CREATING A CARRIER OIL BY MACERATION

Fat-soluble components of medicinal plants can be extracted by macerating the plants in vegetable oil. Selected parts of the plants are chopped up and added to a vat of basic carrier oil (often sunflower). The mixture is agitated gently for some time before being placed in strong sunlight for several days. This transfers all the oil-soluble compounds (including the chemical constituents of the essential oil) to the oil in which the material is macerating. The mixture is then filtered to remove the unwanted plant material.

Purchasing and storing carrier oils

It is important to use high-quality carrier oils, preferably ones that have been produced by cold-pressing without the use of chemicals. The more highly processed an oil, the fewer vitamins it will retain. Refining removes the elements most liable to deterioration, but these include the nutritious skin-restructuring elements.

Carrier oils are perishable so it is wise to buy them frequently and in small quantities. Store them in airtight containers in a cool place, away from sunlight and moisture. The oils will deteriorate if they are exposed to air, heat, water and light, and will develop a rancid smell. Once exposed to the air, a carrier oil will last for up to six months.

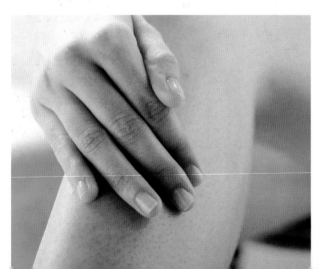

In massage, an essential oil is blended with a carrier oil to dilute it and help it penetrate the skin. Carrier oils also have their own therapeutic properties (see pages 47–49).

Commonly used carrier oils

Like essential oils, carrier oils have individual characters and uses.
Here are details of those most commonly used.

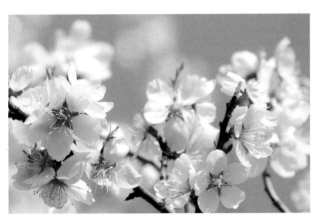

Sweet almond blossom (*Prunus amygdalis* var. *dulcis*)

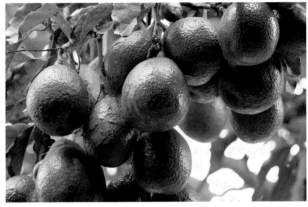

Avocados (*Persea americana*)

Almond (sweet) (*Prunus amygdalis* var. *dulcis*)

The large *Prunus* family includes peach and apricot which, although different in culinary terms, are botanically very close (almonds are contained within fleshy apricot-like fruit, and peach/apricot stones and the kernels within them, are very similar to almonds). Their essential oils are largely interchangeable.

Constituents Rich in vitamins A, B1, B2 and B6. The small amount of vitamin E it contains helps it keep well.

Character Pale-coloured but fairly rich in feel, with a slight but characteristic odour.

Skin types Almond is especially good for dry skin, while peach and apricot kernel suit younger skins.

Therapeutic properties Good for irritated skin, such as eczema. Protects and nourishes.

Comments Occasionally causes an allergic reaction. (NB: if there is any concern over a nut allergy, remember this will apply to peach/apricot kernel oil as well.)

Apricot kernel *see Almond*

Avocado (*Persea americana*)

The rich flesh of this pear-shaped subtropical fruit is first dried and then pressed to produce the oil for aromatherapy. The oil is sold in both unrefined and refined versions. Avocado oil is said to be most like the body's own natural oil.

Constituents Rich in lecithin and vitamins A, B1, B2 and D.

Character Pale yellow in colour, rich and heavy, especially when unrefined.

Skin types Despite viscosity, penetrates upper layers of skin well, so good for dry and wrinkled skin.

Therapeutic properties Moisturizing and anti-wrinkle; also said to have skin-healing properties.

Comments Best used diluted 50:50 with another, lighter carrier oil.

Calendula (*Calendula officinalis*)

Calendula (pot marigold) should not be confused with French marigold (*Tagetes* spp.). The oil, which includes volatile elements, is produced by macerating the flowers in a fixed oil, so it is not truly a fixed oil itself.

Constituents Carotenoids, which give the flowers their characteristic orange and yellow colours, are the precursors of vitamin A and have excellent antioxidant properties. Also contains vitamins A, B, D and E.

Character Light-coloured with a good texture.

Skin types Effective for chapped skin, ulcers, broken veins, bruises and rashes.

Therapeutic properties Anti-inflammatory and wound-healing properties make it useful for varicose veins and gum inflammation after tooth extraction. Excellent for dry eczema and general skin repair.

Comments No known contraindications or allergic reactions. Makes a good synergistic blend with hypericum (see box, page 49).

Coconut (*Cocos nucifera*)

The oil in the coconut's white flesh can be extracted by cold pressing but is often obtained by solvent extraction.
Constituents Glycerides, trimyristin and caproic acids, among others.
Character Rich but fine. Colourless when liquid, but turns white and solid when cooled.
Skin types All skin types.
Therapeutic properties Excellent emollient.
Comments Frequently used in massage creams, makes the skin smooth and satin-like but has been known to cause skin rashes. Needs to be mixed at least 50:50 with another oil to prevent solidification.

Evening primrose (*Oenothera biennis*)

Although a native of North America (the native North American medicine men were the first to recognize its potential as a healing agent), this willowy yellow-flowered biennial is now naturalized in many countries as a wayside flower.
Constituents Rich in fatty acids and has the second highest content of gamma linolenic acid (GLA) after borage oil (see opposite). It is rich in linoleic acid and oleic acid.
Character A yellow oil with a light texture that oxidizes on exposure to air.
Skin types Good for all skin types, especially dry, ageing, inflamed or damaged skin.
Therapeutic properties Accelerates wound-healing by repairing and maintaining skin tissue. Good for eczema and psoriasis. GLA helps to reduce blood cholesterol and maintain the hormonal balance in the body.
Comments The GLA is biologically important as it affects much of the enzyme activity in the body, including the production of prostaglandins, an imbalance or deficiency of which results in a wide range of disorders, such as poor skin, and reproductive and circulatory problems.

Grapeseed (*Vitis vinifera*)

Grapeseed oil is not available cold pressed, and may be refined to improve clarity.
Constituents Vitamin E, linoleic acid, among others.
Character Pale, light and fine, very stable and with a high penetration.
Skin types All skin types.
Therapeutic properties Leaves skin smooth without feeling oily.
Comments The refined oil keep fairly well and has no known contrindications. Although there is a popular cheaper oil available which is unrefined, it is not recommended for aromatherapy use.

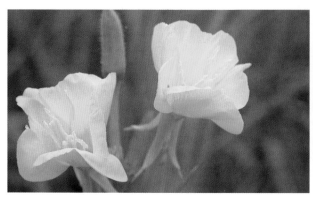

Evening primrose (*Oenothera biennis*)

Hazelnut (*Corylus avellana*)

Hazelnut oil is often used as a substitute for almond oil, especially when considering skin types.
Constituents Oleic acid and small amount of linoleic acid.
Character Amber-yellow in colour and is cold pressed
Skin types Its stimulating, astringent effect good for acne and oily/combination skin.
Therapeutic properties Stimulating to the circulation and has good penetration.
Comments Be aware of a possible nut allergy. Is often diluted with other carrier oils.

Jojoba wax (*Simmondsia sinensis*)

Jojoba (pronounced approximately as a gutteral ho-ho-ba) is a leathery-leaved native of California and Mexico. Its fruit hulls turn from green to brown before cracking to reveal seeds similar in appearance to coffee beans.
Constituents Composed not of triacylgyceroles but of esters high in vitamin E, making it more stable and unlikely to deteriorate.
Character A golden liquid wax, which solidifies on cooling. It does not oxidize easily.
Skin types Good for all skin types as it combines with sebum, which makes it useful for unblocking clogged pores. It is also balancing, and is good for dry scalps and hair products. It contains a waxy substance that mimics collagen and is a natural moisturizer.
Therapeutic properties Excellent for acne, psoriasis and eczema. It contains myristic acid, an anti-inflammatory agent that is beneficial for conditions such as arthritis and rheumatism.
Comments The consistency of jojoba makes it a useful ingredient for lip balms and many other cosmetics. It can be added to a blend to extend its life. Its resistance to oxidation means that it does not require any chemical preservatives.

Macadamia nut (*Macadamia ternifolia*)

This native of the subtropical forests of Australia is now also cultivated in Hawaii. The creamy kernel is contained within a very hard brown shell that has a green outer husk.

Constituents Oleic acid and also very high in palmitoleic acid, which is also found in human sebum. Its substantial amounts of saturated fat give it greater stability.

Character A cold-pressed oil that is available either refined or unrefined. No solvents are used in either case so the oil retains its natural properties. It is pale in colour, with a light odour and a light texture.

Skin types Good for all skin types but particularly recommended for older skins that start to dry as sebum production diminishes. Highly nourishing, easily absorbed.

Therapeutic properties Particularly pleasant as a skin lubricant. It also helps to prevent sunburn.

Comments Added to blends not only for its therapeutic properties but also because it stops the blend going rancid. Skin tests indicate that it has no toxic effects and does not cause any irritation or allergic reactions.

Peach kernel *see Almond*

Wheatgerm oil (*Triticum sativum* var. *vulgare*)

Derived from the germ of wheat grain.

Constituents High in antioxidant vitamin E. Also contains phytosterols, vitamins A and B complex and lecithin.

Character Deep orange, paling to yellow if more refined. It has a heavier texture than most carrier oils, and the strong odour has reduced its popularity.

Skin types Good for all skin types and especially recommended for dry, ageing or damaged skin.

Therapeutic properties Can be used in a sports-massage blend for tired muscles, improves circulation and helps relieve symptoms of dermatitis.

Comments As no cold-pressing, solvent extraction or vacuum extraction methods are used in its production, this oil is a natural antioxidant and a good stabilizer for other carrier oils. Best used 5–10 per cent in another carrier oil. May cause skin reactions in people allergic to gluten, so test before use. Regular facial use may cause hair growth.

LESS COMMONLY USED CARRIER OILS

FIXED OILS

Borage (starflower) oil (*Borago officinalis*) – very high in GLA, an essential fatty acid. Good for skin irritations. May be used in a small quantity for eczema and psoriasis.

Camelina oil (*Camelina sativa*) –an emollient, used mainly in cosmetics such a. skincare creams.

Castor oil (*Ricinus communis*) – used therapeutically for sores and abscesses, also in bath products.

Cherry kernel oil (*Prunus avium*) – a long-lasting emollient, used in cosmetics.

Cocoa butter (*Theobroma cacao*) – used as a massage lubricant, but mainly in ointments and cosmetics.

Corn oil (*Zea mays*) – used mainly in emollient creams and toothpastes.

Kukui nut oil (*Aleurites moluccans*) – easily absorbed and helps many skin conditions. Also provides good skin protection against the weather.

Linseed (or flaxseed) oil (*Linum usitatissimum*) – very soothing for skin.

Palm kernel oil (*Elaeis guineesis*) – similar to coconut oil both in its properties and application.

Peanut oil (*Arachis hypogaea*) – good for arthritis.

Rosehip (*Rosa rubiginosa*) – golden-red oil with high vitamin C content, good for regenerating ageing or damaged skin and healing wounds.

Tamanu oil (*Calophyllum inophyllum*) – helpful for hair and scalp problems, and for shingles.

Walnut oil (*Juglans regia*) – thought to be good for eczema but used mostly in Indian head massage.

MACERATED OILS

Carrot oil (*Daucus carota*) – rich in vitamins A, B, C, D and F, and beta-carotene. Soothing and helps skin to heal.

Meadowsweet oil (*Filipendula ulmaria*) – anti-inflammatory and analgesic, for arthritic conditions.

Hydrocotyle oil (*Centella asiatica*) – thought to regenerate the skin's elasticity in cases of stretch marks.

Lime blossom oil (*Tilia cordata*) – good for wrinkles, soothes rheumatic pain, relaxing so can help with sleep problems.

Passion flower oil (*Passiflora incarnata*) – a good relaxant, said to help insomnia.

St John's wort (hypericum) oil (*Hypericum perforatum*) – soothing on burns and inflammations, antiseptic and analgesic; makes good blend mixed 50:50 with calendula.

Blending essential oils

The art of the aromatherapist lies in combining various essential oils in order to treat specific conditions. This is a highly individual skill and results in the creation of a unique organic mixture.

Why blend?

Essential oils are complex substances that work in harmony with the body and have potentially far-reaching effects. One oil on its own will have certain properties and medicinal uses, but when two or more oils are blended, a chemical reaction occurs and the oils combine to form a new compound. In an appropriate blend each oil's properties are enhanced and the new composition may also be able to help another set of conditions.

Blending aromatherapy oils allows you to make a product specifically suited to the client. At the beginning of an aromatherapy treatment, the consultation will highlight the client's needs. You can then match these needs to the relevant essential oils, and then blend them to create an individual prescription to get the best therapeutic effect. It is not an exact science so there is room for fine-tuning the formula.

Synergy

Synergy is the effect of blending essential oils that complement each other so that their overall effect is enhanced. Essential oils that blend well together are known as synergists.

Using this principle, oils can be blended and modified from treatment to treatment according an individual's requirements on a particular day. To create a powerful synergy, the therapist needs to take into account not only the symptoms being treated but also the underlying cause of the condition (see page 119).

Discovering notes

The volatility of an essential oil, in other words how quickly it evaporates, is described in terms of 'notes'. Each essential oil has its own range of top, middle and base notes, although one will tend to dominate, but this individuality means that the emergence of notes will vary considerably. Some essential oils can also contribute more than one note to a blend. Neroli, for example, can provide an uplift when used as a top note, but act as a fixative if used as a base note. Similarly, although ylang ylang provides a base note, it will lift up a heavy blend and make it smell much more pleasant.

Characteristics of base, middle and top notes

	Top notes	Middle notes	Base notes
Volatility	Most volatile	Moderately volatile	Least volatile
Action	Fast-acting on the body and mind Provide first impressions of a blend, but do not linger for long	Moderate rate of action on the body and mind Add body to a blend	Slowest acting on the body and mind 'Fix' a blend, giving it staying power
Effects	Stimulate the body and mind with uplifting effects	Affect bodily functions, e.g. digestion and menstruation	Sedating and relaxing effects Benefit nervous conditions
Examples	Eucalyptus, citrus oils, sage, thyme, basil	Lavender, geranium, rosemary	Jasmine, sandalwood, ylang ylang, gums, woods and resins

The Joanna Hoare method of blending

Blending essential oils is a creative process, and experience will guide you to personal preferences and effective combinations. There are, however, some tools and guidelines that can help in preparing balanced and satisfying blends.

'Listening through the nose'

Blending involves both chemistry and aesthetics, and it is experience that will make you a good blender, so spend time discovering the odours of different oils. Don't attempt to evaluate more than six essential oils in a session, and clear your nose between each one. Some essential oils are very persistent and can linger on long after you have closed the bottle. Also, some essential oils can be harmful to the mucous tissue (see Oil directory, page 108–109).

Choose an area moderately warm and free from draughts; also make sure it is free from food or household smells. Collect together the bottles of oil you are going to smell, a number of tester strips (readily available from suppliers of essential oils), pen and notebook.

Clear your nose before you start. A good way is to breathe rapidly in and out several times.

Take a strip and write the name of the oil on it. Dip the clear end into the oil to a depth of about 5 mm (¼ in). Hold it just beneath your nose and smell repeatedly – be careful not to let the blotter touch your nose.

Write down your impressions of the smell, using descriptive words that are meaningful to you (see box). If you also note down its origin, supplier and any other relevant information you will later be able to compare the quality of oils from different sources and soon become expert in recognizing differences.

If you have difficulty at first, select your favourite aromas and gradually add in any unusual smelling oils. One of the most difficult oils to identify to begin with is rosemary because of its camphorous top note. Many students mistake it for thyme.

DESCRIBING AROMAS

Our perception of smells is essentially a subjective experience. In perfumery, as in the wine industry, certain terms have been adopted to describe the main characteristic of an aroma, words such as 'warm', 'rich', 'light', 'heavy', 'fresh', 'diffusive', 'dry' and 'harmonious'. Aromas are also described according to their type. Obvious examples are 'spicy', 'citrus' and 'floral', and below are a few more (the entire range runs into hundreds), but aromatherapists in training find it useful to create their own personal vocabulary.

Note	description
balsamic	sweet and soft, like resins
camphoraceous	clean, fresh and medicinal
forest	woody
green	grass-like
powdery	rather indistinct
woody	more leaf-like than forest
sweet	reminiscent of vanilla, coconut, peach and strawberry

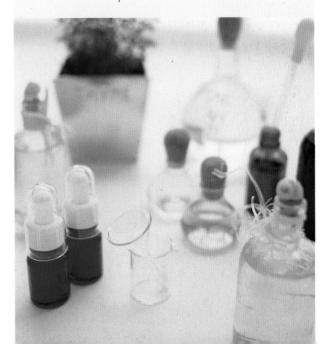

Before blending arrange your selection of oils and blending tools so you have everything in place. Do not evaluate more than six essential oils in a session.

Correct proportions

For therapeutic purposes, essential oils are usually diluted in a carrier oil before being applied to the skin. Between 3 and 6 drops of essential oil will be added to the base of 10 ml of carrier oil. A total of 5 drops in 10 ml of carrier oil makes a 2½ per cent blend.

Some ailments demand a stronger concentration of essential oils than, for example, that required for emotional or nervous conditions. Some oils also have greater power than other oils – the high-quality florals such as rose and jasmine, for example, have more diffusive power than most other essential oils, which means that a very small percentage is all that is needed to have a powerful effect or to influence the character of an entire blend.

Choosing a carrier oil

During a consultation, you will establish the skin type of the client by observation and conversation. Sometimes, when the skin is very dry, it is necessary to use a very rich fixed carrier oil. If the skin is young and inclined to be oily, a different carrier oil will be suitable.

You also need to take into account the condition of the skin, noting, for example, inflammation or bruising that could be helped by adding a proportion of macerated carrier oil to a suitable blend of essential oils.

Formulating a blend

Begin by making a note of your aims. For each blend you should take into account:

- the condition you want to treat
- the odour intensity of the oils
- the medicinal properties of the oils
- the psychological effects of the oils
- the age of the person (choose gentler oils and lower dilutions for the elderly and children)
- the time of day the oil will be used.

Next, draw up a suitable 'shortlist' of suitable oils. A card in chart form is helpful for this.

In this example, rosemary is discounted because it is unsuitable for someone with high blood pressure. The final recipe, which provides the right therapeutic qualities and creates a pleasing aroma for the client, combines lemon, juniper, lavender and ylang ylang.

CLIENT	AROMATHERAPIST		DATE
Condition(s)	**Top note**	**Middle note**	**Base note**
arthritis (main condition)	lemon, eucalyptus	black pepper, Roman chamomile, lavender, juniper, sweet marjoram, ~~rosemary~~	ginger
high blood pressure	lemon, clary sage	juniper, sweet marjoram, melissa	ylang ylang
varicose veins	lemon, peppermint	juniper, cypress, ~~rosemary~~	sandalwood

BODY RECIPE		FACE RECIPE
Top	2 drops lemon	1 drop lavender or ylang ylang, depending on preference
Middle	1 drop juniper, 1 drop lavender	
Base	1 drop ylang ylang	
carrier oil (10 ml) 5 ml jojoba (for arthritis) / 5 ml avocado (for penetration)		**carrier oil (5 ml)** sweet almond for mature, dry skin, or calendula

Some common questions about blending

Q Do all essential oils blend well together?
A No, some oils work against each other, producing an unpleasant aroma and different effects from those expected; for example, rose otto and lemon.

Q How many different essential oils can be used in one blend?
A Opinions on this point vary. Some aromatherapists (Marguerite Maury, for example) recommend the use of up to five essential oils in one blend, while others (such as Shirley Price) recommend a maximum of four.

Q Are there any 'rules' to help produce good blends?
A Oils of the same botanical family blend well together, as do oils with a similar chemical composition. Floral oils blend well together, as do woods and citrus oils. When you have selected the oils that are most appropriate for your client's needs, check how well they blend: rose or peppermint, for example, may overpower all other odours, and should either be used alone or in low concentrations.

Q Are the same blends of essential oils suitable for use all over the body?
A Some essential oils are not suitable for use on the face because they are too strong, so it is necessary to have a separate blend for the face. If different oils are being used on the face, it is recommended that no more than five different essential oils be used on one person in one day.

Q Is it acceptable to use only one essential oil?
A If one essential oil meets the client's needs and the client likes the smell of the oil, then use only one oil.

Q What should I do if I accidentally add too much essential oil to the carrier oil?
A Add more of the carrier oil to dilute the blend to the required strength.

Q How much should I mix up at one time?
A You will only need 10 ml of carrier oil for a complete body massage; if you wish to mix more (for example, for the client to take home), then you will need to adjust the number of drops of essential oils accordingly, to maintain the same proportions. Remember to drop the top note in first, followed by the middle note and then stir them together. This will help you decide if the base note is suitable.

SOME SAMPLE BLENDS

Here are some starter recipes, each to be added to 10 ml of carrier oil, to make a 2½ per cent blend.

A refreshing blend
1 drop geranium
2 drops bergamot
2 drops palmarosa

An energising blend
2 drops peititgrain
1 drop lavender
2 drops rosemary

For fluid retention
2 drops grapefruit
1 drop juniper
1 drop sweet fennel
1 drop patchouli

For muscle pain
1 drop bergamot
1 drop Roman chamomile
2 drops lavender
1 drop plai

A pampering blend
1 drop jasmine
2 drops geranium
1 drop rose
1 drop neroli

For a sore throat
1 drop lemon
1 drop ravemsara
2 drops frankincense
1 drop sweet thyme

SOME BASIC RULES

- Don't over-complicate a blend: begin with a maximum of three essential oils
- Don't blend oils that have opposite effects – such as a stimulating oil with a calming one
- Work on the principles of top, middle and base notes to obtain a good balance
- Keep in mind the odour of the finished blend.

Caution: Check that the client is not allergic to nuts before using any nut-based carrier oils.

Mixing a blend

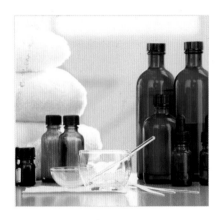

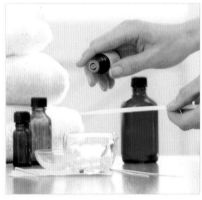

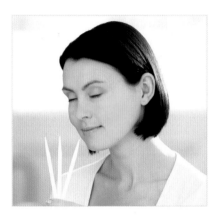

1 Gather all your utensils together before you open the bottles of essential oils. This will minimize the exposure of the oils to the air. You will need two clear glass measuring cups or beakers (one for the face blend and one for the body blend), a glass stirring rod, a pipette for each oil (so you do not transfer the character of one oil to another) and some testing strips. All should be very clean and dry, and kept covered when not in use.

2 Select the oils that you wish to blend, bearing in mind any medical condition or emotional factors that you have noted from your client. Keep things simple: even three oils will allow you to create a blend with a top, middle and base note.

3 After selecting the essential oils, put a drop or two of each of them on a testing strip. Waft the testing strips under your nose. This will give you an idea of how the finished blend will smell.

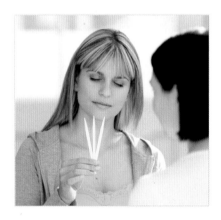

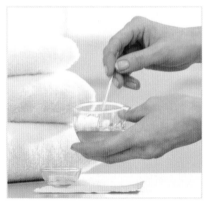

PROPORTIONS

As a practical guide, appropriate measures of essential oils for treating an adult are:

- **General massage** 5–6 drops in 10 ml of carrier

- **Facial massage** 1 drop in 5 ml of carrier

- **Localized massage** up to 6 drops in 10 ml of carrier.

4 Ask your client to smell any oils or your blend, to get feedback. This will help you build up a picture of what the client prefers. Remember there is a strong association between scent and memory, so avoid an essential oil that conjures up unpleasant associations. It may be necessary to start fine-tuning the mix by substituting one oil with another.

5 When your client is happy with the blend and you are ready to begin treatment, you can measure out the carrier oil and add the essential oils in appropriate proportions (see below). Add the top notes first, followed by the middle notes, then the base notes. Add each essential oil very carefully, so the drops can be precisely counted. Stir with a glass rod and cover the container to prevent evaporation.

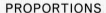

ESSENTIAL OILS AND AILMENTS

T = top note
M = middle note
B = base note

Note	Frankincense	Ylang ylang	Cedarwood	Roman Chamomile	Neroli	Petitgrain	Lemon	Grapefruit	Mandarin	Orange (sweet)	Myrrh	Cypress	Eucalyptus	Jasmine	Juniper berry	Lavender	Melissa	Peppermint	Basil	Marjoram	Geranium	Pine	Black pepper	Patchouli	Rose otto	Rosemary	Clary sage	Sandalwood	Plai	Ginger
	T	M	B	M	TM	MB	T	B	T	M	B	B	M	M	T	T	M	M	B	B	T	B	TM	T	M	B	M	T	B	B
Mental fatigue														✓	✓			✓								✓	✓			
Anxiety		✓		✓	✓									✓	✓	✓	✓			✓	✓				✓		✓	✓		
Depression		✓		✓				✓						✓		✓			✓		✓				✓		✓	✓		
Insomnia		✓		✓								✓		✓	✓	✓	✓			✓					✓			✓		
Sex-drive problems		✓												✓											✓		✓	✓		
Headaches				✓									✓			✓	✓	✓		✓						✓				
Migraine				✓												✓		✓		✓						✓				
Throat infections			✓				✓						✓			✓					✓							✓	✓	
Colds and flu		✓					✓						✓			✓					✓		✓			✓				
Sinusitis													✓			✓														
Bronchitis / Asthma		✓											✓			✓				✓		✓						✓		
Eczema				✓							✓				✓	✓	✓				✓							✓		
Acne		✓	✓			✓									✓	✓														
Stretch marks	✓								✓							✓														
Herpes simplex							✓						✓			✓	✓													
Athlete's foot																✓														
Hair loss		✓	✓													✓										✓				
Heartburn							✓											✓							✓					
Indigestion				✓											✓	✓		✓	✓	✓						✓			✓	✓
Irritable bowel syndrome				✓	✓			✓										✓												
Mouth ulcers							✓			✓						✓		✓			✓									
Diarrhoea				✓								✓				✓		✓			✓									
Nausea							✓										✓	✓							✓	✓			✓	✓
Constipation				✓				✓	✓											✓					✓	✓			✓	
Palpitations		✓			✓		✓									✓	✓													
Low blood pressure																										✓				
High blood pressure		✓					✓									✓	✓			✓							✓			
Fluid retention								✓				✓			✓	✓					✓									
Cellulite								✓				✓			✓	✓					✓			✓		✓				
Detox							✓	✓				✓			✓															
Varicose veins							✓					✓			✓						✓					✓	✓			
Cramp				✓				✓		✓										✓										
Sprains																✓				✓										
Muscular pains				✓												✓							✓			✓			✓	✓
Rheumatism / arthritis				✓		✓									✓	✓				✓			✓			✓			✓	✓
Pre-menstrual syndrome				✓													✓				✓				✓	✓	✓	✓		
Menstrual pain				✓								✓		✓		✓				✓					✓		✓			
Irregular periods				✓										✓		✓	✓				✓				✓		✓			
Menopausal problems				✓			✓			✓	✓			✓		✓					✓	✓			✓		✓	✓		
Cystitis													✓		✓	✓								✓				✓		
Infantile colic				✓												✓				✓								✓		
Diaper / nappy rash				✓												✓												✓		

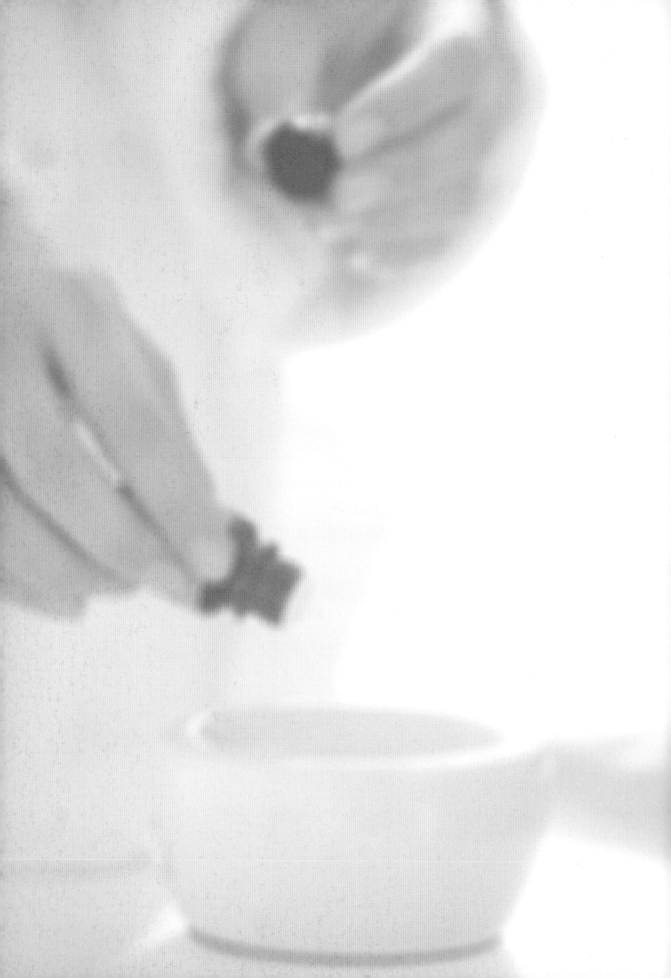

Directory of essential oils

The term essential oil is generally used to describe all the aromatic oils used by aromatherapists, and can be extracted from every conceivable part of the plant, including flowers, leaves, seeds, herbs, bark, resin and roots. Aromatherapists use around 60 essential oils, and need to be aware of the source, characteristics, healing properties and safety precautions for every oil that they use. This directory is an invaluable reference for all that an aromatherapist needs to know about a particular oil. The concluding section on safety will help you choose and apply your oils with confidence.

How to use the directory 58

At-a-glance guide to plant families 60

The directory 61

Safety guidelines 108

How to use the directory

This directory provides details of 47 of the essential oils most commonly found in aromatherapy: how they are obtained, how they work and the principal ways in which they can be used.

Classification

There are several ways of classifying essential oils, such as by the botanical family or by type of plant from which it is extracted, or the part of the plant from which the oil is derived. Other less common methods include classification according to yin and yang qualities and astrological charts.

For easy reference the oils listed here are in alphabetical order by botanical name, from *Achillea millefolium* (yarrow) to *Zingiber cassumunar* (plai), although the main heading is the common name by which the oil is best known. The oil usually has the same name as the plant from which it originates, but there are a few exceptions: the bitter orange (*Citrus aurantium*), for example, yields both neroli and petitgrain.

Each entry includes any alternative names for the oil and also the botanical family to which it belongs, for example Myrtaceae (tea tree) or Cupressaceae (Cypress). Like humans, plants have a family resemblance, and these family groups can be a useful guide to the nature of the oil a plant yields: see the At-a-glance guide to plant families, page 60.

Each entry consists of:

- a description of the plant from which the essential oil is obtained
- the parts of the plant that are used and the extraction process
- the principal chemical constituents of the oil
- the country where the plant originated, together with details of where it is now cultivated for oil extraction
- the characteristics of its odour, including its notes (or scent characteristics), i.e. whether it has a top, middle or base note, and its intensity
- a list of other oils with which it blends well
- a summary of the healing properties of the oil
- the conditions for which it is most commonly used and the way it works.

DIRECTORY OF ESSENTIAL OILS **77**

Coriandrum sativum
Coriander

Coriander is one of the more gentle of the spicy essential oils. A highly fragrant annual herb, Coriander grows to a height of about 1 m (3 ft) and has delicate, bright green leaves and white flowers, followed by a mass of round green seeds that eventually turn brown. The oil is colourless to pale yellow, with a sweet musky-woody odour. In Chinese medicine the whole herb is utilized and the seeds are used widely for culinary purposes, particularly for flavouring curries. Psychologically, Coriander is reviving and good for stimulating low energy, and is also comforting.

Botanical family Apiaceae (Umbelliferae).

Part of plant used Seeds.

Extraction process Steam distillation of the crushed ripe seeds.

Principal chemical constituents Linalol (55–75 per cent), decylaldehyde, borneol, geraniol, carvone, anethole and others.

Country of origin Native to Europe and western Asia. The essential oil is produced mainly in Russia, Romania, Croatia, Serbia and Bosnia.

Note Top.

Odour intensity Medium.

Blends well with Bergamot, Jasmine, Neroli, Petitgrain, Clary sage, Cypress, Pine, Ginger, Sandalwood.

Properties Analgesic, aperitif, anti-spasmodic, bactericidal, depurative, digestive, diuretic, carminative, revitalizing, stimulant (cardiac, circulatory, nervous) and stomachic.

Most common uses

Circulatory system, muscles and joints Arthritis, gout, muscular aches, poor circulation and fluid retention.
Action Said to help detoxification and rheumatic pain and to boost the immune system.

Digestive system Colic, dyspepsia, flatulence and nausea.
Action Recommended for digestive disturbances and can help with griping pains and other intestinal upsets.

Nervous system Migraine, neuralgia and nervous exhaustion.
Action Said to clear the head and revitalize the nervous system.

Safety Non-toxic, non-irritant and non-sensitizing. Use this oil in moderation (it is stupefying in large doses).

The nature of essential oils

Essential oils are generally light, clear and non-greasy, although a few are viscous or coloured. They all dissolve in fatty oils or in alcohol, but will not dissolve in water.

Each essential oil has a number of properties and medicinal uses. Lavender, for example, has a gentle sedative effect, and is often used to help insomnia. Below are the medical terms used to describe the healing characteristics listed in the directory. As the section on blending explains (see page 50), when two oils are mixed together a new composition is created, which may have properties that neither oil alone possesses.

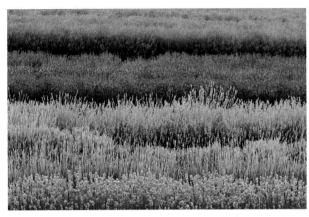

Lavender works as a gentle sedative and can help insomnia.

Explanation of terms (plant properties)

analgesic	Relieves pain	**hepatic**	Tones and aids liver function
anti-anaemic	Combats anaemia	**hypnotic**	Induces sleep
anti-inflammatory	Combats inflammation	**hypotensive**	Lowers blood pressure
anti-spasmodic	Eases spasms or convulsions	**lymphatic**	Acts on the lymph system
astringent	Contracts and tightens body tissue	**nervine**	Strengthens and tones the nerves
cicatrizant	Promotes healing by formation of scar tissue	**restorative**	Strengthens and revives the body systems
cytophylactic	Increases leucocyte activity in defence of the body/Boosts immune system/promotes cell regeneration	**rubefacient**	Causes redness of the skin
		sedative	Has calming effects
		stomachic	Aids and stimulates digestion
digestive	Promotes or aids digestion	**sudorific**	Promotes sweating
diuretic	Promotes urination	**tonic**	Strengthens and boosts whole or parts of the body
emmenagogue	Induces or assists menstruation		
emollient	Softens and soothes the skin	**vasodilator**	Dilates the blood vesels
expectorant	Promotes removal of mucus from the respiratory sytem	**vermifuge**	Expels intestinal worms
		vulnerary	Heals wounds
febrifuge	Reduces fever		

At-a-glance guide to plant families

Anonaceae
Oils featured here:
Ylang ylang (page 64)

Apiaceae (Umbelliferae)
Oils featured here:
Coriander (page 77)
Sweet fennel (page 82)

Asteraceae (Compositae)
Oils featured here:
German chamomile (page 87)
Roman chamomile (page 66)
Yarrow (page 61)

Burseraceae
Oils featured here:
Frankincense (page 63)
Myrrh (page 76)

Cupressaceae
Oils featured here:
Cypress (page 78)
Juniper berry (page 84)

Geraniaceae
Oils featured here:
Geranium (page 94)

Lamiaceae (Labiatae)
Oils featured here:
Basil (page 92)
Clary sage (page 101)
Melissa (page 90)
Lavender (page 85)
Patchouli (page 97)
Peppermint (page 91)
Rosemary (page 100)
Sweet marjoram (page 93)
Thyme (page 104)

Lauraceae
Oils featured here:
Brazilian rosewood (page 62)
May chang (page 86)

Myrtaceae
Oils featured here:
Eucalyptus (page 81)
Niaouli (page 89)
Tea tree (page 88)

Oleaceae
Oils featured here:
Jasmine (page 83)

Pinaceae
Oils featured here:
Atlas cedarwood (page 65)
Pine (page 95)

Piperaceae
Oils featured here:
Black pepper (page 96)

Poaceae (Graminae)
Oils featured here:
Lemongrass (page 79)
Palmarosa (page 80)
Vetiver (page 105)

Rosaceae
Oils featured here:
Rose absolute (page 98)
Rose otto (page 98)

Rutaceae
Oils featured here:
Bergamot (page 71)
Bitter orange (page 68)
Grapefruit (page 73)
Lemon (page 72)
Lime (page 67)
Mandarin (page 74)
Neroli (page 69)
Petitgrain (page 70)
Sweet orange (page 75)

Santalaceae
Oils featured here:
Sandalwood (page 102)

Styracaceae
Oils featured here:
Benzoin (page 103)

Zingiberaceae
Oils featured here:
Ginger (page 107)
Plai (page 106)

Achillea millefolium
Yarrow

This perennial herb has a single stem up to 1 m (3 ft) high, with fine, lacy leaves and pinky-white flowerheads. The essential oil is dark blue or greenish, with a slightly sweet, herbaceous odour. It has been used for a variety of complaints since the days of ancient Greece – Achilles is said to have used it for injuries during the Trojan wars. Today it is used in China for menstrual problems and haemorrhoids.

Botanical family Asteraceae (Compositae).

Alternative common name Milfoil.

Part of plant used Dried leaves and flowerheads.

Extraction process Steam distillation.

Principal chemical constituents Chamazulene, borneol acetate, borneol, cineol, camphene, penene and tricydene.

Country of origin Found in most temperate zones. Distilled mainly in Germany, Hungary and France; also in the USA and Africa.

Note Middle.

Odour intensity Medium.

Blends well with Bergamot, Chamomile, Clary sage, Juniper, Lavender, Lemon, Neroli and Rosemary.

Properties Anti-inflammatory, anti-rheumatic, antiseptic, astringent, anti-spasmodic, carminative, cicatrizant, digestive, expectorant, hypotensive, stomachic and tonic.

Most common uses

Skin conditions and hair Acne, burns, eczema, inflammation, rashes, scars, varicose veins and wounds.
Action Anti-inflammatory and astringent action helps with capillary network in varicose veins. Also said to help promote hair growth if used as a hair rinse.

Circulation, muscles and joints Arteriosclerosis, high blood pressure, rheumatoid arthritis and thrombosis.
Action A hypotensive so helps to regulate high blood pressure.

Digestive system Constipation, cramp, flatulence, haemorrhoids and indigestion.
Action A carminative and stomachic, which aid digestion.

Genito-urinary system Amenorrhea, dysmenorrhea, cystitis and other infections.
Action Helps menstrual problems and boosts the immune system to help fight colds, flu and fevers.

Nervous system Hypertension and insomnia.
Action Helps all stress-related conditions.

Safety Generally non-toxic and non-irritant but it may cause sensitization in some individuals. Do not use this oil on pregnant women or young children.

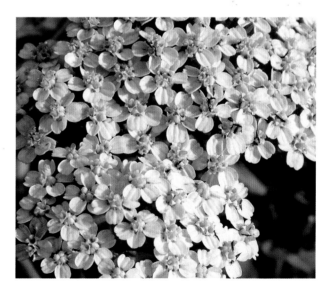

Aniba rosaeodora var. *amazonica*
Brazilian rosewood

This is a medium-sized, tropical evergreen tree with a reddish bark and heartwood and yellow flowers, The essential oil, which has only been introduced to aromatherapy relatively recently, is pale yellow with a sweet, woody-floral and slightly spicy odour. The Brazilian Rosewood tree is used extensively for timber and furniture-making and is being extensively felled in the Amazon rainforest, so legislation now requires distilleries to plant a new tree for each one cut down. Rosewood oil is used in perfumery. It is balancing, uplifting and fortifying, and is an effective anti-depressant. The Brazilian Rosewood is now an endangered species, so the International Federation of Aromatherapists recommends using oils from a chemotype of Howood leaf (*Cinnamomum camphora*), which has a very camphoraceous odour, or from Linaloe (*Bursera glabrifolia*, which has a similar odour and is non-hazardous.

Cinnamomum camphora

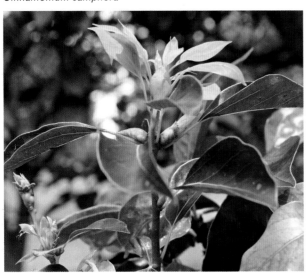

Botanical family Lauraceae.

Alternative common name Bois de Rose.

Part of plant used Wood chippings.

Extraction process Steam distillation of the heartwood chippings.

Principal chemical constituents Linalol (80-90%), cineol, terpineol, geraniol, citronellal, limonene and pinene.

Country of origin Native to the Amazon region. Brazil and Peru are the main producers.

Note Middle.

Odour intensity Medium.

Blends well with Bergamot, Cedarwood, Frankincense, Geranium, Lavender, Neroli, Palmarosa, Patchouli, Petitgrain, Rose, Sandalwood, Vetiver and Ylang ylang.

Properties Analgesic, anti-depressant, bactericidal, deodorant, cephalic, insecticide and tonic.

Most common uses

Skin conditions Dull combination oily/dry skin, scars, wounds and wrinkles.
Action Mild, antibacterial and safe to use so good for sensitive or inflamed skin and makes a good deodorant.

Immune system Colds, fevers and infections.
Action Said to stimulate the immune system.

Nervous system Frigidity, headaches, nausea and nervous tension.
Action Enlivening and uplifting, and has the effect of balancing the emotions and helping with mood swings, especially when weary or stressed.

Safety Non-toxic, non-irritant and non-sensitizing.

Boswellia carteri
Frankincense

A small tree or shrub with many feathery leaves and small white or pink flowers. Frankincense yields a natural oleo gum resin. The essential oil is obtained from the resin. It smells sweetly balsamic and is often burned in churches to aid meditation and prayer. According to the Bible, frankincense, together with gold and myrrh, were gifts for the baby Jesus, although this would have been the resin not the essential oil as we know it. It is used as incense in India and China, traditionally being burned as an offering to the gods. It is also used as a fixative in perfumery. There are reports of Frankincense being used to alleviate the pains associated with arthritis. It is emotionally balancing, producing a wonderful sense of calm.

Botanical family Burseraceae.

Part of plant used Drops of oleo gum resin.

Extraction process Steam distillation. An absolute is also produced.

Principal chemical constituents Monoterpene hydrocarbons, thujone, and octyl acetate in censole.

Country of origin Oman, Somalia, Ethiopia and China. The gum resin is usually distilled in Europe and India.

Note Base.

Odour intensity High.

Blends well with Geranium, Grapefruit, Lavender, Orange, Melissa, Patchouli, Pine, Rose and Sandalwood.

Properties Anti-inflammatory, antiseptic, cytophylactic and expectorant.

Most common uses

Skin conditions Mature or dry complexions, scars and blemishes.
Action Said to stimulate cell regeneration and also thought to help with stretch marks.

Respiratory system Asthma, bronchitis, catarrh, coughs, laryngitis and shortness of breath.
Action A good pulmonary oil so helps with breathing, as well as helping the immune system to fight colds and flu.

Nervous system Anxiety, anger, nervous tension and insecurity.
Action Slows and deepens the breathing, so is thought to have cleansing and purifying properties that help the mind release emotional blockages. Can also help meditation.

Safety Non-toxic, non-irritant and non-sensitizing. Do not use this oil on pregnant women during the first trimester.

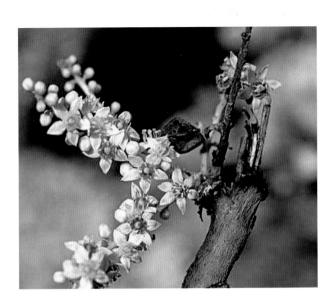

Cananga odorata var. *genuina*
Ylang ylang

This tall tropical tree has large fragrant flowers, usually yellow but occasionally pink or mauve. The yellow flowers are considered the best for the extraction of essential oils. The oil is pale yellow with an intensely sweet odour that is very soothing, hence its popularity in the perfume industry. Ylang ylang was used in Victorian times as a hair treatment and to soothe insect bites. In Indonesia, the flowers are spread on the beds of newlyweds on their wedding night because they are thought to be an aphrodisiac. It is used extensively in the perfumery industry for its exotic fragrance. Ylang ylang has a euphoric effect, helping to boost positive emotions, and calming in times of stress.

Botanical family Anonaceae.

Part of plant used Fresh flowers.

Extraction process Steam or water distillation. The first distillate is the top-grade Ylang ylang extra; the successive distillates are Ylang ylang 1, 2 and 3. Solvent extraction yields an absolute with long-lasting floral odours.

Principal chemical constituents Linalol, geranyl acetate, caryophyllene, benzyl acetate, methyl benzoate and other sesquiterpenes. (Ylang Ylang Extra is high in esters.)

Country of origin Indonesia, Philippines and Madagascar.

Note Base.

Odour intensity High

Blends well with Grapefruit, Bergamot, Orange, Jasmine, Geranium, Sandalwood and Vetiver.

Properties Anti-depressant, anti-infectious, aphrodisiac, euphoric, hypotensive, nervine, sedative (nervous) and tonic (uterine).

Most common uses

Skin conditions and hair Acne, general skincare, insect bites, irritated skin and lifeless hair.
Action Said to have a balancing effect on sebum, making it effective on both oily and dry skins. Used as a rinse, it promotes healthy hair.

Circulatory system High blood pressure, palpitations and tachycardia.
Action Reduces blood pressure, and is recognized for its regulatory and calming effect on the heart.

Nervous system Anxiety, depression, frigidity, insomnia and nervous tension.
Action A reassuring essential oil that boosts confidence and helps with stress-related disorders. It is also useful for anger and insecurity.

Safety Generally non-toxic and non-irritant, although a few cases of sensitization have been reported. Use in moderation because the strong odour can cause headaches and nausea.

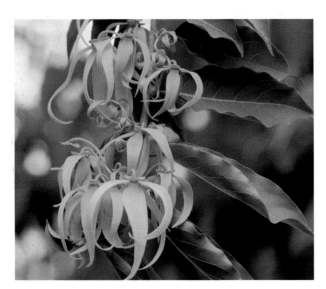

Cedrus atlantica
Atlas cedarwood

This tall, strongly aromatic evergreen tree grows to over 33 m (100 ft) and lives for more than a thousand years. The essential oil was used by the ancient Egyptians for embalming, cosmetics and perfumery. In Tibet, it is still used in traditional medicine and as incense in the temples. The essential oil is a deep amber colour with a warm camphoraceous and woody balsamic odour. It is used in antiseptic ointments and perfumes and has fortifying, calming and opening qualities.

The Atlas cedarwood is now an endangered species, so the International Federation of Aromatherapists recommends oil from the Himalayan cedarwood (*C. deodorata*), a close relative, as an alternative. The Texas cedarwood (*Juniperus ashei*) and the Virginian cedarwood (*J. virginiana*) belong to a different botanical family and produce a quite different essential oil.

Botanical family Pinaceae.

Alternative common names Atlantic Cedar, Moroccan cedarwood (oil).

Part of plant used Wood and sawdust.

Extraction process Steam distillation of the wood, stumps and sawdust. A resinoid and absolute are also produced.

Principal chemical constituents Atlantone, caryophyllene, cedrol and cadinene.

Country of origin Native to the Atlas mountains of Algeria. The oils are mostly produced in Morocco.

Note Base.

Odour intensity Medium.

Blends well with Bergamot, Cypress, Frankincense, Jasmine, Juniper, Lemon, Neroli, Clary sage, Vetiver, Rosemary, Ylang ylang and Patchouli.

Properties Antiseptic, astringent, diuretic, expectorant, fungicidal, insecticide, sedative (nervous) and tonic.

Most common uses

Skin conditions Acne, seborrhoea, dandruff, alopecia, dermatitis, psoriasis and ulcers.
Action Has astringent and antiseptic properties said to benefit oily conditions of the skin and scalp, and hair loss.

Respiratory system Bronchitis, coughs and catarrh.
Action An expectorant, eases congestion and coughs.

Genito-urinary system Cystitis and leucorrhoea.
Action May be helpful in the treatment of kidney and bladder disorders, and infections like cystitis.

Nervous system Nervous tension, anxiety, exhaustion and stress-related conditions.
Action Warming, comforting, and harmonizing.

Safety Non-toxic, non-irritant and non-sensitizing. Do not use this oil on pregnant women.

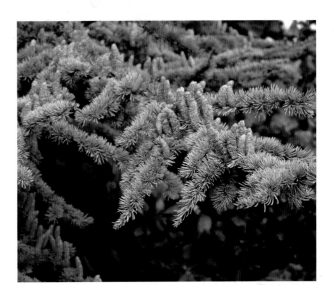

Chamaemelum nobile (syn. *Anthemis nobilis*)
Roman chamomile

One of the oldest known medicinal herbs, Roman chamomile is calming and a good all-round oil. A perennial herb that has been used in Europe for over two thousand years, the plant has delicate feathery leaves and small, daisy-like flowers. It was used by the ancient Egyptians and the Moors, and was one of the Saxons' nine sacred herbs (known as 'maythen'). There are many varieties of chamomile but Roman chamomile is the only one commonly used in medicine. The essential oil is pale blue but turns yellow when stored and has a warm, sweet odour.

Botanical family Asteraceae (Compositae).

Part of plant used Flowerheads.

Extraction process Steam distillation of 'past their peak' flowerheads.

Principal chemical constituents Esters, 85 per cent chamazulene, pinene, farnesol and cineol.

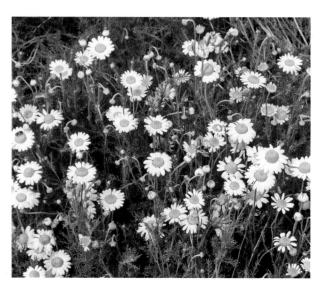

Country of origin Southwestern Europe, Britain, Belgium, France, Hungary, USA.

Note Middle.

Odour intensity High.

Blends well with Bergamot, Clary sage, Geranium, Jasmine, Lavender, Neroli and Rose.

Properties Analgesic, anti-anaemic, anti-inflammatory, carminative, cicatrizant, digestive, emmenagogue, febrifuge, hepatic, hypnotic, nerve sedative, stomachic, sudorific, tonic, vermifuge and vulnerary.

Most common uses

Skin conditions Acne, allergies, burns, cuts, eczema, inflammation, insect bites and rashes. Also hair care, earache, toothache and teething pain.
Action Reduces inflammation.

Circulation, muscles and joints Arthritis, inflamed joints, muscular pain, rheumatism and sprains.
Action Reduces inflammation, especially where there is also swelling.

Digestive system Dyspepsia, colic, indigestion and nausea.
Action Helps particularly with indigestion, helping to calm and soothe.

Genito-urinary system Dysmenorrhea and menopausal problems.
Action Helps whenever there is pain.

Nervous system Headache, insomnia, nervous tension and migraine.
Action Has many soothing and calming properties and is particularly helpful in stress-related conditions.

Safety Generally non-toxic and non-irritant, although it may cause dermatitis in some individuals.

Citrus aurantifolia (syn. *C. medica* var. *latifolia*)
Lime

There are several species of the Lime, which is a small evergreen tree, up to 4.5 m (15 ft) high, with drooping branches, smooth oval leaves, small white flowers and small bitter fruit. The fruit is green and the essential oil is pale yellow or green with a fresh, sweet citrus-peel aroma. The distilled oil is paler, with a fresh but sharp fruity-citrus odour. The Moors introduced the Lime to Europe and it was then taken to North America by the Spanish and Portuguese at some time around the 16th century. Psychologically, it is refreshing and uplifting.

Botanical family Rutaceae.

Part of plant used Fruit.

Extraction process Cold expression of the fruit peel. Steam distillation of the whole ripe fruit.

Principal chemical constituents Monoterpene hydrocarbons, pinene, sabine, myrcene, limonene, camphene, and citral, cineols and linalol. The expressed oil also contains coumarins. Distilled lime oil contains most of the above plus traces of neryl acetate and geranyl acetate.

Country of origin Originally from Asia but naturalized in many other regions of the world, mainly Italy, Florida, the West Indies, Cuba and Mexico.

Note Top.

Odour intensity High.

Blends well with Neroli, Lavender, Rosemary, Clary Sage, Geranium, Grapefruit, Mandarin, Palmarosa, Petitgrain, Vetiver, Ylang ylang – and may take over the blend with its strong, but pleasant odour.

Properties Antiseptic, antiviral, aperitif, bactericidal, febrifuge, haemeostatic, restorative and tonic.

Most common uses

Skin conditions Oily or congested skin, brittle nails, boils, chilblains, cuts, insect bites and mouth ulcers.
Action Has antiseptic and astringent properties that can help these conditions.

Circulatory system Cellulite, varicose veins and immune system.
Action Helps mainly by detoxifying and reducing fluid retention.

Digestive system Dyspepsia, poor appetite and nausea.
Action A digestive stimulant that helps to stimulate the appetite after illness or in anorexia.

Nervous system Mental fatigue, anxiety and depression.
Action Very refreshing and uplifting, helping where there is fatigue and apathy.

Safety Non-toxic, non-irritant and non-sensitizing. The expressed oil is phototoxic (but not the steam-distilled 'whole fruit' oil).

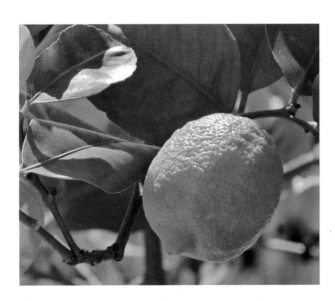

Citrus aurantium var. *amara* (syn. *C. vulgaris*, *C. bigardia*)
Bitter orange

An evergreen tree that grows up to 10 m (33 ft) high, with glossy, dark green oval leaves, with long spines. There are many different varieties. It has very fragrant white flowers and the fruit is smaller and darker than the Sweet orange. The dark yellow oil has a fresh, dry citrus odour with sweet undertones. The dried bitter orange peel is used as a tonic and carminative in the treatment of dyspepsia. In Chinese medicine, it is used internally to treat prolapse of the uterus, although reports suggest that the peel is toxic when ingested in large amounts.

Botanical family Rutaceae.

Alternative common name Seville Orange.

Part of plant used Fresh fruit, leaves and blossom.

Extraction process Cold expression (by hand or machine) of the outer peel of the almost ripe fruit. Distillation of the leaves for Petitgrain and of the blossom for Neroli oil (see pages 70 and 69).

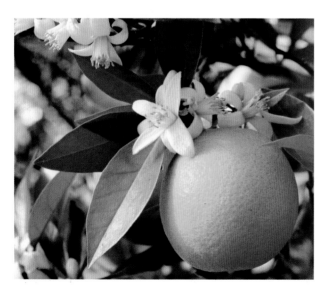

Principal chemical constituents Montoterpenes (90 per cent), pinene, limonene, myrcene, camphene, and small amounts of alcohols, aldehydes and ketones.

Country of origin Native to China. Cultivated in the USA and Mediterranean. The expressed oil is mainly produced in Israel, Cyprus, Brazil and North America. The distilled oil mainly comes from the Mediterranean and North America.

Note Top.

Odour intensity Medium.

Blends well with Clary sage, Cypress, Lavender, Neroli, Myrrh, Frankincense, Petitgrain, Rose, Rosewood, Sandalwood, Ylang ylang and all the spice oils.

Properties Anti-inflammatory, antiseptic, astringent, bactericidal, carminative, fungicidal, sedative (mild), stomachic and tonic.

Most common uses

Skin conditions Mouth ulcers.
Action Used in a mouthwash. Sometimes recommended for dull, oily complexions, but can be too strong for the face.

Circulation and immune system Obesity, fluid retention and colds and flu.
Action Helps to reduce swollen tissue, has antiseptic properties and boosts the immune system.

Digestive system Dyspepsia, constipation and irritable bowel syndrome.
Action Stimulates the digestive tract and gall bladder.

Nervous system Nervous tension, anorexia, anxiety and depression.
Action Has a delightfully fresh and uplifting odour that seems to help people to relax and unwind.

Safety Non-toxic, non-irritant and non-sensitizing. The oil is phototoxic, so clients should avoid exposure to strong sunlight or ultraviolet light after treatment.

Citrus aurantium var. *amara*
Neroli

Like Bitter orange and Petitgrain, Neroli oil is obtained from the Bitter orange (see opposite). Neroli is among the finest of the flower essences (the flowers of the Sweet orange also yield an essence but it is of inferior quality). Neroli essential oil is pale yellow with a light, sweet-floral odour. Neroli takes its name from Anna-Marie, Princess of Nerola in 16th-century Italy, who used it as a perfume and in bath water. It is used in perfumery and, psychologically, it is the best choice for the treatment of anxiety and emotional problems.

Botanical family Rutaceae.

Alternative common names Bitter orange, Seville orange, Orange blossom (oil), Orange flower (oil), Neroli bigarade (oil). 'Neroli bigarade' indicates the oil has been extracted by distillation rather than solvent extraction.

Part of plant used Fresh flowers.

Extraction process Steam distillation (essential oil, plus orange flower water and an absolute). Solvent extraction (a concrete and an absolute).

Principal chemical constituents Linalol (approx 34 per cent), linalyl acetate, limonene, pinene, nerolidol, geraniol, nerol, methyl anthranilate, indole, citral and others.

Country of origin Native to the Far East, it has adapted well to the Mediterranean. Major producers include France, Italy, Tunisia, Morocco, Egypt, and the USA.

Note Essential oil – top. Absolute – base.

Odour intensity High.

Blends well with Nearly every other essential oil, but particularly with Benzoin, Frankincense, Geranium, Lavender and Rose.

Properties Aphrodisiac, anti-depressant, antiseptic, anti-spasmodic, bactericidal, carminative, cicatrizant, cytophylactic, stimulant (nervous) and tonic.

Most common uses

Skin conditions Dry, sensitive and mature skins and broken capillaries.
Action An excellent regenerative oil for all skin types since it does not irritate and can help combat stretch marks and scars.

Circulatory system Poor circulation and palpitations.
Action Has antispasmodic properties.

Digestive system Colic, flatulence, chronic diarrhoea and irritable bowel syndrome.
Action Can help to relax the muscles of the small intestine, especially in cases of nervous tension.

Nervous system Anxiety, depression, nervous tension and premenstrual syndrome.
Action Can help with all emotional problems and is thought to be a natural tranquillizer for anxiety and shock. Valuable for insomnia caused by anxiety.

Safety Non-toxic, -irritant, -sensitizing and -phototoxic.

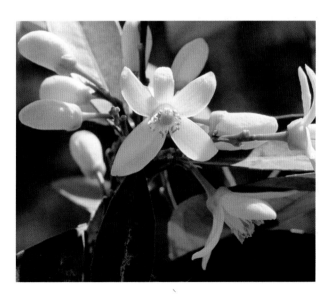

Citrus aurantium var. *amara*
Petitgrain

Petitgrain is distilled from the Bitter orange, an evergreen tree with dark green leaves and fragrant white flowers. The essential oil is steam-distilled from the leaves and twigs, unlike Bitter orange essential oil, which is distilled from the fruit, and Neroli, which is distilled from the flowers. The essential oil is pale yellow to amber in colour, with a very fresh, citrus and woody herbaceous undertone. The name means 'little grains', as Petitgrain was originally distilled from the small unripe fruit. Its refreshing aroma makes it popular as one of the traditional ingredients of eau de cologne, and it is often used in skincare products. Psychologically, Petitgrain is revitalizing, balancing and nourishing.

Botanical family Rutaceae.

Alternative common names Bitter orange, Seville orange.

Part of plant used Leaves and twigs

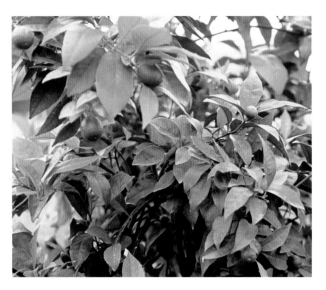

Extraction process Steam distillation.

Principal chemical constituents Esters (40–80 per cent), linalyl acetate, geranyl acetate and also geraniol, linalol and nerol.

Country of origin Native to China and India. The best oil is produced in France. Also produced in North Africa, Paraguay and Haiti.

Note Middle to top.

Odour intensity Medium.

Blends well with Rosemary, Lavender, Geranium, Jasmine, Palmarosa, Sandalwood, Ylang ylang and other citrus oils.

Properties Anti-depressant, antiseptic, anti-spasmodic, deodorant, nervine and sedative.

Most common uses

Skin conditions Acne, oily and combination skins.
Action Has a toning effect on oily skins and may be used on the face as it is non-sensitizing and non-phototoxic.

Nervous system Insomnia, stress-related conditions and palpitations.
Action Has a sedative effect on the nerves, helping insomnia and digestive problems caused by nervous exhaustion.

Safety Non-toxic, non-irritant, non-sensitizing and non-phototoxic.

Citrus bergamia
Bergamot

The bergamot tree is about 4.5 m (15 ft) high with smooth, oval leaves. The tree bears small round fruit that resemble miniature oranges but is too sour to eat. The essential oil is the finest of the citrus oils, with a light greenish-yellow colour and a fresh, delicate, spicy lemony aroma with slight floral overtones. Bergamot has been used in Italian folk medicine for centuries, primarily for treating fever and worms. It is used to flavour Earl Grey tea and is a very popular in perfume. Bergamot is reviving, soothing and balancing.

Botanical family Rutaceae.

Part of plant used Peel of the small yellow fruit.

Extraction process Cold expression of the peel of nearly ripe fruit.

Principal chemical constituents About 300 compounds, but mainly: linalyl acetate (30–60 per cent), linalol, sesquiterpenes, limonene, pinene and myrcene; also furocoumarins (including bergapten).

Country of origin Native to tropical Asia. Cultivated in southern Italy.

Note Top.

Odour intensity Medium

Blends well with Basil, Chamomile, Cypress, Eucalyptus, Geranium, Jasmine, Lavender, Lemon, Juniper, Lime, Marjoram, Neroli, Orange, Palmarosa, Patchouli, Petitgrain, Rosemary, Sandalwood and Ylang ylang.

Properties Analgesic, anti-depressant, anti-septic, anti-spasmodic, antiviral, carminative, cicatrizant, digestive, febrifuge, stomachic, tonic, vermifuge and vulnerary.

Most common uses

Skin conditions Acne, oily congested skin, herpes and psoriasis.
Action Has strong antiseptic properties,and in low dilutions is good for treating skin conditions.

Digestive system Dyspepsia, flatulence, colic and loss of appetite.
Action Carminative and digestive, so should help in cases of indigestion and can have a stimulating effect on the liver, stomach and spleen.

Respiratory system Mouth infections, sore throat and tonsillitis.
Action Can be used as an inhalant for throat infections.

Genito-urinary system Cystitis, pruritis and thrush.
Action Good as antiseptic hip bath in very weak dilutions.

Nervous system Anxiety, depression, anger and stress-related problems.
Action Sedating and soothing, yet can uplift the spirits.

Safety Non-toxic and non-irritant. Can increase the photosensitivity of the skin, so warn your client to avoid ultraviolet light or direct sunlight after applying this oil.

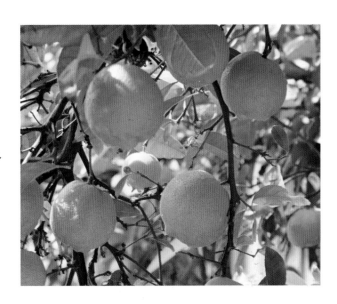

Citrus limon (syn. *C. limonum*)
Lemon

The Lemon is a small evergreen tree, up to 6 m (20 ft) high, with serrated oval leaves and very fragrant flowers. The essential oil is a pale greeny-yellow colour with a refreshing, sharp citrus odour. The lemon is highly regarded as a 'cure-all' for infectious conditions. The fruit contains high levels of vitamins A, B and C. Lemon protects and stimulates the body's systems and lifts the emotions.

Botanical family Rutaceae.

Part of plant used Fruit peel.

Extraction process Cold expression of the outer parts of the fresh peel.

Principal chemical constituents Limonene (about 70 per cent), pinene, bisapolene, sabinene, myrcene, citral, linalol, geraniol, citronellal and nerol.

Country of origin Native to Asia but grows well in the Mediterranean. Also grown in California and Florida.

Note Top.

Odour intensity Medium to high.

Blends well with Benzoin, Chamomile, Eucalyptus, Geranium, Ginger, Juniper, Fennel, Lavender, Neroli, Sandalwood and Ylang ylang.

Properties Anti-anaemic, antiseptic, anti-microbial, anti-rheumatic, anti-spasmodic, astringent, bactericidal, carminative, cicatrizant, depurative, diuretic, febrifuge, haemostatic, hypotensive, insecticidal, rubefacient, tonic and stimulates leucocytosis (production of white blood cells).

Most common uses

Skin conditions Oily skin, cuts and boils.
Action Antiseptic and astringent, with excellent cleansing properties.

Circulatory system Poor circulation, low immunity, colds and flu, and infections.
Action Good for treating varicose veins and reducing high blood pressure. It can also help rheumatism.

Digestive system Dyspepsia, bloated condition and liver congestion.
Action Improves the functioning of the digestive system

Respiratory system Asthma, bronchitis, catarrh and sore throats.
Action Antiseptic so helps with respiratory infections, especially if used early.

Nervous system Mental fatigue and worry.
Action Helps to improve concentration, lift the spirits and clear the mind.

Safety Non-toxic but may cause skin irritation or sensitization in some individuals. The expressed oil is phototoxic so you should advise clients to avoid exposure to strong sunlight or ultraviolet light after treatment.

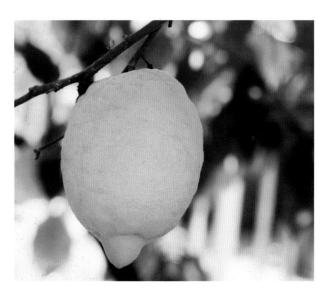

*Citrus paradisi (*syn. *C. racemosa, C. maxima* var. *racemosa)*
Grapefruit

This large tree, often over 10 m (33 ft) high, has glossy leaves and large yellow fruits, which are familiar to most people. It is believed to have been first cultivated in the West Indies some time in the 18th century, when it was known as Shaddock fruit. It has significant nutritional qualities as it is rich in vitamin C, which helps to combat infectious diseases. The essential oil is yellow or greenish with a fresh, sweet, citrus aroma, and has a short shelf-life. Grapefruit is refreshing and reviving, and lifts the spirits, helping to combat depression and fatigue.

Botanical family Rutaceae.

Part of plant used Fruit peel.

Extraction process Cold expression of the fresh peel.

Principal chemical constituents Limonene (90 per cent), cadinene, pinene, sabinene, myrcene, neral, geraniol, citronellal, esters, coumarins and furocoumarins.

Country of origin Native to tropical Asia and the West Indies. Cultivated in California, Florida, Australia, Brazil and Israel.

Note Top.

Odour intensity Medium

Blends well with Basil, Bergamot, Chamomile, Sweet fennel, Frankincense, Juniper, Geranium, Lavender, Lime, Palmarosa, Patchouli, Rose and Ylang ylang.

Properties Antiseptic, astringent, depurative, diuretic, disinfectant, stimulant and tonic.

Most common uses

Skin conditions Acne and congested oily skin.
Action Although helpful for these conditions on the body, the oil should not be used on the face.

Circulatory system Cellulite, colds and flu.
Action Boosts the immune system by stimualting the lymphatic system, reduces fluid retention and helps to detoxify the system.

Digestive system Constipation and flatulence.
Action Stimulates the digestive system.

Nervous system Stress, depression, headaches and nervous exhaustion.
Action Has an uplifting and reviving effect, helping to clear the head and improve low confidence often associated with stress.

Safety Non-toxic, non-irritant and non-sensitizing, although exposure to strong sunlight or UV light within 24 hours of treatment may result in skin irritation.

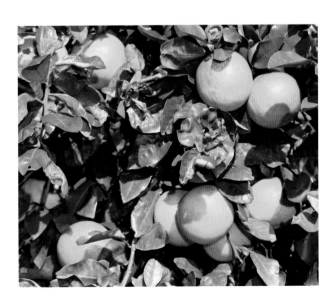

Citrus reticulata (syn. *C. nobilis, C. madurensis, C. unshiu*)
Mandarin

An evergreen tree, up to 6 m (20 ft) high, with glossy leaves, the Mandarin tree is smaller than the Orange tree and has fragrant flowers and fleshy fruit that is slightly flattened at both ends. The fruit was a traditional gift to the mandarins of China, hence its name. The Mandarin is generally preferred for aromatherapeutic purposes. The oil is a yellowy orange colour and has an intensely sweet, fresh tangy aroma. It is one of the safest oils and is recommended for treating children and the frail or elderly, and for use during pregnancy. In France it is considered a safe remedy for the digestive system, especially for children and the elderly. Overall, it is uplifting and soothing. The most usual form is red mandarin, although green and yellow are also occasionally sold.

Botanical family Rutaceae.

Alternative common name Tangerine, Satsuma.

Part of plant used Fruit peel.

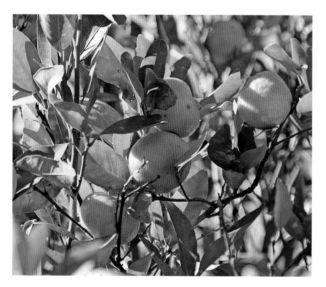

Extraction process Cold expression from the outer peel.

Principal chemical constituents Limonene, pinene, myrcene, geraniol, citral, citronellal and geranial.

Country of origin Native to southern China and the Far East. Also cultivated in Brazil, Spain, Italy and California.

Note Top.

Odour intensity Medium.

Blends well with Basil, Black Pepper, Chamomile, Jasmine, Lavender, Sweet marjoram, Palmarosa, Rose, Sandalwood, Ylang ylang, and other citrus oils.

Properties Antiseptic, anti-spasmodic, carminative, cytophylactic, digestive, diuretic (mild), laxative, sedative and tonic.

Most common uses

Skin conditions All skin types, stretch marks and scarring.
Action Has cell-regenerating properties. This oil is considered safe during pregnancy and is usually recommended from the first trimester in high dilutions (1 per cent).

Digestive system Flatulence, colitis and constipation.
Action Helps to regulate the bile and calms the intestines. A dilution of ½ per cent is useful for babies suffering from colic and can be used on the skin.

Nervous system Insomnia, anxiety, depression and nervous tension.
Action A mild sedative for the nervous system and helps to uplift the spirits in times of stress.

Safety Non-toxic, non-irritant and non-sensitizing. However, it may be phototoxic, so clients should avoid strong sunlight or ultraviolet light after treatment.

Citrus sinensis (syn. *C. aurantium* var. *dulcis*)
Sweet orange

There are two types of Orange tree: Sweet orange (*C. sinensis*) and Bitter orange (*C. aurantium*). The Sweet orange is an evergreen tree, smaller than the Bitter orange and less hardy, it has dark green shiny leaves, fragrant white flowers and fruit with a pitted skin. The oil is a yellowy-orange colour with a sweet, light orange-peel odour. Oranges are often used with spices, such as cinnamon and cloves, to flavour traditional drinks, such as mulled wines, to make pomanders (an orange stuck with cloves and dried), or to soak the logs used on open fires at Christmas. Psychologically, Sweet orange oil is cheering and uplifting, and is often referred to as the 'smiley oil'.

Botanical family Rutaceae.

Part of plant used Fresh ripe or almost ripe peel.

Extraction process Cold expression (hand or machine) from the outer peel. Essential oil can be distilled from the fruit but oxidizes very quickly.

Principal chemical constituents Limonene (over 90 per cent) linalol, citronellae, neral, geranial, esters and coumarins.

Country of origin Native to China. Cultivated in the USA and Mediterranean. The expressed oil is mainly produced in Israel, Cyprus, Brazil and North America. The distilled oil comes mainly from the Mediterranean and North America.

Note Top.

Odour intensity Medium.

Blends well with Clary sage, Cypress, Lavender, Neroli, Myrrh, Frankincense, Petitgrain, Rose, Rosewood, Sandalwood, Ylang ylang, and all the spice oils.

Properties Anti-depressant, antiseptic, anti-spasmodic, carminative, cholagogue, digestive, febrifuge, fungicidal, hypotensive, sedative (nervous), stimulant (digestive and lymphatic), stomachic and tonic.

Most common uses

Skin conditions Mouth ulcers.
Action Sometimes recommended for oily complexions, but can be too strong for the face.

Circulation and immune system Obesity, fluid retention and colds and flu.
Action Helps to reduce swollen tissue, has antiseptic properties and boosts the immune system.

Digestive system Dyspepsia, constipation and irritable bowel syndrome.
Action Stimulates the digestive tract and gall bladder, so helpful for constipation and all digestive disorders.

Nervous system Nervous tension, anorexia, anxiety and depression.
Action Has a delightfully fresh and uplifting odour that seems to help people to relax and unwind.

Safety Non-toxic, non-irritant and non-sensitizing.

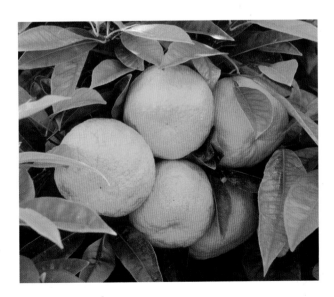

Commiphora myrrha
Myrrh

This plant's name is derived from the Arabic word 'mur', meaning 'bitter'. It is a small tree or shrub with gnarled branches, aromatic leaves and white flowers. The resin is a yellow-brown viscous mass with a warm, rich and spicy balsamic odour. Myrrh was a well-known ingredient of the incense used for religious ceremonies by the ancients and was an ingredient of embalming and the Egyptian perfume kyphi. Its healing reputation stretches back thousands of years (Greek soldiers carried it for first aid). The Chinese use this crude myrrh for arthritis and menstrual problems. In the West it is considered good for respiratory problems. Myrrh inspires peace and tranquillity, and is a great healer.

Botanical family Burseraceae.

Part of plant used Crude myrrh, resinoid.

Extraction process Steam distillation of crude myrrh. Solvent extraction of resinoid to produce an absolute. A tincture is produced for pharmaceutical products.

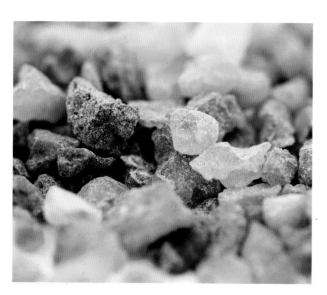

Principal chemical constituents Heerabolene, limonene, eugenol, cuminaldehyde and pinene.

Country of origin Northeastern Africa and southwestern Asia, especially the Dead Sea region (Ethiopia, Somalia and Yemen).

Note Base.

Odour intensity High.

Blends well with Benzoin, Lavender, Orange, Patchouli and Sandalwood.

Properties Anti-catarrhal, anti-inflammatory, antiseptic, carminative and cicatrizant.

Most common uses

Skin conditions Athlete's foot, chapped, cracked and mature skin, eczema and ringworm.
Action Reduces inflammation, soothes irritation and helps with infection.

Circulation, muscles and joints Arthritis.
Action Said to have warming qualities that are especially good for rheumatoid arthritis.

Respiratory system Asthma, bronchitis, gingivitis, catarrh, coughs, sore throat and voice loss, mouth ulcers.
Action A good pulmonary oil and expectorant, helping to clear congestion. Also good for the immune system, helping to clear head colds.

Digestive system Diarrhoea, dyspepsia, flatulence and loss of appetite.
Action Helps to clear the whole system.

Genito-urinary system Amenorrhea, leucorrhea, pruritis, thrush and menopause.
Action May improve menstrual problems.

Safety Non-irritant and non-sensitizing but toxic in high concentrations. Do not use this oil on pregnant women.

Coriandrum sativum
Coriander

Coriander is one of the more gentle of the spicy essential oils. A highly fragrant annual herb, Coriander grows to a height of about 1 m (3 ft) and has delicate, bright green leaves and white flowers, followed by a mass of round green seeds that eventually turn brown. The oil is colourless to pale yellow, with a sweet musky-woody odour. In Chinese medicine the whole herb is utilized and the seeds are used widely for culinary purposes, particularly for flavouring curries. Psychologically, Coriander is reviving and good for stimulating low energy, and is also comforting.

Botanical family Apiaceae (Umbelliferae).

Part of plant used Seeds.

Extraction process Steam distillation of the crushed ripe seeds.

Principal chemical constituents Linalol (55–75 per cent), decylaldehyde, borneol, geraniol, carvone, anethole and others.

Country of origin Native to Europe and western Asia. The essential oil is produced mainly in Russia, Romania, Croatia, Serbia and Bosnia.

Note Top.

Odour intensity Medium.

Blends well with Bergamot, Jasmine, Neroli, Petitgrain, Clary sage, Cypress, Pine, Ginger, Sandalwood.

Properties Analgesic, aperitif, anti-spasmodic, bactericidal, depurative, digestive, diuretic, carminative, revitalizing, stimulant (cardiac, circulatory, nervous) and stomachic.

Most common uses

Circulatory system, muscles and joints
Arthritis, gout, muscular aches, poor circulation and fluid retention.
Action Said to help detoxification and rheumatic pain and to boost the immune system.

Digestive system Colic, dyspepsia, flatulence and nausea.
Action Recommended for digestive disturbances and can help with griping pains and other intestinal upsets.

Nervous system Migraine, neuralgia and nervous exhaustion.
Action Said to clear the head and revitalize the nervous system.

Safety Non-toxic, non-irritant and non-sensitizing. Use this oil in moderation (it is stupefying in large doses).

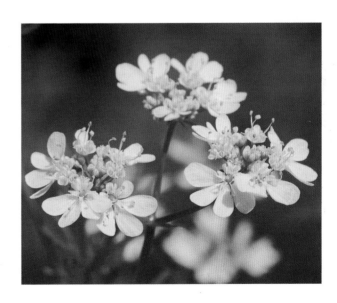

Cupressus sempervirens
Cypress

A tall, conical evergreen tree, with slender branches and needle-type leaves. It bears small flowers and round, brownish-grey cones or nuts. Cypress has spicy, resinous top notes and balsamic undertones, giving it a clean, fresh, woody aroma. It is thought to benefit the urinary system as the cones are very drying and binding. Ancient civilizations valued cypress as a therapeutic medicine and also as a purifying incense.

Botanical family Cupressaceae.

Part of plant used Needles, twigs and cones.

Extraction process Steam distillation of needles and twigs. A concrete and absolute are also produced in small quantities.

Principal chemical constituents Pinene, camphene, sylvestrene, cymene and sabinol.

Country of origin Mediterranean region plus North Africa and Britain. Distilled mostly in France, Spain and Morocco.

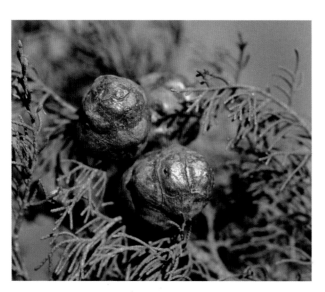

Note Middle to base.

Odour intensity Medium.

Blends well with Benzoin, Bergamot, Clary Sage, Juniper, Lavender, Lemon, Orange, Pine, Rosemary and Sandalwood.

Properties Anti-rheumatic, antiseptic, anti-spasmodic, astringent, deodorant, diuretic, hepatic, styptic (stops bleeding), sudorific, tonic and vasoconstrictive.

Most common uses

Skin conditions Haemorrhoids, varicose veins, oily and over-hydrated skin, excessive perspiration and wounds.
Action An astringent, so helps with excessive perspiration. It can also be used as an insect repellent and possibly to help with bedwetting in older children. It can help to constrict varicose veins when used with Lemon.

Circulation, muscles and joints Rheumatism, cellulitis, muscular cramp, oedema, and poor circulation.
Action A diuretic so helps with fluid retention, and may improve the look of 'orange-peel' skin (cellulite), which is caused by water-logged tissues.

Respiratory system Asthma, bronchitis and coughing.
Action Can help with mucous although there are more suitable essential oils for this.

Genito-urinary system Dysmenorrhea and menopausal problems.
Action Said to work on hormones, stimulating oestrogen production and and helping during the menopause and with premenstrual pain.

Nervous system Nervous tension.
Action Helps with stress-related problems, overwork and anxiety. Thought to be helpful with emotional issues, such as bereavement or the ending of a close relationship.

Safety Non-toxic, non-irritant and non-sensitizing. Do not use this oil on pregnant women.

Cymbopogon citrates (syn. *Andropogon citrates*)
Lemongrass

A tall aromatic perennial grass that grows up to 1.5 m (5 ft) high, there are several species of Lemongrass but those from eastern India and the West Indies are the most common. It has a strong fresh lemony odour and is used to flavour food, as well as in perfumery and to fragrance rooms. It has been used in traditional Indian medicine for infectious illnesses and fever, and recent research in India shows that it also acts as a sedative on he central nervous system. After distillation, the remains of the grass are used to feed cattle. Lemongrass is cooling, refreshing and stimulating

Botanical family Poaceae (Gramineae).

Part of plant used Grass and leaves.

Extraction process Steam distillation of the fresh and partly dried leaves (grass), which are finely chopped.

Principal chemical constituents Citral, limonene, linalol, citronellol, geranyl acetate, geraniol, nerol and farnesol.

Country of origin Native to Asia. Cultivated mainly in the West Indies, Africa and tropical Asia. Main producers are Guatemala and India.

Note Top.

Odour intensity High

Blends well with Basil, Bergamot, Black pepper, Cedarwood, Grapefruit, Geranium, Lavender, Marjoram, Palmarosa, Petitgrain and Rosemary.

Properties Analgesic, anti-depressant, anti-microbial, anti-oxidant, astringent, bactericidal, carminative, febrifuge, fungicidal, insecticidal, nervine, sedative (nervous system) and fatigue.

Most common uses

Skin conditions Athlete's foot and excessive perspiration.
Action Although this oil can be good for acne, it appears to be a skin irritant and should not be used on the face. It can also act as an insect repellent.

Circulation, muscles and joints Poor circulation and muscle tone.
Action Considered an excellent tonic with a beneficial effect on aching muscles, helping them to become more supple, especially after a minor sports injury.

Digestive system Colitis, indigestion and flatulence.
Action Said to help the digestion and boost the immune system to combat cold and flu infections.

Nervous system Nervous exhaustion, headaches and stress-related problems.
Action Has invigorating properties, said to help revive and energize. Good for jet-lag and fatigue, and also helps with lack of mental clarity and focus, especially where there is nervous exhaustion.

Safety Non-toxic but may cause irritation or sensitization. Use this oil with care, especially in skin preparations.

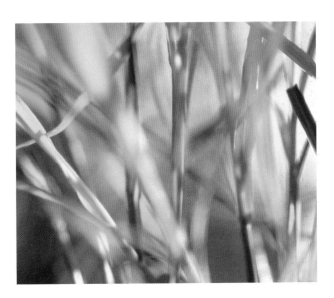

Cymbopogon martini (syn. *Andropogon martini*)
Palmarosa

A tall, grass-like herbaceous plant that grows naturally in the wild, Palmarosa has a long stem with a flowering top. The leaves are very fragrant and the pale yellow essential oil smells sweet and floral. It has also been known as Gingergrass, Indian or Turkish Geranium oil, Russa Grass and East Indian Geranium oil. This last name dates back to when the oil was shipped from Bombay then transported overland to Bulgaria, where it was used for the adulteration of Rose oil. Palmarosa has a calming yet uplifting effect on the emotions.

Botanical family Poaceae (Gramineae).

Part of plant used Fresh or dried grass, and sometimes the leaves.

Extraction process Steam or water distillation.

Principal chemical constituents Geraniol, linalol, myrcene, geranyl acetate, citronellol, dipentene and limonene.

Country of origin Native to India and Pakistan. Now cultivated in the Comoro Islands and Madagascar.

Note Top.

Odour intensity Low to medium.

Blends well with Bergamot, Geranium, Jasmine, Lavender, Lime, Melissa, Neroli, Orange, Petitgrain, Rose, Sandalwood and Ylang ylang.

Properties Antiseptic, antiviral, cytophylactic, febrifuge, stimulant (digestive and circulatory) and tonic.

Most common uses

Skin conditions Dry and mature skins, minor skin infections and scars.
Action Rehydrating and moisturizing, stimulating the secretion of sebum and cell regeneration.

Digestive system Sluggish digestion and intestinal infections.
Action Acts as a tonic for the digestive system and is said to have an adverse effect on intestinal pathogens, particularly E. coli and organisms causing dysentery.

Nervous system Anxiety, depression and anorexia.
Action Has a calming yet uplifting effect on the emotions and is particularly helpful when feeling lost or listless.

Safety Non-toxic, non-irritant and non-sensitizing.

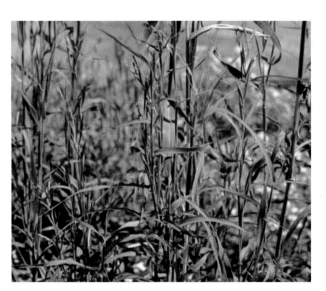

Eucalyptus radiata (also *E. globulus*, *E. smithii*, *E. citriodora*)
Eucalyptus

There are over 700 species of Eucalyptus. The most common species used in aromatherapy is *E. globulus* (Blue Gum). They are tall, evergreen trees, up to 90 m (295 ft) high. The young trees have bluish green leaves while the mature trees develop long, narrow, yellowish leaves with creamy-white flowers. The essential oil is colourless, with a strong, clear camphoraceous odour and woody undertones. *E. radiata* var. *australiana* has a much lighter, fresher odour and is often used as it is rich in cineol. *E. smithii*, is the oil often recommended for children to inhale during epidemics and for infectious illnesses. *E.citriodora is* said to particularly help the immune system. Eucaplyptus is stimulating and purifying, and can protect the body against disease and viruses by strengthening the immune system.

Botanical family Myrtaceae.

Part of plant used Leaves.

Extraction process Steam distillation of the fresh or partly dried leaves and young twigs.

Principal chemical constituents Cineol (70–80 per cent in most except Eucalyptus citriodora, which has a high proportion of citronellol), pinene, limonene and globulol.

Country of origin Australia and Tasmania. Cultivated in Spain and Portugal, Brazil, Russia and the USA.

Note Top.

Odour intensity High.

Blends well with Basil, Benzoin, Cedarwood, Frankincense, Juniper, Lavender, Lemon, Marjoram, Melissa, Rosemary and Thyme.

Properties Analgesic, antiseptic, anti-bacterial, anti-spasmodic, antiviral, carminative, detoxicant, diuretic, cicatrizant, expectorant, febrifuge, stimulant and vulnerary.

Most common uses

Skin conditions Infections, wounds, ulcers and bites.
Action A good remedy for any condition where there is an infection. It is also a good insect repellent.

Circulation, muscles and joints Muscular pains, rheumatoid arthritis, poor circulation and cellulite.
Action Said to be warming and anti-inflammatory.

Respiratory system Asthma, bronchitis, catarrh, coughs, sinusitis and sore throats.
Action A powerful oil for respiratory conditions. It is a traditional remedy for asthma, colds and flu.

Nervous system Debility and headaches.
Action Can help with psychological problems and can also clear a headache.

Safety Externally non-toxic, non-irritant (in low dilution) and non-sensitizing. Do not use in conjunction with homeopathic remedies. THIS OIL MAY BE FATAL IF TAKEN INTERNALLY.

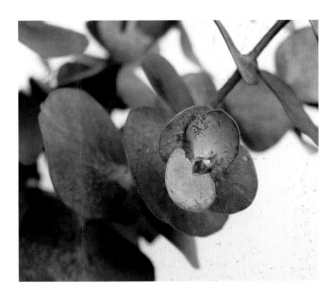

Foeniculum vulgare (syn. *F. vulgare* var. *dulce*)
Sweet Fennel

Sweet fennel grows up to 2 m (6 ft) high and has feathery leaves and golden-yellow flowers. The essential oil is pale yellow with a very sweet herbal anise-like odour. Sweet fennel is widely used in aromatherapy but Bitter fennel (*F. vulgare* var. *amara*) is considered too toxic. Fennel has long been associated with detoxification and was thought to encourage longevity, courage and strength. Fennel is a natural diuretic and depurative, helping get rid of water retention and constipation. Overall, it is deeply cleansing, purifying and revitalizing.

Botanical family Apiaceae (Umbelliferae).

Part of plant used Crushed seeds.

Extraction process Steam distillation.

Principal chemical constituents Anethole (50–60 per cent), limonene, myrcene, pinene, phellandrene, anisic acid, anisic aldehyde and cineole. (Note: Bitter Fennel contains fenchone (18–22 per cent).

Country of origin Indigenous to South Europe, now also cultivated in India, Argentina, China and Pakistan.

Note Middle to top.

Odour intensity High.

Blends well with Basil, Clary sage, Cypress, Geranium, Grapefruit, Lavender, Lemon, Orange, Rosemary, Sandalwood.

Properties Antiseptic, aperitif, anti-spasmodic, anti-inflammatory, carminative, depurative, detoxicant, diuretic, emmenagogue, expectorant, galactagogue, stimulant, stomachic, tonic and vermifuge.

Most common uses

Circulatory system Poor circulation and cellulite.
Action A strong diuretic that can help to treat fluid retention and detoxify the body. It is especially helpful for improving the lymphatic system.

Digestive system Flatulence, indigestion, nausea.
Action Said to be one of the best digestive remedies because, according to Chinese medicine, it has warming and drying qualities.

Respiratory system Asthma, bronchitis and whooping cough.
Action Used as an anti-spasmodic. A good pulmonary oil.

Genito-urinary system Urinary tract infections, menopausal problems, amenorrhea, premenstrual syndrome and insufficient milk production in nursing mothers.
Action Known to have a significant oestrogenic potency due to plant hormones so can be useful in regulating the menstrual cycle. It is also thought to help in reducing the symptoms caused by fluctuating hormone levels.

Safety Non-irritant and relatively non-toxic. Can cause sensitization in some individuals. Use in moderation. Do not use this oil on pregnant women and people with epilepsy, oestrogen-dependent cancers or endometriosis.

Jasminum grandiflorum (syn. *J. officinale*)
Jasmine

Jasmine is a creeping vine, with a mass of delicate, star-shaped white or yellow flowers. Jasmine is known for its wonderfully uplifting sweet aroma, which some people can find overpowering. Revered for centuries in the East, both as a medicine and perfume, Jasmine is called 'queen of the night' in India, as its scent is stronger after sunset. Associated throughout history with goddesses of the Moon, Jasmine grew along the banks of the Nile and was represented by Isis, the Egyptian mother goddess who held the secrets of fertility, magic and healing. Jasmine was used as a general tonic for the whole body in Europe during the Middle Ages. It is now used extensively in perfume and toiletries. Jasmine is soothing, relaxing and uplifting.

Botanical family Oleaceae (Jasminaceae).

Part of plant used Flowers.

Extraction process Solvent extraction which produces an absolute, which is then steam distilled. The traditional method is known as enfleurage.

Principal chemical constituents Over 100 constituents, including benzyl acetate, linalol, jasmere, geraniol and benzyl alcohol.

Country of origin China, northern India, Egypt, France and the Mediterranean.

Note Base.

Odour intensity High.

Blends well with Clary sage, Frankincense, Geranium, Orange, Mandarin, Melissa, Neroli, Palmarosa, Sandalwood and Ylang ylang.

Properties Anti-spasmodic, anti-depressant, sedative, aphrodisiac, galactagogue, lactogenic, relaxing and tonic.

Most common uses

Skin conditions Inflamed, dry and sensitive skin, dermatitis, redness and itching.
Action Encourages skin regeneration and helps heal scar tissue, hydrates and soothes dry skin, and increases elasticity.

Reproductive and endocrine systems
Childbirth, labour pains, menstrual pain and lactation.
Action Helps to balance hormones during premenstrual syndrome and the menopause. Its antispasmodic properties help to ease childbirth and speed up delivery.

Nervous system Depression, emotional repression, impotence, frigidity, lethargy, lack of confidence and prostatitis.
Action Warms and relaxes the body, helping to strengthen and restore the sexual organs. It also improves self-confidence and optimism, eases depression, clams nerves and warms emotions.

Safety Non-toxic, non-irritant and non-sensitizing. It is best not to use this oil during early pregnancy.

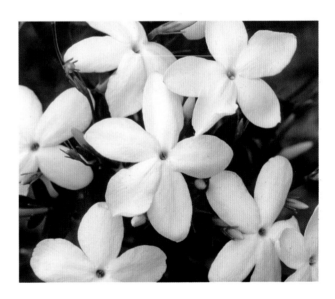

Juniper communis
Juniper berry

An evergreen tree that grows up to 6 m (20 ft) with distinctive bluish-green needles. It has small flowers and berries that are green in the first year and black in the second and third years. The oil is pale yellow and has a fresh, woody odour. Known for its purifying qualities, juniper has been used medicinally for many years, notably against the plague in the 15th and 16th centuries. French hospitals used to burn Juniper and Rosemary twigs to cleanse the air. It was traditionally burned for protection against evil spirits.

Botanical family Cupressaceae.

Part of plant used Berries, resin.

Extraction process Steam distillation of the fresh ripe berries and sometimes the needles and wood. A small amount of absolute is produced from the resin.

Principal chemical constituents Mainly momoterpenes: pinene, turpinene, thujene, camphene and limonene.

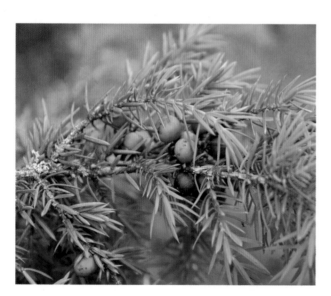

Country of origin The northern hemisphere – Canada, northern Europe and northern Asia. The essential oil is produced mainly in Italy, France, Austria, Spain and Canada.

Note Middle.

Odour intensity Medium.

Blends well with Benzoin, Bergamot, Cypress, Fennel, Frankincense, Geranium, Grapefruit, Orange, Lavender, Lemon, Lime, Rosemary and Sandalwood.

Properties Anti-rheumatic, antiseptic, anti-spasmodic, anti-toxic, astringent, carminative, cicatrizant, diuretic, emmenagogue, nervine, stomachic, tonic and vulnerary.

Most common uses:

Skin conditions Acne and oily congested skin.
Action Known as a 'cleansing' oil and can help unblock clogged pores.

Circulation, muscles and joints Accumulation of toxins, gout, obesity and rheumatism.
Action A valuable diuretic so helps as most of these conditions are due to build-up of fluid and/or toxins.

Genito-urinary system Amenorrhea, cystitis, dysmenorrhea and leucorrhea.
Action Thought to help regulate menstruation and also good for fluid retention.

Nervous system Anxiety and nervous tension.
Action Can help with stress-related problems and is good for clearing negative energy.

Immune system Colds, flu and infections.
Action Helps because of its antiseptic qualities.

Safety Non-sensitizing and non-toxic but may be slightly irritating. Do not use this oil on pregnant women because it stimulates the uterus, nor on people with kidney disease.

Lavandula angustifolia (syn. *L.vera, L. officinalis*)
Lavender

One of the most versatile essential oils, Lavender is said to be effective in treating over 70 conditions and its reputation goes back thousands of years. A perennial bushy shrub with spiky leaves and purple-blue flowers, it has been used as a herb and essential oil for thousands of years. The plant is noted for its fresh, distinctive floral scent, and the best essential oil comes from France. It was a popular bath oil with the Romans, who were responsible for its spread across Europe. It is soothing and relaxing, a good all-rounder that is useful for treating a range of conditions.

Botanical family Lamiaceae (Labiatae).

Part of plant used Flowers.

Extraction process Steam distillation. Solvent extraction produces an absolute.

Principal chemical constituents Over 100 constituents including linalyl acetate (up to 40 per cent), pinene, limonene, linalol and lavandulol. Alpine Lavender is always higher in esters than plants grown at lower altitudes.

Country of origin Native to the Mediterranean. Now grown all over the world, particularly in England, France, Yugoslavia, Bulgaria, Morocco, Australia and Tasmania.

Note Middle.

Odour intensity Middle to high.

Blends well with most oils but especially citrus and florals, also Clary sage, Geranium, Patchouli and Vetiver.

Properties Anti-depressant, anti-inflammatory, antiseptic, anti-spasmodic, anti-bacterial, anti-viral, balancing, calming, decongestant, relaxing, sedative, soothing and tonic.

Most common uses

Skin conditions Acne, boils, cold sores, dermatitis, eczema, lice, rashes, ringworm and sunburn.
Action Stimulates the healing process and promotes cell growth, speeding up the formation of new, healthy skin. It is also an effective way of dealing with skin parasites.

Respiratory system Asthma, bronchial congestion, colds, influenza and sore throats.
Action Works as an anti-spasmodic, relaxing breathing.

Circulation, muscles and joints Muscular aches and pains and rheumatism.
Action Has soothing and anti-inflammatory properties.

Nervous system Headaches, insomnia, mood swings and nervous tension.
Action Soothing, balancing and calming. Can help strong emotions, such as frustration, irritability, nervous anxiety, panic and insomnia. If used in too high a concentration, it has the opposite effect, and stimulates into wakefulness.

Safety Non-toxic, non-irritant and non-sensitizing. This is one of the few essential oils that can be used neat on the skin – applying it carefully to the area to be treated. Do not use it on pregnant women during the first trimester.

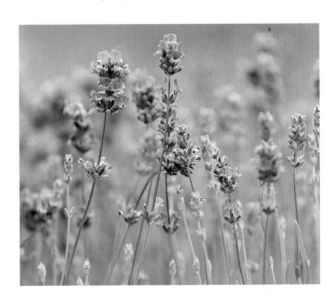

Litsea cubeba
May chang

A small deciduous tree, growing to about 5–8 m (16–26 ft), May chang has small, lemon-scented leaves and flowers, and fruit shaped like peppers, from which the name 'cubeba' derives. The essential oil is pale yellow with a fresh, intensely sweet, lemony, fruity odour. May chang is relatively new to the essential oil market, but has a long history of use in traditional Chinese medicine, where the root and stem of the tree are used to treat dysmenorrheal problems and for common ailments. Recent research shows that it may help in the treatment of some heart disorders. May chang is very versatile, with a cheering, uplifting effect.

Botanical family Lauraceae.

Part of plant used Fruit.

Extraction process Steam distillation of the small fresh aromatic fruit.

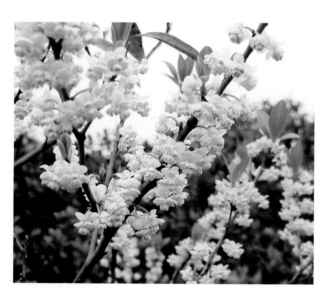

Principal chemical constituents Geraniol, neral, citronellal, linalol, limonene, linalyl acetate, and geranyl acetate.

Country of origin Native to China, Indonesia and South-eastern Asia. Now cultivated mainly in China, Taiwan and Japan.

Note Top.

Odour intensity Medium to high.

Blends well with Basil, Bergamot, Geranium, Ginger, Jasmine, Lavender, Neroli, Orange, Petitgrain, Rose and Ylang ylang.

Properties Antiseptic, anti-inflammatory, anti-depressant, anti-spasmodic (bronchia), anti-viral, digestive, insecticidal, stomachic and tonic.

Most common uses

Skin conditions Acne, oily skin, excessive perspiration and athlete's foot.
Action Has a toning and astringent effect on skin.

Circulatory system Arrhythmia and hypertension.
Action According to Chinese research, a good tonic for the heart and helps to reduce high blood pressure.

Respiratory system Asthma, bronchitis, coughs and colds.
Action Said to be an effective respiratory tonic and bronchial antispasmodic with a pronounced antiseptic and anti-viral action. It has also been used as a bronchodilator and may be helpful for asthmatic conditions.

Nervous system Nervous tension and stress-related conditions.
Action Uplifting and stimulating, helping to lift the spirits and relieve stress and tension, especially when there is a history of depression and worry.

Safety Non-toxic and non-irritant, but may cause sensitization in some individuals.

Matricaria recutica var. *chamomilla*
German chamomile

A well-established medicinal herb, this strongly aromatic annual has tall, hairless branching stems, delicate feathery leaves and simple, daisy-like white flowers on single stems. The flowers are smaller than those of Roman chamomile. It is versatile, calming and soothing, and particularly good for treating children and the elderly. This herb has traditionally been used for stress-related problems, especially tension headaches. It has greater anti-inflammatory properties Roman chamomile. The essential oil is an inky-blue colour and has a strong, easily identified odour.

Botanical family Asteraceae (Compositae).

Part of plant used Flowerheads.

Extraction process Steam distillation. An absolute is also produced.

Principal chemical constituents Chamazulene, farnesene and bisabolol oxide. (Note: chamazulene is only produced during distillation).

Country of origin Native to Europe but cultivated extensively in Eastern Europe, particularly Hungary. (Despite the name, it is no longer grown in Germany.) Also found in North America and Australia.

Note Middle.

Odour intensity Very high.

Blends well with Benzoin, Bergamot, Clary sage, Geranium, Jasmine, Lavender, Marjoram, Melissa, Patchouli, Rose and Ylang ylang.

Properties Analgesic, anti-inflammatory, anti-allergenic, anti-spasmodic, carminative, cicatrizant, digestive, emmenagogue, febrifuge, fungicidal, hepatic, stomachic, sudorific and vulnerary.

Most common uses

Skin conditions Acne, allergies, burns, cuts, eczema, inflammation, insect bites, and rashes. Also haircare, earache, toothache and teething pain.
Action Reduces inflammation.

Circulation, muscles and joints Arthritis, inflamed joints, muscular pain, rheumatism and sprains.
Action Reduces inflammation, especially where there is also swelling.

Digestive system Dyspepsia, colic, indigestion and nausea.
Action Helps with indigestion, calming and soothing.

Genito-urinary system Dysmenorrhea and menopausal problems.
Action Helps whenever there is pain.

Nervous system Headache, insomnia, nervous tension and migraine.
Action Has many soothing and calming properties and is particularly helpful in stress-related conditions.

Safety Generally non-toxic and non-irritant but may cause dermatitis in some individuals. Use in moderation.

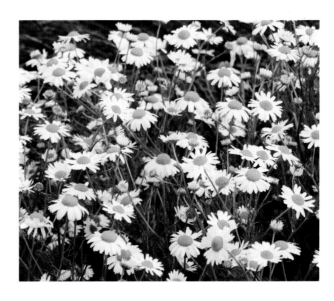

Melaleuca alternifolia
Tea tree

A small tree or shrub native to Australia, the Aborigines have long used this plant for its antiseptic qualities. It is also known as the Ti Tree. The leaves are needle-like and the flowers are yellow or purplish. Tea tree is a general name for members of the *Melaleuca* family, including Cajeput (*M. cajeputi*) and Niaouli (*M. viridiflora*). The essential oil is pale yellowy green in colour and has a pungent antiseptic aroma. It is the most 'medicinal' of the essential oils and is effective for all-round first aid. It is also unique among essential oils in that it has been found to be active against all three categories of infectious organism: bacteria, viruses and fungi. *Ravensara aromatica* is a less well-known oil that has many of the same properties as tea tree but does not smell as strongly. It is in particular a very effective antiviral oil.

Botanical family Myrtaceae.

Part of plant used Leaves and twigs.

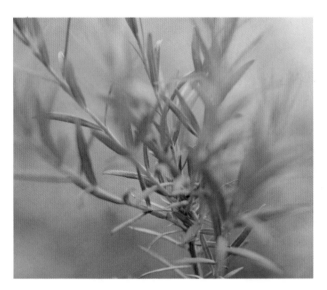

Extraction process Steam or water distillation.

Principal chemical constituents Terpene (at least 30 per cent), cineol (not to exceed 15 per cent), pinene, terpinenes, cymene, sesquiterpenes and sesquiterpene alcohols.

Country of origin Native to Australia. Other species have been cultivated elsewhere but not *M. alternifolia*.

Note Top.

Odour intensity Very high.

Blends well with Cypress, Eucalyptus, Geranium, Ginger, Juniper, Lavender, Lemon, Mandarin, Orange, Rosemary and Thyme but will dominate the blend due to its strong odour.

Properties Antibiotic, anti-microbial, antiseptic, anti-viral, bactericidal, expectorant, fungicidal, insecticide, stimulant and sudorific.

Most common uses

Skin conditions Acne, skin rashes, oily skin, bites and stings, dandruff, head lice and athlete's foot.
Action Can be used (in combination with Lavender) in the treatment of pimples and acne. Applied neat on a cottonwool bud to the centre of the pustule, it will quickly reduce the problem. It can also be applied to insect bites and stings.

Immune system Colds, flu, fever and infections.
Action A very effective stimulant of the immune system, helping to increase the body's defence against invading organisms.

Respiratory system Asthma, bronchitis, coughs and sinusitis.
Action Use in a vapourizer as an inhalant for congested nasal passages and respiratory infections.

Safety Non-toxic and non-irritant, but may cause sensitization in some individuals. Use in moderation.

Melaleuca viridiflora (syn. M. quinquenervia)
Niaouli

This oil is derived from an evergreen tree with a spongy bark and flexible trunk, pointed linear leaves and sessile yellow flowers. When crushed, the leaves have a strong aromatic scent and the essential oil is pale yellow with a sweet, fresh camphoraceous odour. The oil is called gomenol because it was once shipped from Gomen in the French East Indies. It was used to purify water and did not arrive in Europe until the 17th century. It is now used in pharmaceutical preparations such as gargles, toothpaste and mouth washes.

Botanical family Myrtaceae.

Alternative common name Gomenol.

Part of plant used Leaves and young twigs.

Extraction process Steam distillation (usually rectified to remove irritant aldehydes).

Principal chemical constituents Cineole (50–65 per cent), pinene, camphene, terpineol, limonene, linalol and piperitone.

Country of origin Australia and New Caledonia.

Note Top.

Odour intensity High.

Blends well with Basil, Benzoin, Eucalyptus, Sweet fennel, Juniper, Lavender, Lemon, Melissa, Orange and Thyme.

Properties Antiseptic, analgesic, anti-catarrhal, anti-rheumatic, bactericidal, cicatrizant, decongestant, expectorant, stimulant and vermifuge.

Most common uses

Skin conditions Acne, cuts, insect bites and wounds.
Action Aids healing and is especially useful for washing infected wounds.

Immune system Colds, fever and flu.
Action Boosts the immune system.

Respiratory system Catarrh, sinus problems, bronchitis and other infections.
Action An excellent antiseptic.

Genito-urinary system Cystitis.
Action Said to be helpful for urinary infections.

Safety Non-toxic, non-irritant and non-sensitizing. Do not use this oil on clients who are taking homeopathic remedies as it may negate their effect.

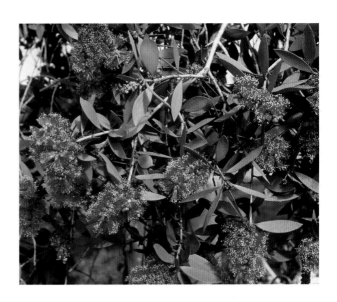

Melissa officinalis
Melissa

A sweet-scented perennial herb that grows to about 60 cm (24 in) high, with green serrated leaves and tiny white or pink flowers. Also known as Lemon balm. The essential oil has a light, fresh, lemony odour with warm overtones. Due to the high price of Melissa it is one of the most frequently adulterated oils and most commercial 'Melissa' contains some Lemongrass or Citronella and is labelled 'nature-identical'. Melissa is uplifting and good for stress-related conditions, acting as a gentle tonic.

Botanical family Lamiaceae (Labiatae).

Alternative common name Lemon balm.

Part of plant used Leaves and flowering tops.

Extraction process Steam distillation.

Principal chemical constituents Citronellol, geranial, nerol, citronellal, caryophyllene, linalol, limonene and geranyl acetate.

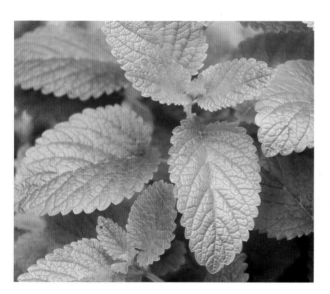

Country of origin Native to the Mediterranean. Found in most parts of Europe, central Asia and North America. Cultivated mainly in Hungary, Egypt, Italy and Ireland.

Note Middle.

Odour intensity Medium to high.

Blends well with Bergamot, Chamomile, Frankincense, Geranium, Ginger, Jasmine, Juniper, Lavender, Marjoram, Neroli, Rose and Ylang ylang.

Properties Anti-depressant, anti-histaminic, anti-spasmodic, antiviral, carminative, emmenagogue, febrifuge, hypotensive, nervine and tonic.

Most common uses

Skin conditions Skin allergies and insect bites.
Action Due to the risk of irritation, use true Melissa oil.

Circulatory system High blood pressure and palpitations.
Action Said to be hypotensive, so may help to reduce high blood pressure.

Digestive system Gastric problems, nausea and dyspepsia.
Action The odour helps upset stomachs. In France, inhaling the oil is recommended for morning sickness, although it is an emmenagogue (stimulates the uterus).

Nervous system Nervous tension, nervous disorders, grief, headaches and anxiety.
Action Can lift the spirits, so is useful for all nervous complaints, especially where emotions are involved.

Immune system Influenza, herpes, smallpox and mumps.
Action Has antiviral properties. Thought to be effective in treating cold sores and shingles.

Safety Non-toxic but may cause sensitization and skin irritation. Use this oil in low dilutions only and do not use on pregnant women.

Mentha piperita
Peppermint

A perennial herb up to 1 m (3 ft) high, with underground runners and green leaves; there are many species of Peppermint but the oil used for aromatherapy is easily recognizable for its strong, sharp, piercing menthol fragrance. The Egyptians used it to flavour wine and food and Culpepper advocated this as the best herb for stomach complaints. Peppermint is cool, refreshing and good for the digestion.

Botanical family Lamiaceae (Labiatae).

Part of plant used Leaves and flowering tops.

Extraction process Steam distillation of the flowering herb.

Principal chemical constituents Menthol, menthone, menthyl acetate, menthofuran, limonene, cineol and pulegone.

Country of origin USA, Tasmania, France. Cultivated worldwide.

Note Top.

Odour intensity Medium to high.

Blends well with Basil, Benzoin, Cypress, Lemon, Lime, Lavender, Marjoram, Pine and Rosemary.

Properties Analgesic, anti-inflammatory, antiseptic, anti-spasmodic, antiviral, astringent, carminative, cephalic, decongestant, emmenagogue, expectorant, febrifuge, hepatic, nervine, stimulant, stomachic, sudorific, vasoconstrictor and vermifuge.

Most common uses

Skin conditions Skin congestion and irritation.
Action Relieves itching or irritation, but only use in a 1 per cent dilution to avoid aggravating the condition.

Circulatory and muscular systems Muscular and joint pain.
Action An analgesic that helps to relieve muscle and joint pain (lumbago) and bruising.

Respiratory and immune system Colds and flu.
Action An antiseptic and expectorant so may be helpful with sinus congestion and infections.

Digestive system Colic, cramp, dyspepsia, flatulence and nausea.
Action An effective remedy for nausea and vomiting, and can be helpful for travel sickness.

Nervous system Headaches, migraine and fatigue.
Action Can help to clear headaches, especially if there is difficulty with concentration and clear thinking. In this instance, it is best used in burners.

Safety Non-toxic and non-irritant (except in high concentrations), but the menthol content may cause sensitization. Do not use this oil on pregnant women or on clients who are taking homeopathic remedies. This is a very stimulating oil and should not be used on people who have epilepsy or a history of heart disease.

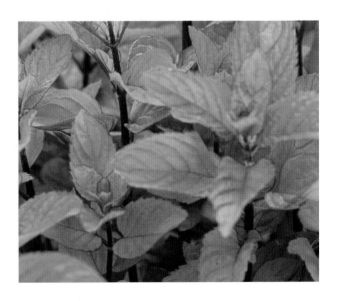

Ocimum basilicum
Basil

A tender, annual aromatic herb with green leaves and small white or pink flowers. There are a number of varieties but the one recommended for aromatherapy is French basil (Sweet basil), which has pale pink flowers and a high percentage of linalol. The essential oil has a very pleasant, sweet, light and refreshing herbaceous fragrance. It is widely used in the ayurvedic tradition, where it is called *tulsi*. Basil is restorative, fortifying and good for clearing the mind and lifting spirits.

Botanical family Lamiaceae (Labiatae).

Part of plant used Flowering tops and leaves.

Extraction process Steam distillation.

Principal chemical constituents Methyl chavicol, linalol, cineol, camphor, eugenol, limonene and citronellol.

Country of origin Native to Asia and Africa. Now widely cultivated in France, Italy, Bulgaria, Egypt, Hungary, Australia and South Africa.

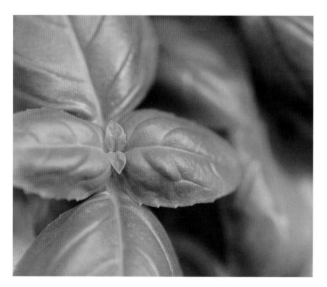

Note Top.

Odour intensity High.

Blends well with Bergamot, Black pepper, Clary sage, Eucalyptus, Geranium, Ginger, Lavender, Melissa, Neroli, Rosemary and Sandalwood.

Properties Analgesic, anti-depressant, antiseptic, anti-spasmodic, carminative, cephalic, digestive, emmenagogue, expectorant, febrifuge and nervine.

Most common uses

Skin conditions Insect bites.
Action Due to possible sensitization, it is better to use with caution and not in the bath.

Digestive system Vomiting, nausea, dyspepsia and hiccups.
Action Said to settle the stomach.

Respiratory system Asthma and bronchitis.
Action An anti-spasmodic that can help to relieve sinus congestion, particularly in whooping cough; also reduces fever and helps to boost the immune system.

Genito-urinary system Irregular periods and menstrual pain.
Action Can help with menstrual problems, especially scanty periods, if gently massaged over the stomach.

Nervous system Anxiety, depression, migraine, headaches and nervous tension.
Action One of the most useful cephalics, relieving mental fatigue and clearing the mind. It is useful for many nervous disorders, especially nervous exhaustion.

Safety May cause sensitization and irritation. Do not use this oil in the bath or on clients with sensitive skin, and avoid prolonged use. Do not use this oil on pregant women. Research has raised concerns over the possible carcinogenic effects of the methyl chavicol contained in the Exotic basil chemotype, therefore it is best to use French basil (Sweet basil).

Origanum marjorana (syn. *Marjorana hortensis*)
Sweet Marjoram

Marjoram is a small bushy perennial plant about 60 cm (24 in) high, with oval, dark green leaves and small, greyish white or purple flowers in clusters. It has a well-established reputation as a herbal medicine, and was used by the ancient Greeks in their fragrances and medicines. It The essential oil is yellow or amber in colour, with a warm, peppery, spicy odour. Marjoram is the great comforter of essential oils, known for its warming and comforting qualities.

Botanical family Lamiaceae (Labiatae).

Part of plant used Dried leaves and flowering tops.

Extraction process Steam distillation. An oleoresin is also produced in smaller quantities.

Principal chemical constituents Terpinenes, terpineol, sabinenes, linalol, linalyl acetate, and citral.

Country of origin Native to the Mediterranean region, Egypt and North Africa.

Note Medium.

Odour intensity Medium.

Blends well with Bergamot, Chamomile, Cypress, Grapefruit, Jasmine, Lavender, Lime, Mandarin, Rosemary and Ylang ylang.

Properties Analgesic, anti-oxidant, antiseptic, anti-spasmodic, antiviral, carminative, cephalic, digestive, emmenagogue, expectorant, fungicidal, hypotensive, nervine, sedative, rebefacient and vulnerary.

Most common uses

Skin conditions Chilblains and bruises.
Action Used for its warming and healing properties.

Circulation, muscles and joints High blood pressure and heart conditions.
Action Reduces blood pressure and relieves the muscular tension that accompanies it. Very comforting and warming when blended with Lavender, especially for stiffness in the joints.

Respiratory system Asthma, bronchitis and coughs.
Action Can be used as an inhalation or diluted in a massage oil for respiratory problems.

Genito-urinary system Premenstrual syndrome and menstrual problems, dysmenorrhea and amenorrhea.
Action May help to treat delayed, scanty or painful periods. Eases menstrual cramps if used as a hot compress over the lower abdomen, especially if used together with Clary sage.

Nervous system Headaches, migraine, insomnia, nervous tension, anxiety and depression.
Action A restorative that helps stress-related problems, which can show up as headaches or insomnia, by calming the nervous system.

Safety Non-toxic, non-irritant, non-sensitizing. Do not use this oil on pregnant women.

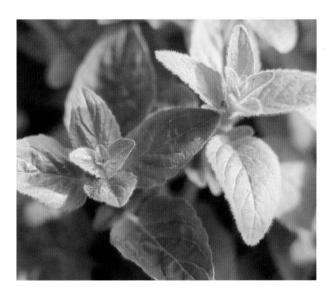

Pelargonium graveolens (syn. *P. odoratissimum*)
Geranium

Used by the ancients to treat wounds and tumours, Geranium is an aromatic perennial shrub about 1 m (3 ft) high, with serrated leaves and small pink flowers. Over 700 varieties of cultivated Geranium are grown for ornamental purposes and some varieties are used in the perfume industry. The essential oil has a sweet, heavy aroma similar to Rose, but with the sharpness of Bergamot. Geranium is well known for its balancing and uplifting properties.

Botanical family Geraniaceae.

Part of plant used Flowers, leaves and stalks.

Extraction process Steam distillation.

Principal chemical constituents Limonene, menthone, geranyl acetate, linalol and citronellol

Country of origin Native to South Africa. Now cultivated worldwide, especially in Spain, Morocco, Egypt, Italy and China.

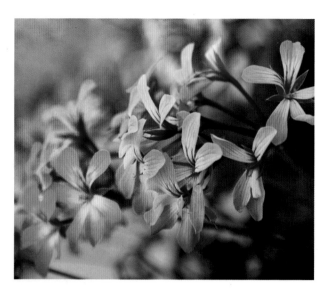

Note Middle.

Odour intensity High.

Blends well with Basil, Bergamot, Grapefruit, Jasmine, Lavender, Neroli, Orange, Patchouli, Petitgrain, Rose, Rosemary, Sandalwood and Ylang ylang.

Properties Anti-depressant, anti-inflammatory, antiseptic, astringent, cicatrizant, cytophylactic, diuretic, haemostatic, tonic (liver and kidneys) and vulnerary.

Most common uses:

Skin conditions All skin conditions, particularly burns, wounds and ulcers.
Action Helps to balance the sebum secreted by the sebaceous glands and keeps the skin supple by moisturizing it. Also good for congested oily skin and has been known to help relieve pain in herpes zoster.

Circulatory system Oedema and cellulite.
Action A diuretic, so helps the lymphatic system by relieving congestion and the fluid retention that leads to swelling.

Genito-urinary and endocrine system
Menopause and premenstrual syndrome.
Action Is considered to have balancing and stimulating qualities on the adrenal cortex, so can help to regulate hormonal conditions associated with the menopause and premenstrual syndrome. It can also help with engorgement during breastfeeding.

Nervous system Nervous tension and stress-related problems.
Action Said to be helpful for anxiety and depression (which is related to hormones), and will lift the spirits.

Safety Generally non-toxic, non-irritant and non-sensitizing, but it may cause irritation to sensitive skins. You can use this oil in a low concentration on pregnant women after the first trimester But do not use it on women with cancer, especially of the breast or ovaries.

Pinus sylvestris
Pine

This tall evergreen tree can grow up to 40 m (131 ft) high and has a flat crown. The long stiff needles grow in pairs and the cones are pointed and brown. It is wise to check the botanical name to make sure you get the right oil. Dwarf pine (*Pinus pumilio*) is classified as a hazardous oil.

The essential oil is colourless with a strong, fresh balsamic fragrance. Pine is invigorating, refreshing and cleansing, and is widely used in air fresheners, deodorants and cleaning products.

Botanical family Pinaceae.

Alternative common names Scotch pine, Forest oine, Pine needle.

Part of plant used Needles.

Extraction process Dry and steam distillation of the needles. Also dry distillation of wood chippings, which produces an inferior essential oil.

Principal chemical constituents Monoterpene hydrocarbons (50–90 per cent), pinene, carene, limonene, myrcene, camphene, also bornyl acetate, cineol, borneol and citral.

Country of origin Northern Europe and Asia, and North America. Cultivated especially in Finland.

Note Middle to top.

Odour intensity High.

Blends well with Cinnamon, Cypress, Lavender, Rosemary, Marjoram and Thyme.

Properties Antiseptic, anti-microbial, antiviral, anti-rheumatic, bactericidal, decongestant, diuretic, expectorant, hypertensive, restorative, rubefacient and stimulant (adrenal cortex, circulation and nervous system).

Most common uses

Circulatory and immune system Poor circulation.
Action Stimulates the circulation and the immune system.

Respiratory system Bronchitis, asthma and laryngitis.
Action Has good antiseptic and expectorant properties so may help generally with chest infections, especially if used in steam inhalations.

Genito-urinary system Cystitis, hepatitis and prostate problems.
Action Said to reduce inflammation of the gallbladder and may help with gout.

Nervous system Nervous debility, mental fatigue and weakness.
Action Known for its cleansing and invigorating properties, so can promote feelings of energy and well-being. Often used before meditation.

Safety Non-toxic and non-irritant (except in high concentrations) but may cause sensitization in some individuals. Do not use this oil on clients with skin allergies.

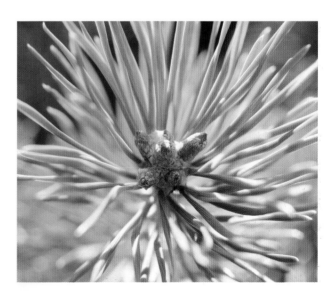

Piper nigrum
Black pepper

A perennial woody vine that grows up to 3 m (10 ft) high, the Black pepper has heart-shaped leaves and small white flowers. The berries turn from red to black as they mature into peppercorns. Black pepper is the dried, fully grown unripe fruit and the essential oil is pale green with a sharp, hot, spicy odour. In ancient Rome, it was so sought-after that citizens paid their taxes with peppercorns. Black pepper warms the blood, helping to relieve aches and pains in the muscles. It is one of the best stimulant essential oils for the digestive system.

Botanical family Piperaceae.

Part of plant used Dried and crushed black peppercorns.

Extraction process Steam distillation. Solvent extraction produces an oleoresin.

Principal chemical constituents Monoterpenes (70–80 per cent), thujene, pinene, camphene, sabinene, myrcene, limonene, sesquiterpenes, thujone and linalol.

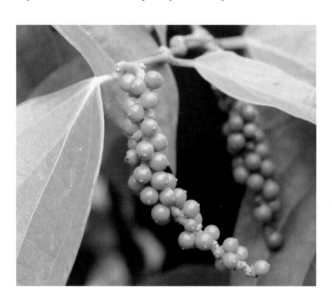

Country of origin Native to south-western India. Produced mainly in India, Indonesia, Malaysia, China and Madagascar.

Note Middle.

Odour intensity High.

Blends well with Basil, Bergamot, Cypress, Frankincense, Geranium, Ginger, Grapefruit, Lavender, Lemon, Orange, Palmarosa, Pine, Rosemary, Ylang ylang and Sandalwood.

Properties Analgesic, antiseptic, anti-spasmodic, carminative, detoxicant, diuretic, febrifuge, laxative, rubefacient and stomachic.

Most common uses

Skin conditions and circulatory system Poor circulation and bruises.
Action Reduces bruising, is generally warming and stimulates the immune system.

Muscular system Aching joints, arthritis and muscle stiffness.
Action A rubefacient with analgesic properties, it can be used to treat these conditions either by massage or in a compress.

Digestive system Colic, constipation, loss of appetite and nausea.
Action Good for bowel problems because it has a stimulating and stomachic effect, encouraging peristalsis and restoring tone to the colon muscles. It also stimulates the appetite and expels wind.

Nervous system Mental fatigue and lethargy.
Action The hot penetrating odour stimulates the nervous system generally and will encourage the mind to move on.

Safety Non-toxic and non-sensitizing. Use this oil in low concentrations as it may cause irritation. Note that excessive use may over-stimulate the kidneys.

*Pogostemon cablin (*syn. *P. patchouli)*
Patchouli

A perennial bushy herb, growing up to 1 m (3 ft) high, with fragrant, furry leaves and white flowers tinged with purple. Its dark orange oil has a sweet, earthy, exotic odour. It is used in perfumery as a fixative due to its persistent long-lasting character. Patchouli is used in the East to scent linen and clothes, and is believed to help prevent the spread of disease so is used as a prophylactic. In Japan and Malaysia it is used as an antidote to poisonous snake bites. It was very popular in the 1960s, when it became associated with the hippy movement – it was used to mask the unpleasant odour of Afghan coats and the smell of marijuana! Patchouli is both a stimulant (in large amounts) and a sedative (used sparingly), and is known as a powerful aphrodisiac.

Botanical family Lamiaceae (Labiatae).

Part of plant used Dried leaves.

Extraction process Steam distillation of the leaves (usually after fermentation). A resinoid is also produced.

Principal chemical constituents Alcohol (40 per cent), patchoulene, pogostol, bulnesol, bulnese and norpatchoulenol.

Country of origin Native to tropical Asia. Cultivated for its oil in India, China, Malaysia and South America.

Note Base.

Odour intensity High.

Blends well with Bergamot, Black pepper, Clary sage, Frankincense, Geranium, Ginger, Lavender, Lemongrass, Neroli, Pine, Rose and Sandalwood.

Properties Anti-depressant, antiseptic, aphrodisiac, astringent, cicatrizant, cytophylactic, diuretic, febrifuge, fungicide, insecticide, sedative and tonic.

Most common uses

Skin conditions Mature or oily skin, scars and sores.
Action Said to stimulate the growth and regeneration of skin cells so can help to repair scar tissue and heal wounds. Astringent so can help oily skin.

Circulatory system Cellulite and fluid retention.
Action Benefits the lymphatic system, especially when used together with other diuretic essential oils, such as Juniper and Sweet fennel. Also conditions and tones.

Nervous system Anxiety, apprehension, indecision and insecurity.
Action Useful when dealing with mood swings and other problems associated with stressful situations.

Safety Non-toxic, non-irritant and non-sensitizing. As Patchouli is very strong-smelling, use it sparingly in a blend.

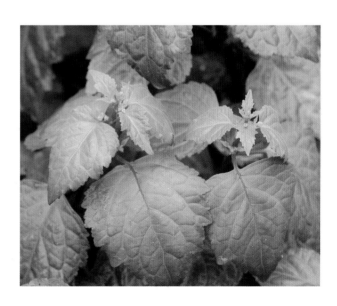

Rosa centifolia

Rose absolute (Cabbage rose)

Rosa damascena

Rose otto (Damask rose)

The rose generally used for production of Rose absolute is a hybrid of *R. centifolia* and *R. gallica*. It grows to a height of 2.5 m (8 ft) and produces flowers with large pink or rosy-purple petals. The essential oil is pale yellow, with a lovely rich, sweet-floral, slightly camphoraceous scent. It is a dark reddish orange in colour, with a deep sweet-scented odour.

Rose otto, known as the 'Queen of Flowers', is thought by many aromatherapists to be the finest of the essential oils. The Damask rose is a small prickly shrub, about 1-2 m (3-6 ft) high ,with fragrant blooms, often pink, and whitish hairy leaves. Rose otto essential oil varies in colour from pale yellow to clear. It has light sweet floral top notes with deep spicy undertones.

Rosa centifolia

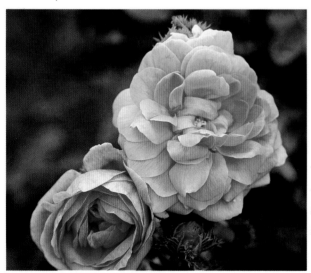

Harvesting of the flowers to make rose oil is done by hand in the morning before sunrise and material is distilled the same day. The oil is one of the most expensive of the essential oils as it takes many pounds of petals to produce the smallest amount of essential oil. Consequently, some rose oil on the market is diluted with Geranium (*Pelargonium graveolens*) or Palmarosa (*Cymbopogon martinii*). Some adulterated rose oils are only 10 per cent actual rose oil.

Rose oil was used to treat a wide range of disorders until the Middle Ages. It was probably the first essential oil to be distilled, in the 10th century in Persia (the birthplace of the cultivated Rose), because Rose water and Rose oil were both known in Arab-speaking countries by the end of that century. In England, the physician and herbalist Nicholas Culpeper used Rose oil as an anti-inflammatory agent.

The symbolism connected with the Rose is probably one of the richest and most complex of any plant. The plant was traditionally linked with Venus, goddess of love, beauty, youth and perfection, and the oil is still used in many cosmetics and perfumes today, although now mainly in a synthetic form. It is also used to flavour food. Damask rose oil is especially effective for emotional and reproductive problems, and is also thought to be an aphrodisiac.

Botanical family Rosaceae.

Alternative common names *Rosa centifolia*: French rose, Rose maroc, Rose de Mai. *Rosa damascena*: Bulgarian rose, Turkish rose.

Part of plant used Fresh flower petals.

Extraction process Water or steam distillation (which produces rose water as a by-product). Solvent extraction (which produces a concrete and an absolute). Enfleurage, the nearly obsolete method used in France (which produces 'attar' used in perfumery.

Principal chemical constituents 300 complex chemical compounds (many still unidentified) consisting mainly of: citronellol, phenyl ethanol, geraniol, nerol, farnesol and stearopten plus other trace elements.

Country of origin *Rosa centifolia*: Believed to originate in ancient Persia. *Rosa damascena*: Native to the Orient. Both roses now cultivated mainly in Morocco, Tunisia, Italy, France and China. The absolute and oil are mainly produced in France, Italy and China.

Note Rose Otto – top. Rose absolute – base.

Odour intensity Very high.

Blends well with Benzoin, Bergamot, Chamomile, Cypress, Frankincense, Geranium, Jasmine, Lavender, Mandarin, Melissa, Neroli, Patchouli, Rosewood, Sandalwood and Ylang ylang.

Properties Anti-depressant, antiseptic, anti-spasmodic, antiviral, aphrodisiac, bactericidal, cicatrizant, depurative, emmenagogue, hepatic, sedative (nervous system) stomachic and tonic (heart, liver, stomach and uterus).

Most common uses:

Skin conditions Broken capillaries, dry skin, mature skin and sensitive skin.
Action Has excellent emollient and hydrating properties, which makes it helpful for mature skins and any inflammatory conditions.

Circulation, muscles and joints Poor circulation and palpitations.

Action Has a tonic effect on the heart. Rose oil has also been shown to reduce high blood pressure.

Digestive system Gastroenteritis, dyspepsia and nausea.
Action Helps to decongest the liver.

Endocrine system Menstrual problems, premenstrual syndrome and uterine disorders.
Action This oil seems to have an affinity for the female reproductive system. Marguerite Maury comments that it has been found to have a purifying and strengthening effect on gynaecological conditions.

Nervous system Depression, insomnia, nervous tension and grief.
Action Invaluable in times of sadness, heartbreak and emotional trauma. According to Micheline Arcier, 'Rose chases away sad thoughts'.

Safety Non-toxic, non-irritant and non-sensitizing. Do not use this oil on pregnant women until 36 weeks, when it can fortify the uterus for labour.

Rosa damascena

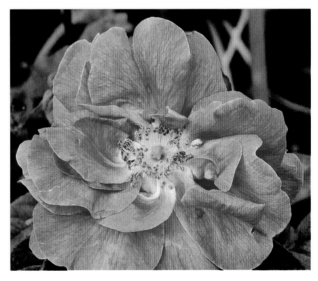

Rosmarinus officinalis
Rosemary

This aromatic evergreen bush grows up to 2 m (6 ft) high, with silvery green, needle-shaped leaves and pale blue flowers. The essential oil is usually colourless or pale yellow, with a strong, penetrating odour that is slightly minty or herbaceous. Rosemary is a good all-round oil and is particularly associated with stimulating the mind, promoting clear thought and inner vision.

Botanical family Lamiaceae (Labiatae).

Part of plant used Flowering tops and sometimes the leaves.

Extraction process Steam distillation.

Principal chemical constituents Pinenes, camphene, limonene, cineol, borneal with camphor, linalol, terpineol, octanone and bornyl acetate. (There are several different chemotypes.)

Country of origin Native to the Mediterranean. The oil is produced mainly in France, Spain and Tunisia.

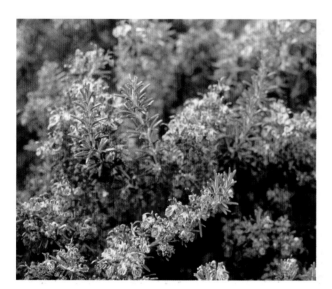

Note Middle.

Odour intensity High.

Blends well with Basil, Bergamot, Frankincense, Geranium, Grapefruit, Lavender, Lemongrass, Lime, Mandarin, Orange, Pine and Petitgrain.

Properties Analgesic, anti-depressant, antiseptic, anti-rheumatic, anti-microbial, astringent, carminative, cephalic, cordial, digestive, diuretic, emmenagogue, hepatic, hypertensive, nervine, rebefacient, stimulant (circulatory), sudorific, tonic and vulnerary.

Most common uses

Skin and hair conditions Acne, dermatitis, dandruff, oily hair and hair loss.
Action Found in shampoos and tonics that stimulate the scalp, it is said to promote hair growth.

Circulatory system, muscles and joints Arthritis, muscle pain, palpitation, poor circulation, rheumatism and varicose veins.
Action Stimulates the circulation, strengthens the heart and can also help to relieve cold feet and hands. It also helps to relieve tired, stiff and overworked muscles. A good analgesic, it may be used in a compress for painful arthritis and rheumatism. It is also a diuretic.

Digestive system Colitis and hepatic disorders.
Action An excellent tonic for the liver and gallbladder.

Respiratory system Asthma, bronchitis and sinusitis.
Action A valuable oil for respiratory problems and is thought to be helpful in cases of whooping cough.

Nervous system Headaches, mental fatigue and nervous exhaustion.
Action Can stimulate the brain. It has long been known to improve the memory and clear the mind.

Safety Non-toxic, non-irritant and non-sensitizing. Do not use this oil on pregnant women or on people with high blood pressure or epilepsy.

Salvia sclarea
Clary sage

Clary sage is a highly aromatic biennial or perennial herb, up to 1 m (3 ft) high, with large, broad, wrinkled hairy green leaves with a hint of purple, and blue flowers. The essential oil is pale yellowy green with a sweet, leafy, nutty aroma. Clary sage is one of the most euphoric essential oils and can even produce a narcotic-like 'high'. It cools inflammation and is warming and relaxing.

Botanical family Lamiaceae (Labiatae).

Alternative common name Muscatel sage.

Part of plant used Flowering tops and leaves.

Extraction process Steam distillation. Solvent extraction produces small quantities of absolute.

Principal chemical constituents Linalyl acetate, linalol, pinene, terpineol, geraniol and germacrene.

Country of origin Native to southern Europe. Cultivated worldwide.

Note Top to middle.

Odour intensity Medium.

Blends well with Bergamot, Cypress, Frankincense, Geranium, Grapefruit, Juniper, Jasmine, Lavender and Sandalwood.

Properties Anti-depressant, anti-spasmodic, carminative, emmenagogue, hypotensive, nervine, sedative, stomachic, tonic and uterine.

Most common uses

Skin conditions and hair Acne, boils, greasy skin, greasy hair and dandruff.
Action Helps to reduce excessive production of sebum. May be used to help greasy hair and dandruff.

Circulation, muscles and joints High blood pressure and joint problems.
Action Reduces blood pressure and relieves muscular pains.

Respiratory system Asthma, bronchitis and infections.
Action Relaxes spasms in the bronchial tubes and helps anxiety in asthmatics.

Digestive system Colic, dyspepsia, constipation, flatulence and intestinal cramps.
Action A carminative and stomachic.

Genito-urinary and endocrine system Premenstrual syndrome, menstrual problems and menopause.
Action Helps with painful or scanty periods and is useful for menopausal and menstrual problems. Can accelerate labour. It is helpful in easing postnatal depression.

Nervous system Migraine, insomnia, debility, depression and paranoia.
Action Helps to lift the spirits. Used for many conditions associated with nervous or stress-related problems

Safety Non-toxic, non-irritant and non-sensitizing. Do not use this oil on pregnant women or individuals who have been drinking alcohol.

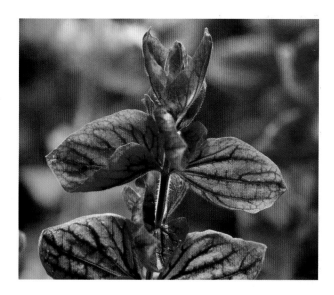

Santalum album
Sandalwood

The Sandalwood is a small, evergreen parasitic tree that grows to a height of 9 m (30 ft), with leathery leaves and small pinky-purple flowers. The oil is extracted from the inner wood, known as heartwood. The oil is a yellow, green or brownish viscous liquid with a deep woody-sweet balsamic odour. It is a relaxing and soothing oil, especially good for calming irritation of the nerves.

The International Federation of Aromatherapists recommends the use of *S. austrocaledonicum* or *S. spicatum* (which has a dry-bitter top note) as *S. album* is now an endangered species.

Botanical family Santalaceae.

Alternative common names East India sandalwood, Mysore sandalwood.

Part of plant used Roots and heartwood.

Extraction process Water or steam distillation of the powdered and dried roots and heartwood.

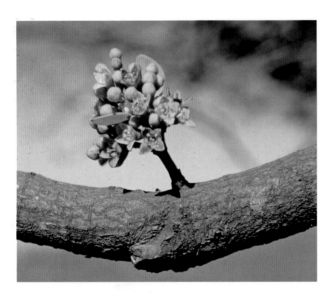

Principal chemical constituents Santalols (about 90 per cent), santyl acetate and santalones.

Country of origin Native to tropical Asia. The best-quality essential oil comes from Karnataka, formerly Mysore, East India.

Note Base.

Odour intensity Medium.

Blends well with Rose, Lavender, Black pepper, Geranium, Benzoin, Vetiver, Patchouli, Myrrh, Jasmine, Basil, Cypress, Lemon, Palmarosa and Ylang ylang.

Properties Anti-depressant, antiseptic, pulmonary, anti-spasmodic, astringent, bactericidal, carminative, diuretic, emollient, expectorant and sedative.

Most common uses

Skin conditions Dry, dehydrated or oily skins, acne and chapped skin.
Action A helpful skincare oil for dehydrated and dry skins, and a mild astringent for oily and combination skins.

Respiratory system Bronchitis, catarrh, dry coughs, sore throat and laryngitis.
Action Helps all the above conditions due to its anti-spasmodic and antiseptic actions.

Digestive system Diarrhoea and nausea.
Action Helps to relieve intestinal spasms and colic.

Genito-urinary system Cystitis.
Action Has a beneficial action on the mucous membranes of the urinary.

Nervous system Depression, insomnia, nervous tension and emotional exhaustion.
Action Helps all stress-related conditions, especially those associated with anxiety, fear and a busy life.

Safety Non-toxic, non-irritant and non-sensitizing. Has no known contraindications.

Styrax benzoin

Benzoin

This is a large tropical tree that grows up to 20 m (65 ft) high and has pale green leaves and hard-shelled fruits. The dark grey gum, streaked with red, is obtained by making a cut in the trunk. The resinoid produced from this gum has the consistency of a fatty oil. One of the classic ingredients of incense, Benzoin was used in ancient times to ward off evil spirits. It is is not strictly speaking an essential oil because pure Benzoin is a resin and has to be melted over hot water before use. It is usually dissolved in ethyl glycol to make it suitable for aromatherapeutic purposes, but ideally the best Benzoin is dissolved in wood alcohol. The oil is orange-brown and viscous with a very rich sweet, vanilla-like balsamic odour. Benzoin creates a feeling of euphoria and has a warming and soothing effect on the whole body.

Botanical family Styracaceae.

Alternative common name Gum benzoin.

Part of plant used Gum from the trunk.

Extraction process Solvent extraction of the crude resin, which produces a 'resin absolute'.

Principal chemical constituents Mainly coniferyl cinnamate, sumaresinolic acid and vanilla.

Country of origin Native to tropical Asia: Sumatra benzoin comes from Sumatra, Java and Malaysia and Siam benzoin from Laos, Vietnam, Cambodia, China and Thailand.

Note Base.

Odour intensity High.

Blends well with Bergamot, Sandalwood, Rose, Jasmine, Frankincense, Orange, Cypress, Juniper, Lemon, Coriander and all spice oils.

Properties Anti-inflammatory, antiseptic, carminative, sedative, tonic (heart) and vulnerary.

Most common uses

Skin conditions Cracked, chapped and inflamed skin.
Action Helps to reduce irritation and soothe inflammation.

Respiratory and immune system Coughs and sore throats, bronchitis and loss of voice.
Action Thought to be an excellent oil for these chesty conditions.

Nervous system Nervous anxiety, depression, despair and grief.
Action Thought to be one of the best oils for relieving stress-related problems.

Safety Non-toxic and non-irritant but may cause sensitization in some individuals.

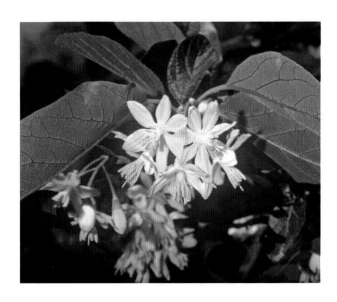

Thymus vulgaris

Thyme

Thyme is a perennial evergreen shrub that grows to about 45 cm (18 in) high. It has grey-green aromatic leaves and pale purple or white flowers. There are two essential oils: Red thyme oil, which is brown or orange with a warm and powerful herbal fragrance, and White thyme oil, which is a clear pale yellow liquid with a sweet green-fresh, milder scent. Thyme is known to be restorative, reviving and stimulating.

Botanical family Lamiaceae (Labiatae).

Part of plant used Fresh or partly dried leaves and flowering tops.

Extraction process Water or steam distillation: Red thyme oil is the crude distillation, White thyme oil is produced by further redistillation.

Principal chemical constituents Red thyme: thymol – thymol and carvacrol (up to 60 per cent), cymene, terpinene, camphene, borneol and linalol. White thyme: contains more linalol and has very few phenolic compounds. Sweet thyme: contains more geraniol and linalol.

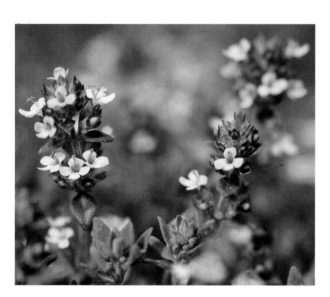

Country of origin Native to Spain and the Mediterranean region. Now found in other countries, including Asia, Russia and the USA.

Note Top to middle.

Odour intensity High.

Blends well with Bergamot, Chamomile, Juniper, Lavender, Lemon, Mandarin, Melissa and Rosemary.

Properties Anti-microbial, anti-rheumatic, antiseptic, anti-spasmodic, cardiac, carminative, cephalic, cicatrizant, diuretic, emmenagogue, expectorant, hypertensive, insecticidal, nervine, rubefacient and stimulates leucocytosis.

Most common uses

Circulatory system including lymphatic system: Low blood pressure, poor circulation and accumulation of toxins.
Action Generally very good for the circulation, especially in helping to raise low blood pressure. White thyme oil is considered ideal to use for children and is more of an immunostimulant and antibacterial.

Digestive system Diarrhoea, dyspepsia and intestinal cramps.
Action A digestive stimulant – helps with digestion.

Respiratory system Coughs, sore throats, tonsillitis, laryngitis and pharyngitis.
Action Red thyme oil has excellent broncho-pulmonary properties and is highly antiseptic, so is particularly recommended for upper respiratory problems, especially loss of voice and sore throat.

Nervous system Anxiety, nervous exhaustion, mental and physical fatigue.
Action Said to strengthen the nerves and help concentration. Both Red and White thyme oils are cephalic and help combat exhaustion in cases of mental overload.

Safety Red thyme oil can cause skin irritation and sensitization. Do not use this oil on pregnant women or on people with high blood pressure. Use it in moderation.

Vetiveria zizanioides
Vetiver

Used since antiquity for its fine fragrance, Vetiver is a tall, tufted and scented perennial grass with long, narrow leaves and many complex fibrous underground roots that are white in colour and highly aromatic. The essential oil is viscous and dark brown or amber in colour, with a deep earthy-woody odour. The earthy fragrance is popular with both men and women, and is a common ingredient of men's aftershave and toiletries. It acts as a fixative for Oriental perfumes, and is known as the 'oil of tranquility' according to Madame Arcier. In the East, the roots are also used to protect domestic animals from vermin, and in India and Sri Lanka, they are woven into fans, screens and mats. Vetiver has a grounding effect and helps relaxation.

Botanical family Poaceae (Gramineae).

Part of plant used Root and rootlets.

Extraction process Steam distillation of roots and rootlets, washed, chopped, dried and soaked. Solvent extraction produces a resinoid.

Principal chemical constituents Benzoic acid, vetiverol, furfurol, vetivone and terpenes (i.e: vetivenes). Country of origin Native to India, Indonesia, Sri Lanka, Haiti and Réunion. Produced mainly in Java.

Note Base.

Odour intensity High.

Blends well with Bergamot, Clary sage, Frankincense, Geranium, Jasmine, Lemon, Lavender, Patchouli, Rose, Sandalwood and Ylang ylang.

Properties Antiseptic, anti-spasmodic, depurative, nervine, sedative, tonic and vermifuge.

Most common uses

Skin conditions Dry skin, mature skin, iritated skin, and cuts and wounds.
Action Considered helpful for all skin types but particularly mature, dry or irritated skins. It helps to tone slack or tired-looking skin.

Nervous system Nervous debility, irritability, anger and hysteria.
Action Helps on an emotional level and used for neurotic behaviour resulting from stress and tension.

Safety Non-toxic, non-irritant and non-sensitizing.

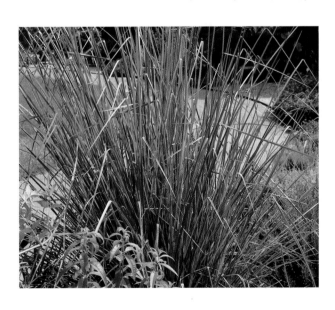

Zingiber cassumunar (syn. *Z. purpureum*)
Plai

This herb is similar in appearance to Ginger (*Zingiber officinale*, see page 107), but the oil has different properties and a more intense action. Plai oil has a cool, green, peppery aroma with a touch of bite but does not possess the classic heat commonly found in the rhizomes. It has long been highly regarded by Thai massage therapists, who consider it a vital addition to their range of oils, mainly to combat joint and muscle problems.

This is a comparatively new essential oil in the West and is included because of its cooling anti-inflammatory properties on muscles and conditions such as rheumatoid arthritis and osteoarthritis. When used instead of Sweet marjoram or Rosemary, both of which affect blood pressure, it can reduce swelling and ease pain. The author has used this oil very successfully in the hospital where she has worked for eight years.

Botanical family Zingiberaceae.

Part of plant used Fresh rhizome.

Extraction process Steam distillation.

Principal chemical constituents Sabine (27-34 per cent), g-terpinene, terpene-4-ol (30–35 per cent) and (E)-1-(3,4-dimethoxyphenyl) and butadiene (DMPBD) (12–19 per cent).

Country of origin Thailand, Indonesia, India.

Note Middle to top.

Odour intensity High.

Blends well with Black pepper, Lemon, Neroli, Cedarwood, Orange, Rosemary, Cypress and Lavender.

Properties Analgesic, anti-neuralgic, anti-inflammatory, antiseptic, anti-spasmodic, anti-toxic, antiviral, carminative, digestive, diuretic, febrifuge, laxative, stimulant, tonic and vermifuge.

Most common uses

Musculoskeletal disorders Osteoarthritis, rheumatoid arthritis, bursitis and tendonitis.
Action Helps to relieve pain and inflammation for the above conditions, including soft-tissue disorders, such as sprains and strains.

Respiratory system Asthma and lung problems.
Action Said to be most helpful in allergic types of asthma, although clients have reported that the aroma is initially a little overwhelming. Just smelling a blend of Plai, Rosemary and Cypress reduces an attack.

Safety Non-toxic and non-irritant (as far as known), but may cause sensitization in some individuals, so start with low concentrations.

Zingiber officinale
Ginger

This tropical perennial herb grows to a height of l m (3 ft) and has a thick, spreading tuberous rhizome and white or yellow flowers that only bloom for about 36 hours. Ginger was introduced to Europe via the Spice Route in the Middle Ages and was then introduced to South America by the Spaniards. In ayurvedic medicine, Ginger is considered a universal medicine for physical and spiritual cleansing. The pale yellow or amber oil has a warm, sharp, spicy odour. Ginger is warming and stimulating, and also calms and settles the stomach.

Botanical family Zingiberaceae.

Part of plant used Roots (dried and unpeeled).

Extraction process Steam distillation. Solvent extraction produces an absolute for use in perfumery.

Principal chemical constituents Gingerin, zingiberene, pinene, camphene, gingerone, linalol, cineol, borneol and geraniol.

Country of origin Native to southern Asia. Cultivated throughout the tropics, especially in Jamaica and the West Indies. Most essential oil is distilled in Britain, China and India.

Note Base.

Odour intensity Medium.

Blends well with Sandalwood, Vetiver, Eucalyptus, Geranium, Patchouli, Rosewood, Coriander, Rose, Neroli, Lime and other citrus oils.

Properties Analgesic, antiseptic, anti-spasmodic, bactericidal, carminative, cephalic, expectorant, febrifuge, laxative, rubefacient, stimulant, stomachic and tonic.

Most common uses

Circulatory system, muscles and joints
Athritis, poor circulation, chilblains, rheumatism.
Action Reduces swelling caused by injury and resulting fluid retention. Warming, so helps arhtiritis and rheumatism.

Respiratory system Catarrh, colds and flu, coughs and sore throat.
Action A comforting oil that may help relieve symptoms.

Digestive system Diarrhoea, colic, indigestion and nausea.
Action A well-known aid to the digestion and an ideal choice for travel sickness. It also helps morning sickness if sniffed from a tissue.

Nervous system Debility, nervous exhaustion and confusion.
Action Stimulates the memory and is also very grounding for the spirit.

Safety Non-toxic and non-irritant, but may cause sensitization in some individuals, so use this oil in low concentrations.

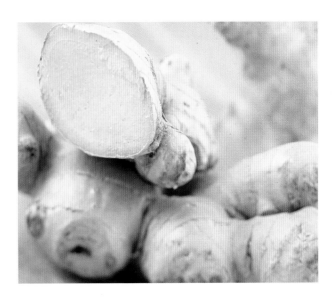

Safety guidelines

Essential oils are potent, highly concentrated plant extracts, which can be 99 times stronger then the oils occurring naturally in plant tissue. At these concentrations, they can cause undesirable side-effects if over-used or wrongly applied.

General safety

As with any concentrated substances, certain basic rules should be observed when using essential oils:

- Keep all essential oils out of reach of children.
- Never apply neat essential oil to the skin, and do not assume that an essential oil has the same properties as the whole plant from which it is extracted.
- Never exceed the recommended dilution.
- Do not use an oil as a food flavouring without expert guidance. **No oil should be ingested without medical supervision of a medical adviser**.

Dilutions

In aromatherapy, essential oils are most commonly used as room fragrances, in a bath, or diluted in a carrier oil for massage. (Only a medically qualified advisor should consider alternative methods.)

As a room fragrance Use neat oil on oil-burners or place up to 6 drops on a radiator (but not on the elements of an electric fire). If anyone in the room shows signs of irritation, ventilate the room and then reduce the amount of oil used.

In the bath

- Adults: 6–7 drops in 10 ml (2 teaspoons) of carrier oil or milk (full-fat or dried) (but see Precautionary notes)
- Babies aged less 18 months **no more than** 1 drop in 5 ml (1 teaspoon) of carrier oil or milk.
- Children aged 18 months to 12 years: **no more than** 4 drops in 10 ml (2 teaspoons) of carrier oil or milk.

For a massage

- Adults: Up to 6 drops in 10 ml (2 teaspoons) of carrier oil (see page 54).
- Babies aged less than 18 months: **no more than** 1 drop in 5 ml (1 teaspoon) of carrier oil.
- Children aged 18 months to 12 years: **no more than** 1–2 drops in 10 ml (2 teaspoons) of carrier oil.

Use of essential oils during pregnancy

All concentrated products, including essential oils, are best avoided during the first trimester of pregnancy, after which there are a number of oils that can helpful during pregnancy (see Chapter Seven, pages 214–219). In all cases, it is advisable to regulate the frequency with which a pregnant woman uses essential oils, for example, by having a week's break after using them every day for three weeks.

Precautionary notes

The majority of essential oils are safe for home use and, if applied correctly, can help to enhance mood, promote relaxation and relieve some ailments. However, there are some oils that should only be used with caution or avoided altogether. (Many oils listed below are not freely available, but are included in case you encounter them for sale.)

Oils that may cause severe irritation, or even burning, if applied to the skin undiluted
Birch, Clove, Ginger, Juniper, Peppermint, Black pepper, Pimento, Thyme and Turpentine.

Oils that may cause skin sensitization if used regularly at high concentrations
Bay, cardomon, citronella, clary sage, fennel, hyacinth, jasmine, juniper, lemon, lovage, may chang (*Litsea cubeba*), mimosa, orange, pine, rose, spearmint and ylang ylang. (These may be tolerated if used just enough to provide a gentle fragrance.)

Oils that may irritate damaged skin, skin sensitive to cosmetics or those with allergic skin conditions
Aniseed, benzoin, camphor (rectified), clove, eucalyptus, ginger, juniper, black pepper, pimento, peppermint, sage, savory, spearmint and thyme.

Oils that should not be used regularly on moles, extensive areas of freckles, sunburned skin, melanoma, premelanoma or other skin cancers
Citrus fruit oils and turpentine.

Oils considered unsafe for general use because of the inherent risks of toxicity, skin irritation or skin sensitization.

Latin name	Common name
Prunus amygdalus	almond, bitter
Peumus boldus	boldo leaf
Acorus calamus	calamus
Cinnamomum camphora	camphor (brown)
Cinnamomum camphora	camphor (yellow)
Cinnamomum cassia	cassia
Cinnamomum zeylanicum	cinnamon (bark)
Saussurea lappa	costus
Croton eluteria	croton
Inula helenium	elecampane
Foeniculum vulgare	fennel, bitter
Armoracia rusticana	horseradish
Pilocarpus jaborandi	jaborandi (leaf)
Artemisia vulgaris	mugwort
Brassica nigra	mustard
Pinus mugo	pine, dwarf
Ruta graveolens	rue
Sassafras albidum	sassafras
Ocotea cymbarum	sassafras, Brazilian
Juniperus Sabina	savine
Artemisia abroanum	southernwood
Tanacetum vulgare	tansy
Thuja occidentalis	thuja (cedarleaf)
Thuja plicata	thuja, western red or Washington
Gaultheria procumbens	wintergreen
Chenopodium anthelminticum	wormseed
Artemesia absinthium	wormwood

NB Some of these cannot be sold legally to the public in some countries.

Oils unsuitable for home use (in addition to those in table above)
Birch (sweet) (*Betula lenta*); bergamot (*Citrus bergamia*) (expressed, furocoumarin-free oil is safe); cade (*Juniperus oxycedrus*); camphor (unrectified) (*Cinnamomum camphorum*); lemon verbena (*Aloysia triphylla*); opoponax (*Commiphora erythraea*); Peru balsam/tolu (*Myroxylon peruiferum* syn. *M. balsamum*); and turpentine (*Pinus palustris*).

Oils that must not be used before sunbed treatment or exposure to strong sunlight
Angelica root, bergamot (expressed), caraway, cedarwood, cumin, ginger, grapefruit, lime (expressed), mandarin, orange (expressed), patchouli, rue and verbena.

Oils that require caution when used in the bath (generally use no more than 1–2 drops)
Aniseed, benzoin, camphor (rectified), clove, eucalyptus, ginger, juniper, black pepper, pimento, peppermint, sage, savory, spearmint and thyme.

FIRST AID

Despite all precautions, the occasional accident does occur. One of the commonest accidents is the transfer of essential oils from the fingers to the eyes or delicate skin (this is why you should always remove neat oil from your fingers by gentle scrubbing with a strong solution of washing-up liquid).

Eyes All essential oils, even when diluted, will cause stinging if they get into the eyes. If this happens, flush the eyes with warm water. If neat oil is splashed into the eyes, flush them immediately with milk (ideally full-fat) or warm water. If this treatment does not alleviate the stinging and irritation, seek medical advice. Common oils that tend to persist on the fingers for a long time and can cause eye irritation are cinnamon and peppermint.

Delicate skin areas Essential oils may also cause stinging and inflammation if they come into contact with delicate parts of the body. If this occurs, wash the affected area with warm soapy water, dry thoroughly and, if necessary, apply hand cream, medicated cream or, if nothing else is available, a small amount of butter, margarine or vegetable cooking oil.

Accidental swallowing If this occurs, you must seek medical assistance. If a person shows signs of distress immediately after swallowing a few drops of oil, this may be a rare, allergic reaction, similar to a bee sting allergy, and will require immediate medical attention.

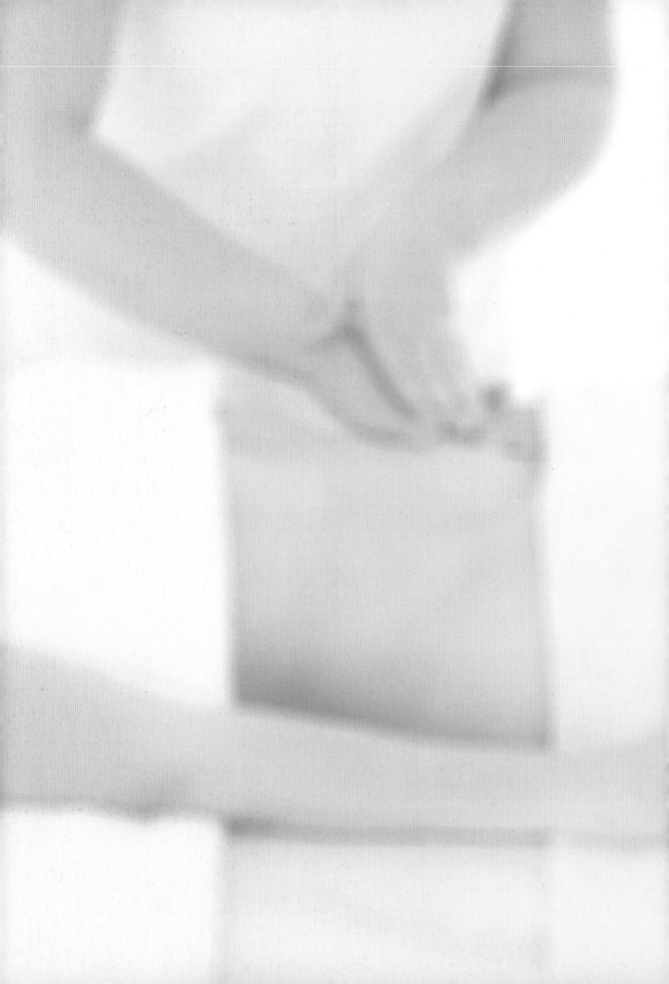

Aromatherapy massage

A professional massage, given in comfortable surroundings, is a deeply relaxing experience and, when combined with the use of essential oils, has great therapeutic value. This chapter looks at basic massage techniques, which are not hard to learn, and takes you step by step through a complete head to foot massage. It also offers advice on how to provide a fully professional service, from initial consultation to advice to clients on how they can continue to benefit from treatment with essential oils at home.

How massage works 112

Swedish massage 113

Other styles of massage 115

Providing an aromatherapy massage 116

Precautions and contraindications 121

A complete step-by-step massage treatment 122

Evaluation and aftercare 148

Home treatments 150

Seated massage 154

How massage works

Massage is much more than simply the manipulation of the soft tissues of the body. It is a healing art and has deep psychological implications. The word massage is derived from the Arabic word *masah*, meaning 'to stroke softly with the hand', and massage is performed by the hands for the purpose of producing effects on the vascular, lymphatic, muscular and nervous systems of the body.

Massage in the past

Records show that ancient civilizations practised massage in various forms before medicine was developed. Greek and Roman physicians used massage as a principal means of healing and relieving pain. In the early 5th century BC, Hippocrates, the 'father of modern medicine', wrote: 'The physician must be experienced in many things, but assuredly in rubbing for rubbing can bind a joint that is too loose and loosen a joint that is too rigid'. Massage features in the *Canon*, work of the Persian physician Avicenna (980–1037) , together with Chinese and other Oriental massage techniques going back 5,000 years. So massage has been firmly established for many years as a therapeutic treatment, and it can relax and release stress in this modern life.

Why we need massage today

Every day, massage therapists improve the lives of many people, from premature babies and children with cerebral palsy to people suffering from cancer, heart disease and stroke. It can also bring a valuable quality to the lives of the elderly, lonely and terminally ill. There are many reasons why people choose to have massage. It is used to relieve muscular aches and pains and to lower blood pressure.

You don't need to feel ill to appreciate massage. After an exercise programme in the gym a massage can help tired muscles. Massage is also good for toning the skin, while the 'hands-on' and caring touch of massage can strengthen relationships and improve general health. There is a great need to understand the power of touch. Learning massage techniques is an excellent way of understanding and being able to use touch to the client's benefit.

Importantly, in this fast-moving, stressful world, not enough time is dedicated to rest, relaxation and repair. People rush about and often find themselves in a constant state of stress. Massage can help in numerous ways. It can have an uplifting effect on anxiety caused by stress and emotional states and. in turn, a relaxed body and mind are better able to deal with stressful situations. Additionally, aromatherapy massage uses specific essential oils that will help with depression and anxiety and the holistic approach incorporates relaxation and advice on diet and exercise.

A relaxing head massage involves putting gentle pressure on the soft tissue of the face, neck and scalp. It can help to release tension and stress.

Swedish massage

Swedish massage was developed early in the 19th century by Professor Heinreich Ling and it is this type of general body massage that is now familiar to most people.

The importance of technique

Correct technique is a basic requirement of massage and is even more important than mastering the routine of movements. You should adopt a correct and comfortable posture, and apply the massage in a calm, rhythmical manner. The pressure can be adjusted according to changes in the amount of muscle and the degree of tension present, and the duration, sequence and intensity of the massage movements should be altered if beneficial.

Most clients will be looking for a massage that relaxes them, and applying the movements at the correct speed will increase the relaxation effect. However, you can create a more stimulating effect by altering the combination of movements, to leave the client feeling toned and invigorated rather than relaxed and sleepy – this may be a helpful adaptation for a sufferer to multiple

THE BENEFICIAL EFFECTS OF MASSAGE

A therapeutic massage has a number of different effects:

Circulation Massage improves the flow of blood through the arteries and veins. (Some massage techniques use chopping, percussive movements that cause the skin to redden with the increased blood supply, but percussion is not used in aromatherapy.)

Skin By increasing the circulation and removal of waste products via the lymphatic system, massage improves skin tone. When done regularly it also increases the elasticity of the skin, making it more supple, and also improves desquamation (shedding of dead skin cells).

Muscles Massage relieves fatigue by removing accumulated lactic acid in the muscles and relaxing tense muscle fibres.

Adipose tissue In conjunction with a weight-reducing diet, regular massage helps to firm the body contours. A very light lymphatic drainage massage will help cellulite.

sclerosis, for example, where increased energy, rather than increased relaxation is required.

Therapists should aim to develop strong, flexible hands that can mould to the contours of the areas to be massaged and, lastly but importantly, empathy and a caring attitude towards clients. An aromatherapy massage can be emotionally draining, as it is not just the laying on of hands but the giving of oneself. A therapist should ensure there is sufficient time between clients to refocus on the next person.

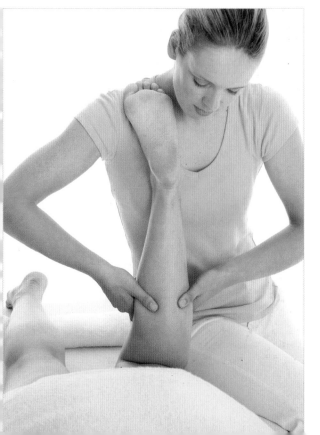

Swedish massage involves the use of different types of massage techniques, including effleurage, a stroking movement that uses the whole hand.

Basic massage techniques

There are many different types of massage movements and it is helpful to know which category each type of movement falls so that you can apply it safely and to best effect. Note that aromatherapy massage does not use percussion movements (tapotement), which include clapping, beating and pounding, as they are very stimulating and not in the spirit of aromatherapy.

Effleurage (stroking)

This is performed with the flat palm of the hand before and after all other movements. It involves the application of both superficial and deep pressures. It stimulates the sensory nerve endings and increases venous and lymph flow locally. It aids arterial circulation by removing congestion in the veins and it also improves the absorption of waste products by the lymphatic circulation (see page 180). It prepares the body for further massage and is also used to link the more active massage movements, thus maintaining contact with the client.

Petrissage (compression)

Petrissage or compression pressure can be applied in several different ways.

Kneading This involves intermittent pressure, using one or both hands. The pressure is smoothly and firmly applied and then relaxed. The effects are to increase circulation, removing waste products and eliminating fatigue. Correctly applied, compression movements produce a toning effect on muscular tissue.

Friction Also a type of compression, friction movements have a different purpose from kneading. They are concentrated movements that exert a controlled pressure on a small area of the surface tissues, moving them over underlying structures. The movements are applied in a circular manner with the thumb or pad of the palm, often along a muscle. The effects are to prevent the formation of skin adhesions and to free adhesions in deeper structures. They also aid absorption of fluid around the joints, particularly in the ankle, provided the oedema is not related to any systemic condition.

Vibration This consists of fine trembling movements performed on or along a nerve path by the fingers. They can be applied either in a static or running form. The effects are to stimulate and clear the nerve paths, bringing about relaxation and relieving tension.

Acupressure

This acts in the same way as acupuncture, a Chinese therapy that involves inserting fine needles into certain points on the skin. The needles stimulate the flow of energy known as *qi* (or *chi*), which circulates from the internal organs to the periphery of the body and back again through channels known as meridians. However, instead of using needles, pressure is applied to the points with the finger or thumb. Aromatherapy makes use of certain acupressure points.

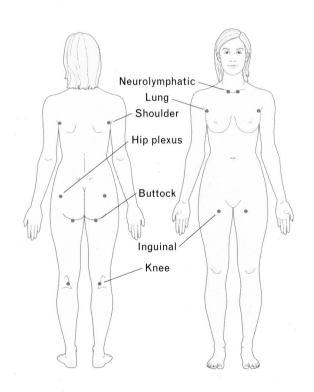

Lymphatic pressure points These points are used in the acupressure style of massage detailed in this chapter. Stimulating each point encourages the flow of bodily energy.

Other styles of massage

There are many styles of massage and, although an experienced therapist should be able to adapt any treatment to meet the needs of the client, some techniques may be more suitable than others.

Oriental massage

Shiatsu Originating in Japan as a therapy for emotional and physical pain, and based on ancient massage techniques, this is often described as 'acupuncture without needles'. Pressure is applied to key points along the body's energy channels to stimulate energy flow.

Tui Na This deep vigorous massage enjoys the same status in China as acupuncture. It aims to prevent and treat diseases of the mind, emotions and spirit, as well as the body. Practitioners manipulate the muscles, joints and soft tissues to rebalance *qi* levels in order to restore health (see Acupressure, left).

Ayurvedic massage This is part of the ancient Indian ayurvedic life system that covers health, emotions and spirituality. The treatment is aimed at improving consciousness and therefore overall health. Massage aims to rebalance the body type, which is defined according to three energetic principles or *doshas*.

Thai massage In this whole body strategy, pressure is applied to stimulate energy flow. Energy lines are called *sen* lines, and this type of massage benefits both the giver and the receiver.

Reiki This Japanese hands-on healing technique transfers healing energy from a giver to a receiver. The word 'reiki' means 'universal life energy'.

Indian head massage One of the oldest known therapies, this has been used in India for nearly 4,000 years. Massaging the head is a wonderful release for any mental or emotional stress.

Western massage

Sports massage This includes deep tissue massage and can be performed before exercise as part of a warm-up routine and after exercise to help drain away waste products and relax tired muscles.

Manual lymphatic drainage (MLD) Developed over 50 years ago by Dr Emil Vodder, this uses specialist techniques to stimulate and rebalance the lymphatic system, which carries waste out of the body and fights illness. MLD uses a gentle, relaxing pumping action to

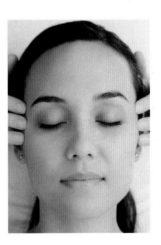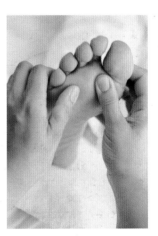

Indian head massage and reflexology are two styles of massage that can be included in a massage routine if appropriate. Indian head massage is good for releasing stress and reflexology for stimulating energy flow.

stimulate the flow of lymph fluid that may have accumulated as a result of illness, injury or poor diet.

Hydro-massage This is an underwater massage performed in a bath, usually in a spa.

Hydrothermic massage In this form of massage, the client floats on two pillows of warm water heated at 35°C (95°F) and remains face up throughout the massage.

Reflexology By applying pressure to specific points, known as reflex points, on the hands and feet, the reflexologist links to organs associated with these different points. Working on a particular point stimulates the flow of energy and encourages healing.

Stress therapy ('on site') massage This involves working over the clothes, often in an office environment, with the client sitting at a desk with the head on a pillow.

Hot stone massage Originating in Arizona in the USA, this type of massage uses special basalt stones heated in water and allows the therapist to address problem areas with deep pressure.

Providing an aromatherapy massage

There is a close relationship between Swedish body massage and aromatherapy massage. All aromatherapists will incorporate some Swedish massage strokes during their massage routines, especially effleurage and some palmar kneading. Aromatherapy is a holistic massage, working mainly on the nervous system as a whole and including, as part of the same treatment, the head and body.

The role of massage in aromatherapy

The purpose of aromatherapy massage is to facilitate the absorption of essential oils. It follows that effleurage is an essential part of aromatherapy massage because it warms the skin by increasing the blood supply. It is also relaxing and makes the client more receptive to treatment. It is a gentle process, with no place for harsh or abrupt movements. Effective aromatherapy massage includes neuromuscular elements, lymphatic drainage and acupressure.

This neuromuscular massage technique is the backbone of aromatherapy massage and uses friction, vibration and pressure point movements to influence nerve pathways and muscles. These can help to release energy blocks by stimulating the nerves and relieving muscular spasms.

An autonomic nerve pathway consist of two neurons. One extends from the central nervous system to a ganglion. The other extends directly from the ganglion to the effector muscle or gland. Aromatherapy massage uses techniques that stimulate the ganglia (reflex points), and often has a profound effect on the body. To understand the full benefits of aromatherapy massage, it is necessary to have an understanding of the autonomic nervous system, which regulates the activity of the muscles and glands (see Nervous system, page 184)

I am privileged to have trained with the late Micheline Arcier (see box page 117) who helped me to understand that aromatherapy massage, drawing its healing powers from the plant world, re-establishes harmony and revitalizes the malfunctioning part of the body. The treatment helps to balance the mind, body and emotions to make people look and feel good.

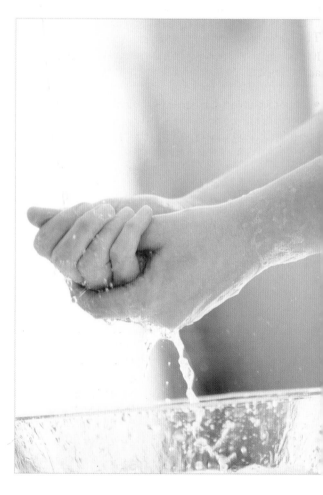

Washing your hands in running water before and after an aromatherapy massage is not only hygenic but helps to remove negative energy.

Aims of aromatherapy massage

The main aims of aromatherapy massage are:

- to ensure thorough oil penetration by good general effleurage
- to stimulate and/or relax the client as required
- to stimulate the lymph flow and blood circulation, which will in turn speed up the elimination of toxic waste from the body
- to act on the nerve supply
- to give the correct pressure point technique (where used) according to the condition of the client.

Fulfilling one or more of these aims – by applying the correct massage technique and using the most appropriate blend of essential oils – will help to keep the client in good general health, or help to relieve the symptoms caused by the general stress of everyday life.

The professional image

It is essential that a therapist presents a professional appearance.

- Maintain a high standard of personal hygiene at all times and, to ensure this, keep soap, a towel, deodorant, toothbrush and toothpaste, and clean clothing to hand at work.
- Your hair should be clean and well-groomed. If you have long hair, tie it back to prevent it from falling into the client's face.
- Your clothing should look professional and be non-restrictive, clean and pressed.
- Wear shoes that are comfortable, supportive, low-heeled and closed-in; never work in bare feet.
- Your hands should be warm and soft (hard, bony hands and very small, thin hands are not the best tools for massaging the body).
- Keep your fingernails short so that they do not disturb the flow of the massage or cause discomfort to the client. They should be unvarnished for reasons of hygiene and in case of client allergy.
- Remove jewellery, such as rings, bracelets and watches, from your hands and wrists, as well as dangling earrings or chains.
- Maintain a good posture throughout the massage, remembering the correct postural stance for the movements and area of the body being treated. This ensures a beneficial massage is provided for the client and helps to prevent fatigue for the therapist.
- Check that the client is comfortable and not too hot or too cold – read the body language.

THE MICHELINE ARCIER MASSAGE TECHNIQUE

Micheline Arcier, born in the south of France, devoted her lifetime to aromatherapy. After learning her craft from Marguerite Maury and Dr Jean Valnet, the pioneers of modern aromatherapy techniques, she practised aromatherapy in London for over 30 years and is considered to have been a leading authority in the field.

Her aromatherapy massage technique uses various holistic principles but works mainly on the nervous system. By applying pressure to the nerve ganglia along the spine the massage works on the autonomic nervous system, having an instant regulating effect. It is interesting to note the similarity between the position of these ganglia and the position of the Chinese acupuncture points. Each *back shu*, or 'associated point' indicates a disharmony in the corresponding meridian and in its associated organ or function.

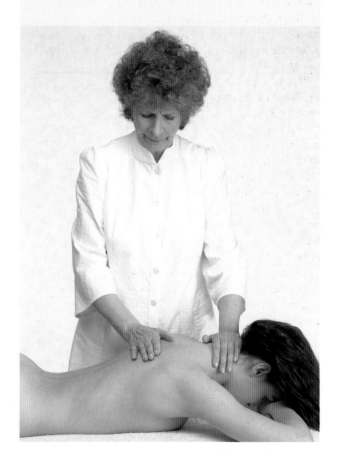

Creating the right environment

An aromatherapy massage will not be a therapeutic success if the ambience is wrong. Providing a peaceful, welcoming environment is a fundamental part of the experience. Look at the setting through the eyes of a client, and you will probably instinctively get things right, but there are also some practical guides in Chapter Eight (see Setting up a Clinic, page 244). A peaceful atmosphere contributes to the success of the treatment. (Clients often fall asleep during the treatment.)

Your own frame of mind is also very important. Massage is a very communicative treatment and some form of energy is transmitted through your fingers to the body you are working on. For the massage treatment to be successful, you must be calm, relaxed, reassuring and focused. If you are tired, angry or tense, or preoccupied with personal matters, the massage will be of little benefit to the client.

Focusing on the client

Clients should be made to feel special. They must like the blend of oils that is finally selected because it will not benefit them if they find the odour too strong or unpleasant.

Different people have different needs and the massage must be tailored to suit the individual. You may choose to change the order of treatment depending on your own and the client's preferences. This could mean performing more effleurage in certain areas, or more work on the shoulders and neck. The Arcier aromatherapy massage movements are usually repeated three to five times. Most clients feel wonderful after treatment and any minor discomfort that does occur usually clears up quickly.

Talking to clients

When talking to clients about aromatherapy, explain the benefits of making a little space in their day to relax with soothing essential oils, away from the stresses and strains of their hectic schedule. Introduce them gradually to essential oils and tell them about the range of unique aromatherapy essential oils that are available to help. You should be knowledgeable about the subject and confident in your ability to explain the properties of essential oils in a simple way. For example, when talking about geranium essential oil (there is no need to use Latin names), you can explain that it works mainly as a balancer for the skin and the mind, that it is excellent in times of stress, especially hormonal stress, and that it is also a slight diuretic and therefore particularly useful for fluid retention associated with pre-menstrual syndrome (PMS), but that it is best not to use it during the first trimester of pregnancy.

The treatment room should be well ventilated and peaceful with a comfortable couch and everything to hand so that there is no interruption to the treatment.

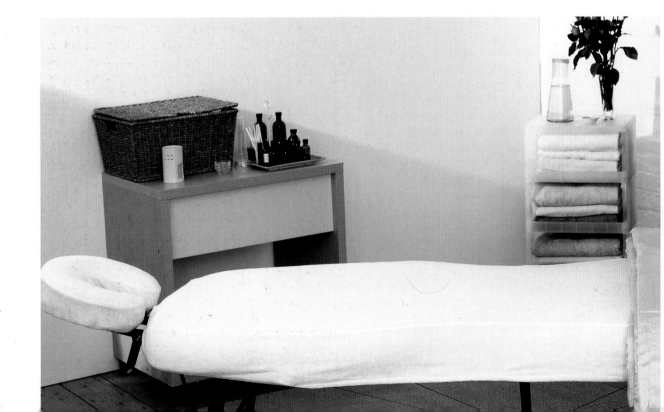

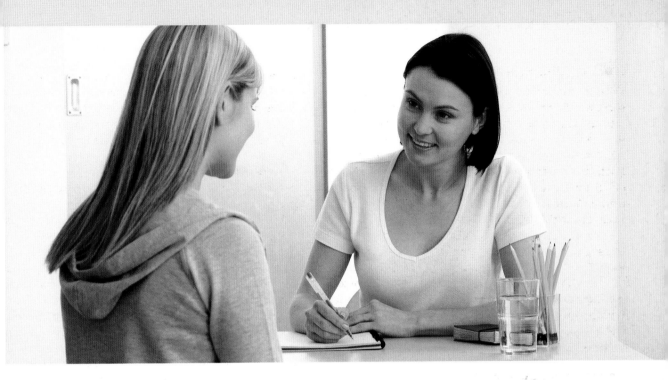

Building a case history

For a consultation to be effective, you must be familiar with each individual client's specific state of health and requirements, including any conditions they have that may prevent them from receiving treatment.

Taking case notes

The initial consultation is devoted to ascertaining the client's personal details, state of health and lifestyle. It is very important because it gives you the opportunity to establish a professional bond with your client and enables you to assess individual needs. It takes place in the treatment area and usually takes about 20–30 minutes.

The details that should be taken during the consultation include:

- the client's problem and details of present therapy or conventional medical treatment
- the medical history of the client, including past and present illnesses, operations and/or accidents, together with any medication that is being taken, prescribed or otherwise
- the relevant family circumstances and lifestyle, including diet, liquid intake, smoking, alcohol consumption, exercise, sleeping pattern, interests, bowel regularity, menstruation, stress levels and causes.

Most therapists find it best to devise a questionnaire on which all the client's details can be noted. An example is shown overleaf, although many therapists produce their own customized versions. It may also be appropriate, or necessary (depending on legal requirements), to ask the client to sign a simple statement giving consent to the treatment and/or their doctor's permission.

You will also need to keep a record of treatment given: see Evaluation and aftercare, page 148.

The completed paperwork should be labelled 'private and confidential' and kept in a safe place where it cannot be read by others. **Remember** to update the medical questionnaire form if further medical information is given, if there is a change in medication or if different symptoms or illnesses are experienced. Remember that a client has the right to see this form at any time. You should keep all personal treatment records for seven years after the final treatment.

If in doubt about the client's medical condition refer them, tactfully and without alarming them, to their medical practitioner.

Consultation notes

Personal details

How did you hear about me?

Name   Age   Date of birth

Sex M/F   Marital status   Occupation

Address

Home tel.   Work tel.   E-mail

Children (no./ages)

Referred by (doctor's name)

Doctor's address   Tel.

Emergency contact details (name, relationship, tel. no.)

Detailed medical history

Medication/Pill/HRT   Vitamins/minerals/self-prescribed supplements?

☐ Anaemia   ☐ German measles   ☐ Chickenpox   ☐ Diphtheria   ☐ Measles   ☐ Mumps   ☐ Pneumonia   ☐ Whooping cough

☐ Rheumatic fever   ☐ Sinuses   ☐ Glandular fever   ☐ Scarlet fever   ☐ Shingles   ☐ Polio   ☐ Other

Operations (appendix, tonsils etc.) incl. dates

Accidents/injuries/falls incl. dates

☐ Insertions (coil/pacemaker)   ☐ Back problems

General state of health

Female clients

Are you pregnant? (affects choice of essential oils)   Do you have any menstrual problems?

Details of any medication:

Details of any complementary medication, such as homeopathic remedies or nutritional supplements

Skin assessment (affects choice of carrier oil):   ☐ dry   ☐ oily   ☐ combination   ☐ sensitive   ☐ dehydrated   ☐ mature

Other details, e.g. allergies, contact lenses, that may affect
the choice of oil (when conducting a facial massage)

Lifestyle

Number of glasses of water consumed daily:

Number of cups of tea/coffee consumed daily:

Do you smoke?

Do you drink alcohol? If so, how many units per week?

Do you eat a balanced diet ?

Do you eat regular meals, eat before going to bed or eat between meals?

Type of exercise undertaken

How many sessions per week lasting approximately how long?

Working hours: ☐ regular   ☐ flexi   ☐ shift   ☐ unspecified

Energy levels: ☐ good   ☐ average   ☐ poor

Sleep patterns: ☐ good   ☐ poor   ☐ restless

Do you make time for recreation/relaxation activities? If so, what do you do?

Are you under any particular stress at home/at work/in relationships?
If so, how well are you coping?

Posture: ☐ straight   ☐ round shoulders

Personality: ☐ confident   ☐ nervous   ☐ mixture

Outlook: ☐ optimistic   ☐ pessimistic

What kind of smells do you prefer: ☐ floral   ☐ fruity   ☐ woody   ☐ herbal

Have you experienced aromatherapy/complementary therapies before?

Signed   Date

*The information I have given about my health in this case history is true to
the best of my knowledge and belief and I hereby give my consent to being
treated by natural therapy.*

Precautions and contraindications

The details that you document during the initial consultation will highlight any precautions you need to take during treatment. If in any doubt always consult the client's medical advisers.

Existing medical conditions

Do not treat any client who is receiving or requires treatment for an existing condition, such as asthma, cancer, diabetes, heart problems or multiple sclerosis, without consulting their medical advisers. Below are a few examples of common conditions of which you should be particularly aware.

Circulatory problems When treating clients with a heart condition, a history of thrombosis or embolism, or high or low blood pressure, choose your oils carefully – the essential oil directory (Chapter Three) includes precautions and safety warnings for oils – and apply only light pressure, avoiding areas that may be affected.

Diabetes Choose oils carefully, as diabetics can have delicate skin (the Directory of essential oils, page 61, gives further guidance).

Epilepsy There are a few oils (rosemary is the most common) that can, in certain cases, bring on an epileptic fit. Check the oil directory. This is a good example of why it is important to have a client's full medical history.

Fevers Avoid treating anyone with a high temperature.

Immunization Do not treat a client within 36 hours of any inoculation or vaccination.

Nervous system dysfunctions The Nervous System in Chapter Six (see page 184) explains conditions of which you should be aware.

Overactive thyroid (hyperthyroidism) Be careful not to overstimulate the client. Use a very light massage only.

Post-operative It is usually safe to give a treatment a week or so after a minor operation (for example, for varicose veins), but it is advisable to avoid treatment for approximately 6–12 weeks after a major operation. In both cases, avoid massaging the affected area and do not massage the reflex areas corresponding to the affected organ or part of the body. If in doubt, always consult the client's medical advisers.

Pregnancy Only an experienced aromatherapist should treat a pregnant client (see Chapter Seven).

Skin disorders In cases of contagious infection and bruising, avoid the affected area. For recent bleeding or swelling either avoid or apply only light pressure using carefully chosen oils.

Sunburn In cases of severe sunburn, avoid the area.

Current treatments

It is important to know what treatments a client is currently receiving, because some essential oils can counteract or magnify their effects.

Chemotherapy Consult the client's medical advisers before giving a treatment. See also Aromatherapy and Cancer, Chapter Seven (page 238).

Complementary therapies Avoid giving treatments on the same day as an any osteopathy or acupuncture treatments. Some oils counteract the effects of homeopathic preparations, so consult the client's homeopath before treatment.

Medicinal drugs Essential oils do not usually affect medication but in some cases they may interact, and the effects of drugs may be magnified by aromatherapy treatment. Consult the client's medical advisers if in any doubt.

Other considerations

There are certain other considerations that need to be taken into account before treating a client.

Age Always obtain the signed, written consent of a parent or guardian before treating a minor (i.e. anyone under the age of 16 years).

Alcohol and recreational drugs Aromatherapy treatment soon after consuming alcohol may have side-effects such as drowsiness or even nightmares, because of the magnifying effect of the essential oils. If you decide to treat, a shorter session or reduced dosages may be advisable. Likewise, no alcohol should be taken for at least six hours after treatment. The magnification effect of aromatherapy treatment may be particularly dangerous in the case of recreational drugs.

Heavy meals Use light pressure and avoid the stomach area if the client has eaten a heavy meal.

Jet lag Often, although a client is suitable to receive aromatherapy massage, there may be a reason why localized massage can be contraindicated. This can be over a limb that has had a thrombosis (DVT) and is an important consideration when massaging after a long air flight. It is worth checking the client's history to assess the risk involved. If in doubt, it is safer to recommend the client postpone the massage.

A complete step-by-step massage treatment

At every stage, your client should feel comfortable and at ease. Take time to explain what he or she can expect, and always explain the order of massage at the beginning of any treatment, especially if this is a client's first visit.

Preparation

If the client is female, ask her to undress and put on a clean towelling robe. A male client will probably be content with a towel. (Note that clients should visit the toilet before the treatment as aromatherapy is very stimulating to the system. They may well need to visit the toilet again when the treatment is over.)

While the client is getting ready, you can prepare the blend of essential oils that is individually tailored to the client's requirements, based on the information you received at the initial consultation.

In the treatment room, ask the client to remove the robe and get on to the couch. You should provide steps if necessary. Then cover the client with warm towels.

In cold climates, therapists often use pre-heated duvets or towels warmed on a radiator in the winter, whereas in hot, humid climates clients generally prefer cool,

darkened treatment rooms. Towels or cotton sheets are usually preferable to heavy blankets, although remember that air-conditioning may make the room feel very cold, in which case blankets may be needed. It is best not to use heated underpads when giving an aromatherapy massage because the client may become too hot and then the essential oils will not penetrate the skin properly. For the same reason it is not advisable for a client to take a sauna or a steam bath before aromatherapy because the body continues to give off heat and perspiration for an hour or two afterwards, and it cannot absorb oils into the tissues at the same time.

Cleansing

Prepare the client by cleansing the face and disinfecting the feet and making sure that the towels are properly draped. You may have to remove the towels during the massage but you should always replace them as soon as possible.

Wash or wipe your hands between each massage sequence, especially after massaging the feet and before massaging the face. Some sequences are performed with dry hands so you will need to remove any traces of oil.

When applying an essential oil, you should pour a little on to the palm of your hand rather than applying it directly to the skin from the container. Use the oil from the palm of the hand like a basin, spreading it with the other hand in upward motions. Unlike Swedish massage, aromatherapy massage uses pressure points and lymphatic drainage movements so the body does not need to be as oily, though a little more oil may be added when working on the shoulder area.

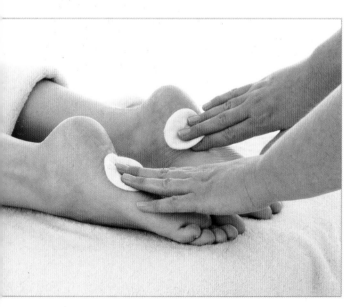

Sanitizing the feet is very important for hygiene reasons. Using tea tree hydrolat on cotton wool pads will enable the therapist to examine the feet while cleansing.

Opening sequences

This first sequence is done with dry hands and used to relax the client and establish a comfortable relationship. The client should be lying face down on the couch. Start by applying deep holistic pressure through the towels, while explaining the sequence of the massage. When you are ready to start the massage you will need to uncover the back.

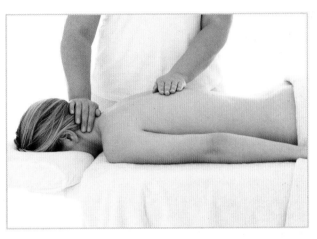

1 Cup one hand on the occipital bone at the base of the skull and keep it there. Place your other hand flat on the fifth thoracic vertebrae for a count of 5–10, then remove.

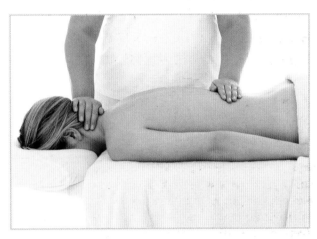

2 Move your hand down the back and place it flat on the 10th thoracic vertebrae for a count of 5–10, then remove.

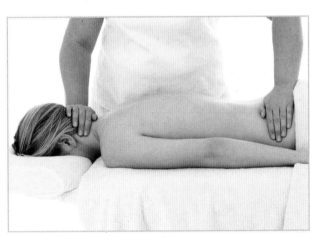

3 Move your hand down to the iliac crest of the pelvis, pushing slightly towards the feet, first on the right side and then on the left. Remove your hand.

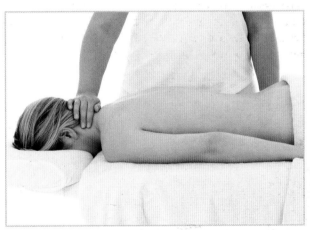

4 Leave your hand on the occipital bone for a count of 5 then slowly release it.

Head and neck

This stage is performed with dry hands and involves stretching and kneading movements at the base of the skull and the neck, working through the hair. The client should be lying face down on the couch. The movements can be performed from the side.

Head

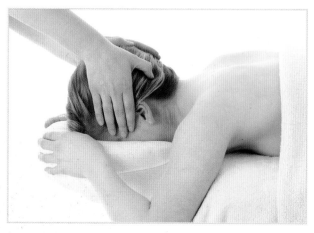

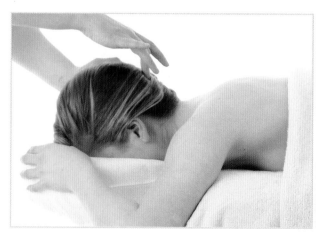

1 Holding the right side of the head with your left hand, use your right thumb to apply pressure along the left side of the skull and under the occipital bone until you reach the centre.

2 With your right middle finger, apply pressure up the centre of the skull towards the top of the head.

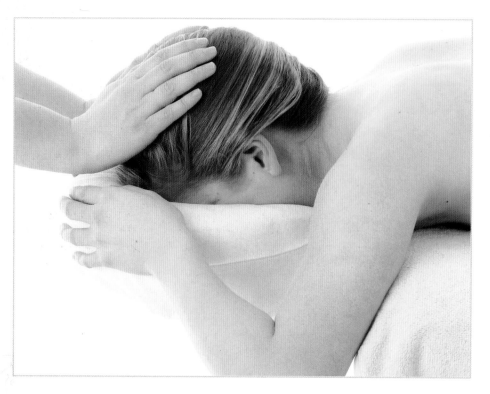

3 Hold the top of the head. Reverse the position so that you are holding the left side of the head with your right hand and repeat the movements with your left thumb and left middle finger. Repeat each sequence three times – more if there is tension – starting with fairly gentle pressure but increasing it if tolerable.

Neck

Scalp

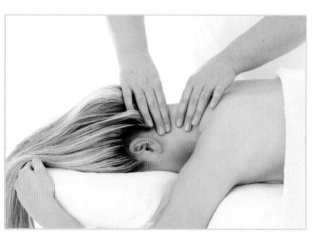

1 With dry hands massage the base of the cranium and the neck.

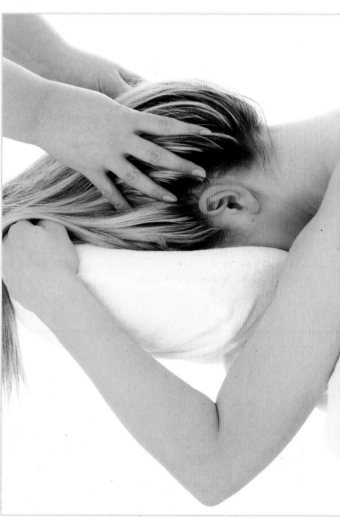

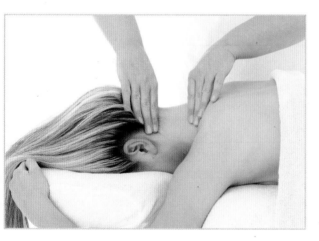

2 Use stretching and kneading movements.

1 Using both hands, perform a deep massage of the scalp, using inward shampooing movements to the top of head in order to shake off negative energy. Repeat three times.

Spine

The client should remain lying face down on the couch throughout this sequence. These massage movements drain the lymph and calm the nervous system. Pour a little of the essential oil body blend on to the palms of your hands.

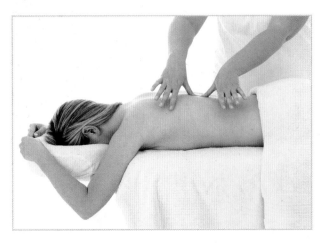

1 To stimulate the spinal nerve ganglia, ask the client to breathe in and out deeply and, on an outward breath, use the tips of both your thumbs to apply pressure along the right side of the spine, starting at the coccyx and working upwards to the neck. Then repeat the movement along the left side of the spine. Repeat three times.

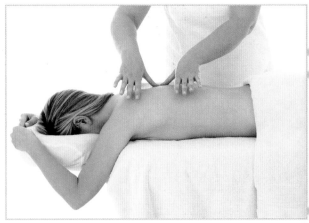

2 To decongest the tissue, work along the left side of the spine, sliding your thumbs from the lower to the upper back. Repeat three times on each side.

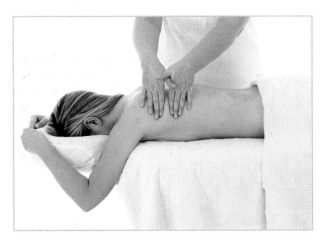

3 Use 'butterfly' movements, catching up the skin between both forefingers. Work from the sacrum towards the head. Then work from the spine out towards the lateral side of the body in three movements. Repeat on the other side, again working from the spine out to the sides and from the sacrum towards the head.

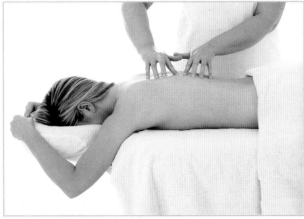

4 To liberate the lymph, apply pressure with the fingertips along the erectus spinus muscle. Flow fingers downwards laterally. Move hands up to repeat pressure and sliding movement at mid-spine and then the top of spine.

Hips and buttocks

These massage movements are used to alleviate problems
associated with the uterus and other sexual organs, and also
the kidney and bladder.

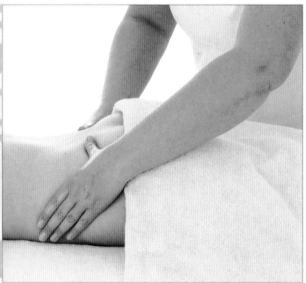

1 Effleurage the hip and buttock area with inward
movements of both hands.

2 Using your thumbs, apply deep circular movements to the
area of the lower (sacral) vertebrae in a V-shape, working
outwards. Repeat three times, then using your thumbs,
apply deep circular movements from the coccyx region to
the hip bone. Repeat three times.

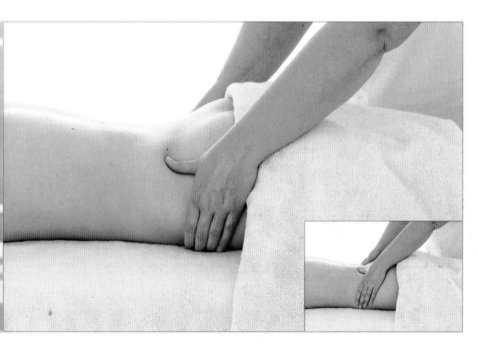

3 Using your thumbs, apply
deep sliding movements
along the spine from the
coccyx region to the hip
bone and bringing hands
out, round and back in a
box shape. Repeat three
times.

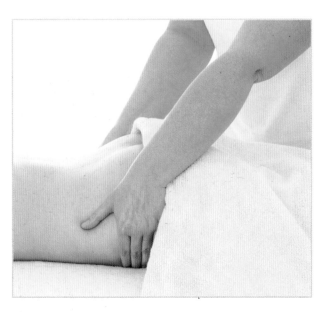

4 Repeat these fanning movements outwards over the buttock area from a central point in the gluteal muscle.

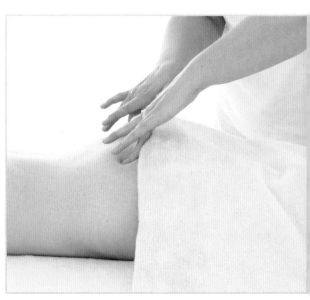

5 Slide back to the acupressure point in the gluteal muscle and press with your middle finger for a count of 4 and then with the flat of your hand for a count of 2.

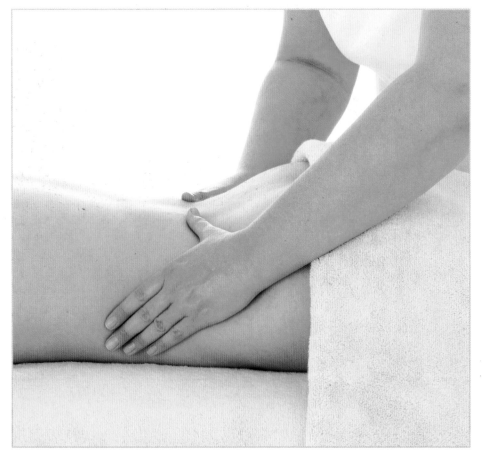

6 Apply deep effleurage inwards over the kidney area, using more oil if necessary. Repeat three times.

Back and arms

The client should be lying face down on the couch. These movements work on the meridian lines to release negative energy.

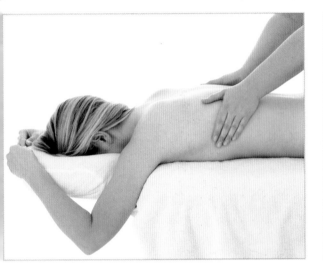

1 First effleurage the entire back. Repeat three times.

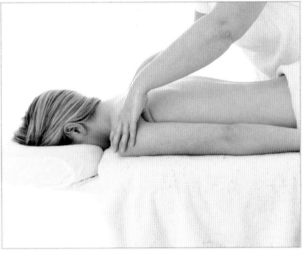

2 On the third effleurage, place the client's arms on the couch alongside the body. Effleurage up the spine and return, applying pressure with your thumbs to the lymph points on the shoulders for a count of 2.

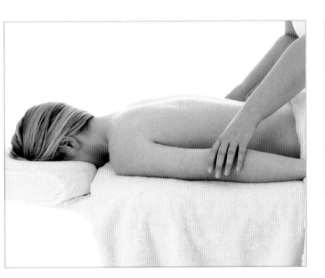

3 Working down the arms, apply pressure to the inside of the elbows (trochlea) and the palms for a count of 2 each. Repeat three times. (These acupressure points affect the lymph nodes, the metabolism and the heart meridians.)

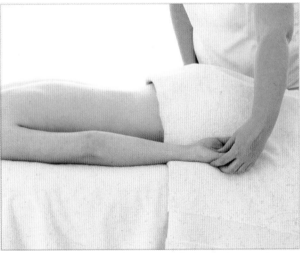

4 Apply pressure to the palms for a count of 2. Repeat steps 3 and 4 three times

Shoulders and neck

The aim of this section of the massage is to relieve tension in an area that is particularly prone to it.

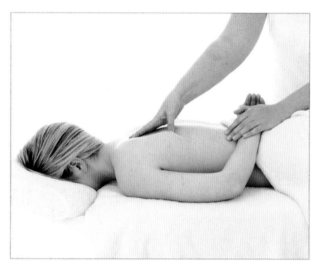

1 Taking the client's left arm, gently fold it back across the body. Using your thumb apply friction movements around the scapula.

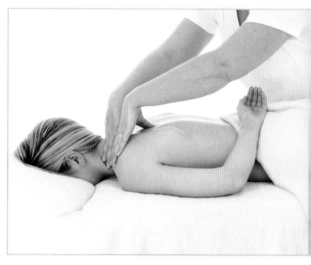

2 Then pinch the trapezius muscles (the triangular muscles of the shoulder and upper back) between finger and thumb.

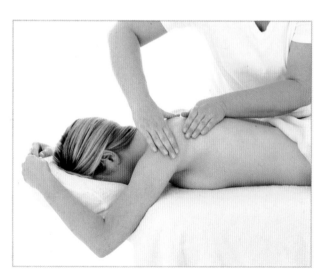

3 Work this area, apply kneading and rolling the movements.

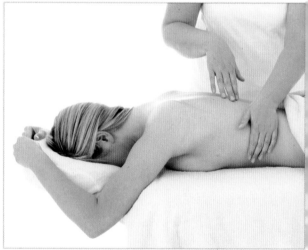

4 Use alternative hands to slowly stroke up to the shoulders, maintaining contact at all times. Repeat three times. Return arm to the side, reposition the right arm and repeat steps 1–4 on the right side.

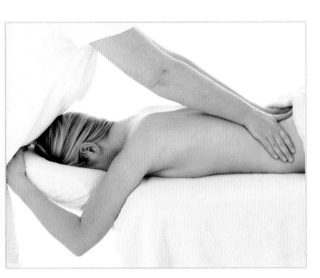

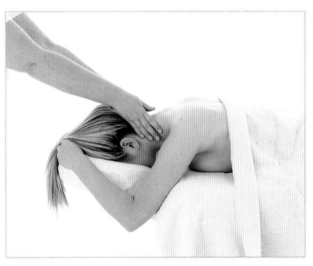

5 Slowly and deeply reverse effleurage down the spine and then up to the lymph point under the arms, and then gently press the shoulders back into position. Repeat three times.

6 Stretch and knead the neck and gently comb fingers through the hair. This 'throws out' negative energy. Repeat three times. Work from the side of the body if possible.

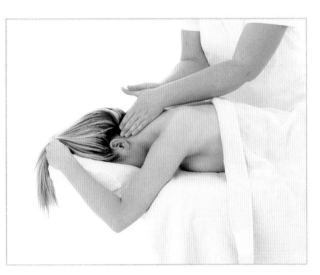

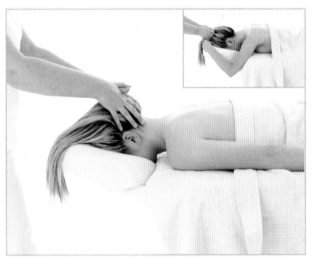

7 Apply deep palmar effleurage along the fibres of the trapezoid muscles.

8 Using small vibrating movements, apply pressure to the skull with the fingers and after a count of 3 throw out through the hair. Repeat three times.

Backs of legs

At this stage, both legs are worked on at the same time. Oil should be applied with an upward effleurage movement only.

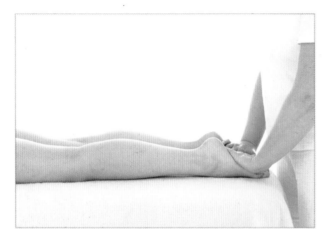

1 Rest your hands on the soles of the feet for a count of 5.

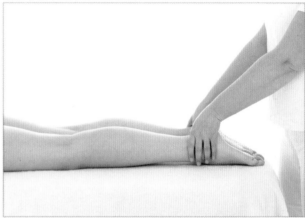

2 Slide your hands up to the ankle bones and rest a count of 2.

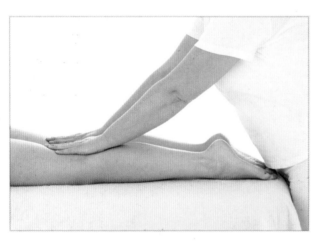

3 Slide your hands up to the backs of the knees and rest for a count of 2.

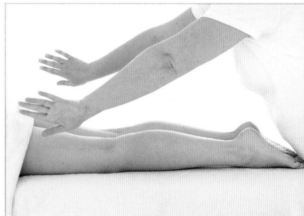

4 Slide your hands up to the thighs and off.

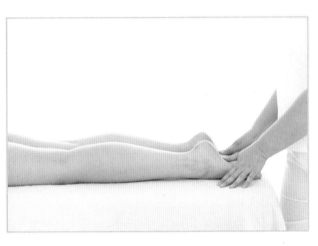

5 Using your thumbs, apply circular movements to the soles of the feet, paying particular attention to the solar plexus reflex point.

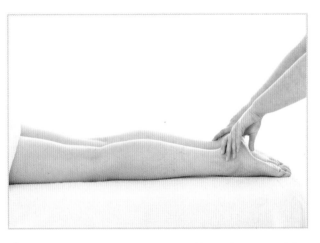

6 Slide the thumbs on to the inner ankle, working around the heel and following the sciatic reflex point.

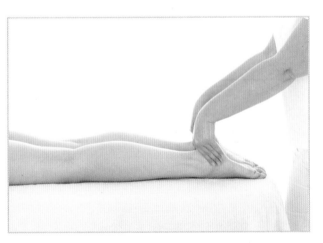

7 Slide your hands up to the ankles and make circular movements around the uterus reflex point (between the heel and the point of the inner ankle bone) and the backs of the legs.

THE SOLAR PLEXUS REFLEX POINT

The solar plexus reflex point on the sole of the left foot is, according to reflexologists, a good indicator of stress in the rest of the body, and working it enhances a feeling of relaxation and well-being.

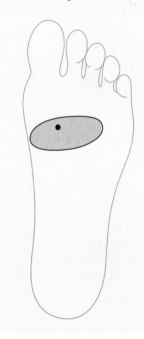

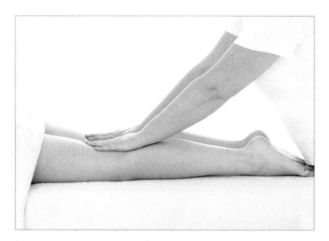

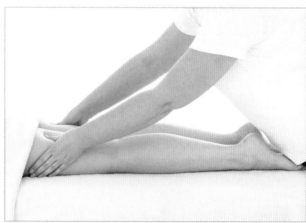

8 Knead the calves, working up to the backs of the knees. Rest your hands on the accupressure point on the backs of the knees (see diagram, page 114) for a count of 2.

9 With your thumbs, slide up to the lymphatic points below the buttocks (see acupressure diagram), hold for a count of 2 and then off. Then repeat steps 1–9 three times.

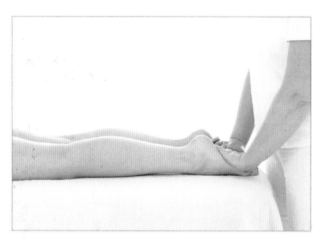

10 Finish by resting your hands on the soles of the feet for a count of 5.

POLARITY THERAPY

This massage is based on polarity therapy, which utilizes the body's magnetic field. It is an 'holistic' health system developed by Dr Randolph Stone and borrowed from Chinese philosophy to describe the forces of Yin and Yang.

Using touch and other methods, polarity therapy is centred on the human energy field and states that the human body, as a living being, emits an electromagnetic energy field of many different frequencies. The body parts are thought to have either a positive or negative charge and, like atoms (see pages 20–21), these seek to balance and restore the natural flow of energy to maintain good health. It is claimed that blockages in the flow of energy can lead to pain, disease or can be shown as lack of vitality and emotional problems. Polarity therapy uses the therapist's own electromagnetic field to help to rebalance that of the client.

In Oriental medicine the negative and positive charges are described in terms of the Chinese words Yin and Yang. The concept implies two forces in opposition. Polarity therapists work with these opposite forces to create a subtle third neutral factor, balance.

Scalp

Ask the client to turn over, to lie face up. The ankles should not be crossed and the arms should not be folded. Clean your hands thoroughly of oil, as this next stage is done with dry hands.

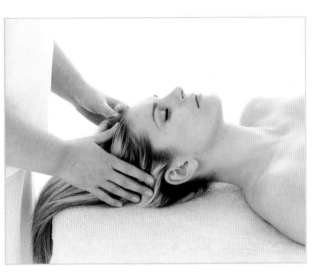

1 Apply pressure with your thumbs over the top of the head along the centre of the scalp. Repeat three times.

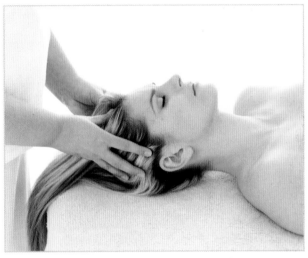

2 Apply circular shampooing movements to the scalp with your thumbs and fingers, to loosen it and eliminate any negative energy.

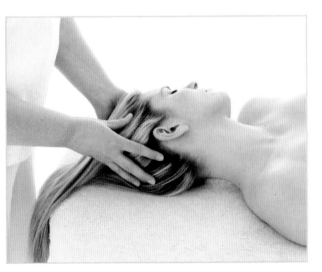

3 Turn the head slowly to one side then the other, and work on the back of the skull to eliminate any negative energy.

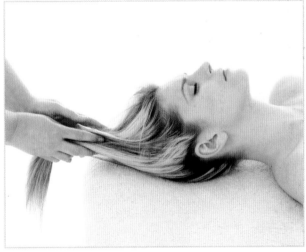

4 Draw your hands through the hair from the roots to the tips. This head drainage movement removes any negative energy.

Face

For this stage you will use the oils specifically blended for the face (see Chapter Three, page 36). The diagram below shows the path the fingers take during each stage of the face massage that follows.

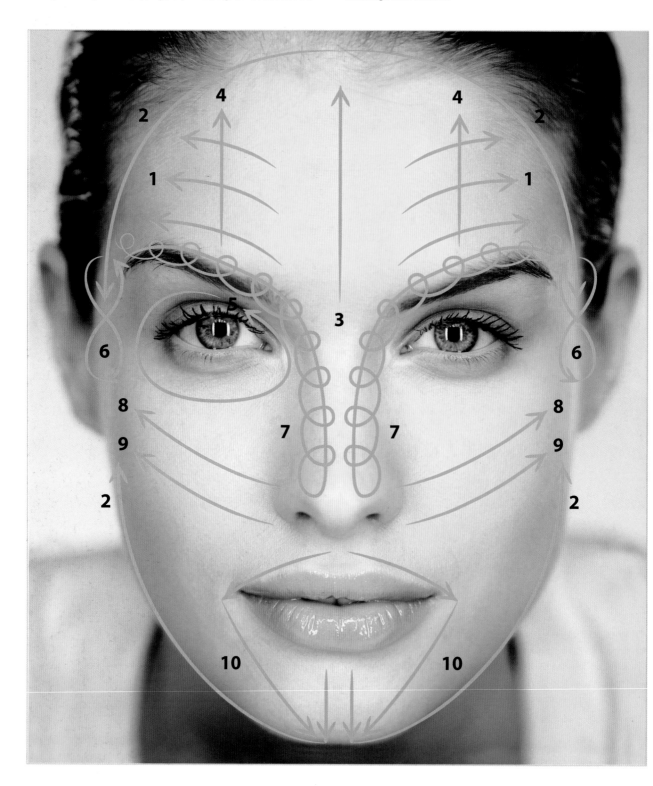

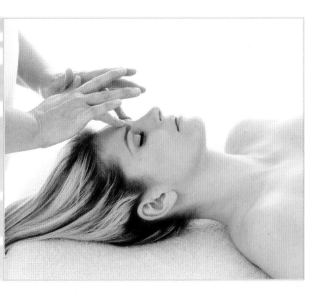

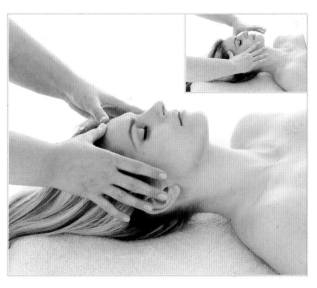

1 Apply a very small amount of oil to the face. Apply pressure above the eyebrows, starting at the centre of the forehead and following the ridges of the brow bone. Reduce the pressure when working on the temples. Repeat the movement in three rows over the forehead up to the hairline. Repeat three times.

2 Using your thumbs, apply deep pressure around the hairline, then reach with your middle fingers to the jawline and work upwards to the ears, and reach again to the centre of the hairline. Repeat three times.

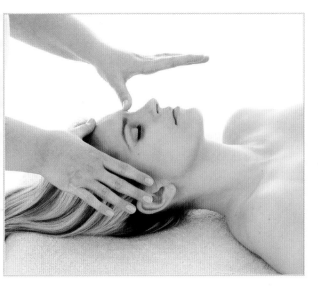

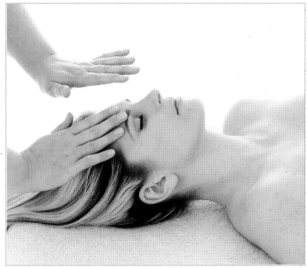

3 With your thumbs parallel, apply pressure along the corrugator (the muscle in the centre of the forehead that wrinkles the brow), then slide your thumbs alternately from between the eyebrows right up to the hairline while slightly decreasing the pressure. Repeat three times.

4 Apply soothing effleurage movements up the forehead towards the hair.

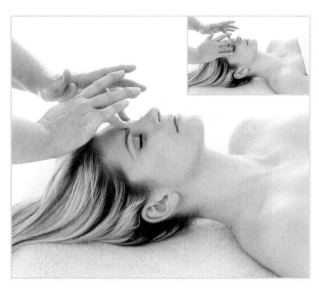

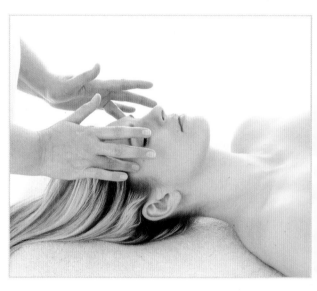

5 With your ring fingers, work around the eye sockets, lifting the eyebrows and applying light pressure inside the bone near the eye. Keep the movement going to form a circle over the eyebrow and under the eye. Then work a further circle across the eyelid and under the eye. Repeat thee times.

6 Perform a figure 8 on the temples with your finger. Repeat thee times (six times for headaches).

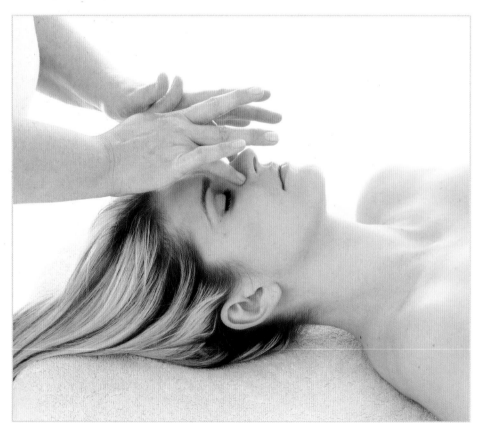

7 To decongest the nose, slide your fingers across each eyebrow and very lightly down the nose, and between the nose and the zygomatic bone (cheek). Return up the face using light circular movements on the sides of the nose and continuing over the brow and through the hairline. Repeat three times.

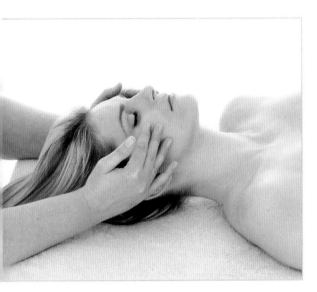

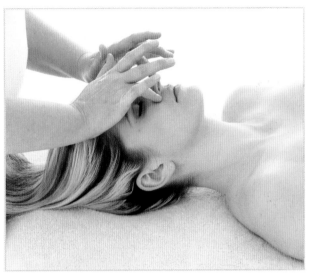

8 To decongest the sinuses, place the pads of your middle fingers on either side of the nose and stroke from the nose outwards over the cheek bones. Repeat three times.

9 With your fingers, apply pressure on the acupressure points near the corners of the nose. Then, using three fingers, make sweeping movements along the cheek bones (zygomatic bones). Repeat three times.

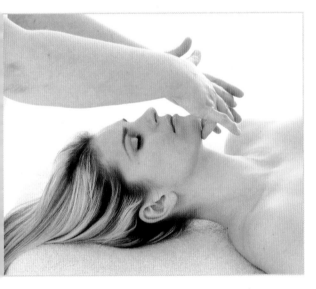

TO PROMOTE LYMPH FLOW AND FINISH

To liberate the lymph, slide your thumbs downwards to the submental nodes in the lower face (see page 136). Repeat three times, then place your hands over the face and vibrate once.

Stimulation of the lymphatic system helps to cleanse the tissues and gives the body a chance to rejuvenate. Regular treatments to liberate blocked lymph can prevent blockages from recurring.

10 Slide your ring ringers from the sides of the nose to the corners of the mouth, then from the corners of the mouth to under the chin, and finally, from the bottom of the lips to under the chin.

Neck and chest

Apply more oil to the throat and shoulders if necessary.

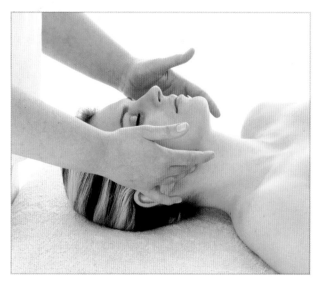

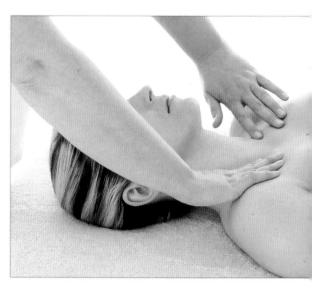

1 Pump the contours of the face by placing two fingers under the jaw bone and working from the chin to the end of the jaw bone. Repeat three times.

2 Using the index fingers massage from the jaw bone down the sides of the neck. This will help to drain the cervical lymph nodes (see page 114). Repeat five times.

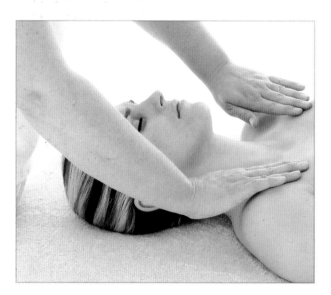

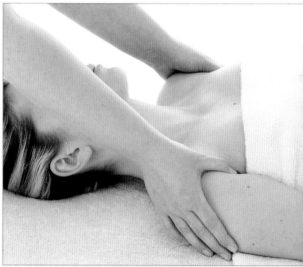

3 Slide down to chest and work four circular pumping movements.

4 Cupping the shoulders, use your thumbs to work the axillary lymph nodes.

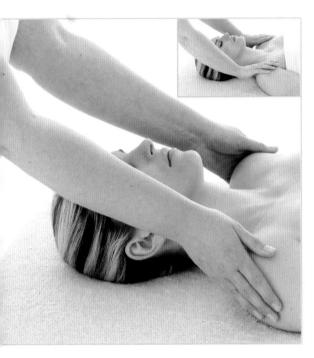

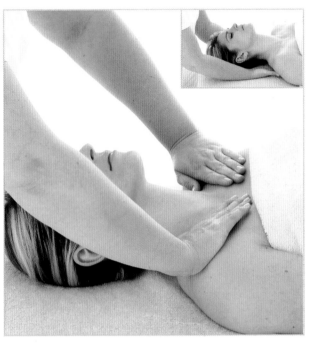

5 Sliding the thumbs under the shoulders, effleurage the deltoid with hands, bringing the thumbs into the trapezius using circular movements. Repeat three times.

6 With your fingers pointing inwards, apply deep pressure to the chest. Then swing outwards over the shoulders and, using the flat of your hand, massage the trapezius muscles using circular movements, with a deep pull either side of the vertebrae to the base of the skull, and vibrate once to finish. Repeat three times.

The Long Journey

The Long Journey is a slow movement which drains the lymph. You travel around the shoulders from front to back, up the back of the neck, along the side of head and out to the tips of the hair. The whole movement should take a count of 20. This also stimulates the lung acupuncture points.

Slide your fingers along the clavicle and around the shoulders, working continuously with deep movements. Continue down to the rhomboid and the erectus spinus muscles, then upwards towards the neck, running your fingers through to the ends of the hair. Repeat five times.

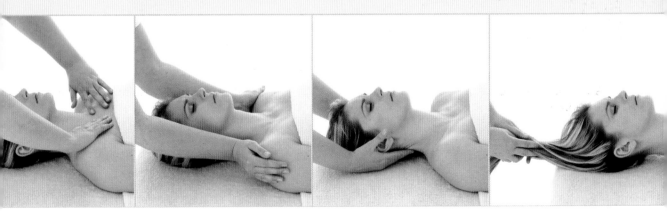

Hands

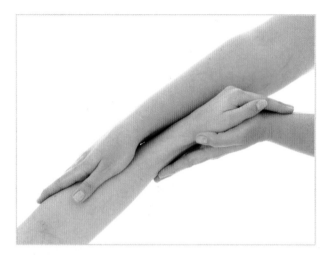

1 Effleurage up the arm.

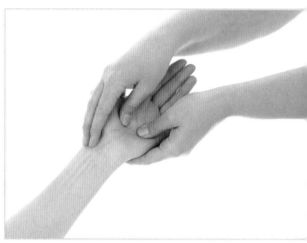

2 Stretch out palm and work in circles.

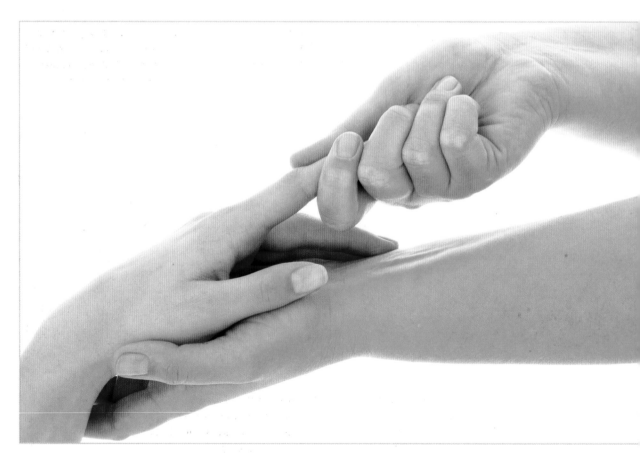

3 Gently pull each finger, flicking out negative energy.

Abdomen

The first three steps aim to calm and revive the diaphragm, and the second three steps are helpful in relieving constipation.

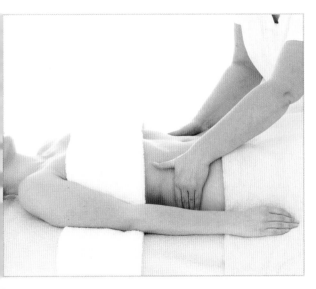

1 Apply oil carefully to abdomen and effleurage inwards. Repeat three times.

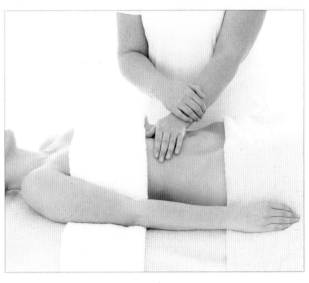

2 Resting your right hand on the left arm, place your left hand over the solar plexus and rotate your hand very gently and slowly, anticlockwise for women and clockwise for men. Repeat five times (more if the client is very tense).

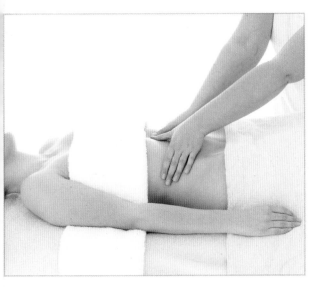

3 Ask the client to breathe deeply. On an outward breath, slide both thumbs down from the solar plexus to the waist and out to the side, then change to your middle fingers and stroke in towards the pressure points at the iliac crests. Repeat three times. If there is too much tension, ask the client to do a few abdominal breathing exercises.

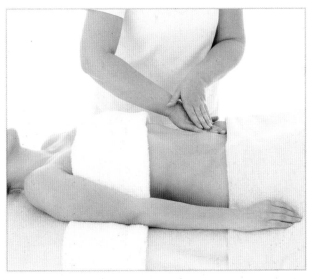

4 Massage the colon using the flats of the fingers, working in small clockwise movements across the lower abdomen, but jump across the central meridian line so as not to block the energy.

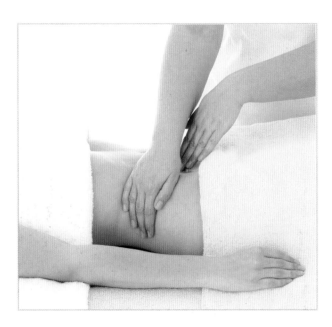

5 Using alternate hands, effleurage upwards and downwards from the waist. Start at the base of the ribs and follow ribs upwards to the solar plexus, return and then slide your whole hand downwards to the iliac crest. Repeat three times.

6 Finish by placing both palms over the solar plexus for a count of 5.

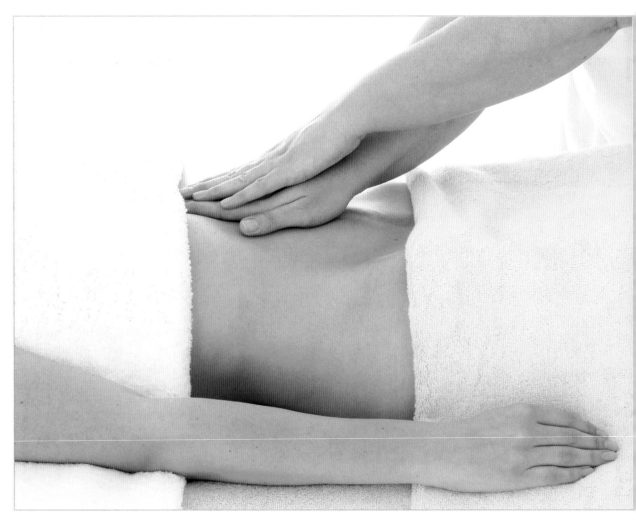

front of feet and legs

Moving to the foot of the client, begin work on the feet. Apply oil with upward effleurage movements only.

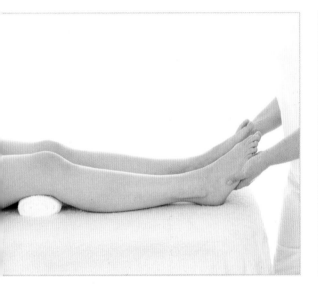

1 Rest your hands on the soles of the feet for a count of 5.

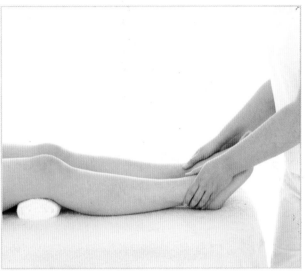

2 Then slide them up to the ankles for a count of 2.

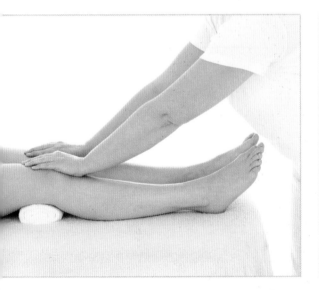

3 Move up to the knees and rest for a count of 2.

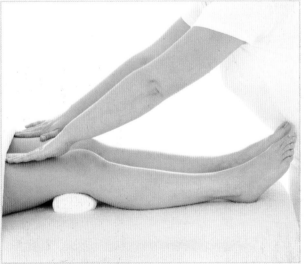

4 Finish with effleurage of the thighs.

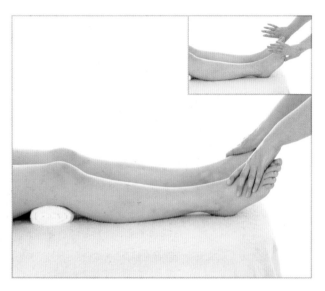

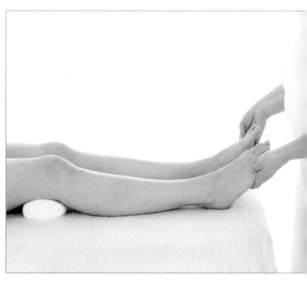

5 To stimulate the flow of lymph in the feet and legs, lightly rest your hands on the top of the feet and, with your wrists tilted forwards, slide your thumbs up the soles of feet four times, each time in line with the gap between one toe and the next, starting with the big toe and finishing with the little toe. This pulls out negative energy.

6 Circle the lymphatic points on the top of the foot, between the toes.

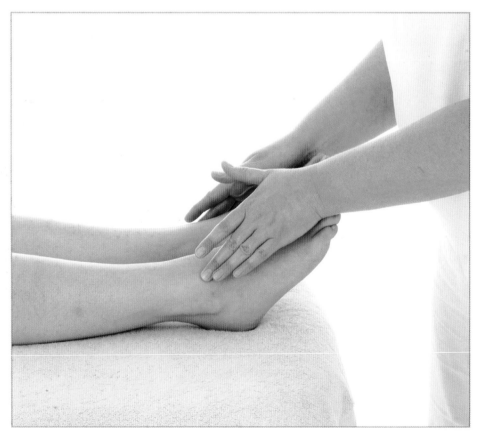

7 Then make circular movements around the outside of the ankles and use light palmar kneading up the legs to the knees.

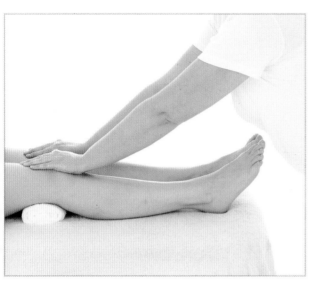

8 Rest your hands over the knees for a count of 2.

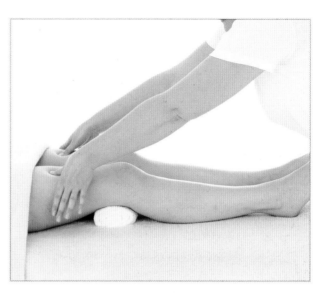

9 Slide your hands up towards the inguinal node pressure point halfway up thigh and apply pressure with your thumbs. Repeat steps 1–9 three times.

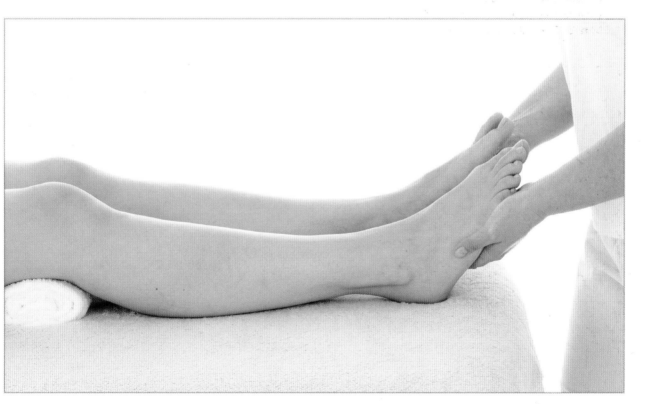

End of treatment

Rest your hands flat on the soles of the feet for a count of 20 to rebalance the flow of energy and shake off any negative energy. Cover the client. Wash your hands to remove any negative energy.

Evaluation and aftercare

Your own observations and the client's response will help you evaluate the effectiveness of the treatment you are giving, and to advise on aftercare.

Learning during treatment

The first treatment after the initial consultation allows you to verify the information the client has given you during the consultation.

Working directly on the body provides a lot of information. Is the skin fine or coarse? Is it well balanced or dehydrated, combination or oily? Is it congested? Is the muscle tone good? Are the blood and lymphatic circulations working well? Are some of the nerve points tender? Are there any blockages? Is the spine in good condition? Is the client suffering from tension? Does the skin turn red when pressure is applied to certain areas? Working on the back, in particular, is like reading a map, and following the different reactions in various reflex zones can give the skilled therapist a good understanding of the client's general state of health.

At each treatment you should observe the client carefully and take note of the following:

- posture, ease of movement, breathing and weight
- attitude – whether it is positive, negative, relaxed, stressed, tense, nervous, outgoing, withdrawn, confident and so on
- skin condition, including texture, tone, colour, temperature, any hot or cold spots, dryness, oiliness or flakiness
- contraindications to treatment, for example, areas of the body that you cannot work on and why (varicose veins, perhaps, or a wound) and areas of the body that the client does not wish to be touched.

Record of oils used

Always keep a note of which essential oils you used and how. You may find it most convenient to use a record card like the one below. (On page 52 is a completed example.) In some clinics several therapists may work on the same client so a record of previous treatments and oils is essential.

CLIENT	AROMATHERAPIST		DATE
condition(s)	top note	middle note	base note
BODY RECIPE		FACE RECIPE	
top			
middle			
base			
carrier oil (10 ml)		carrier oil (5 ml)	

Remember

- Use a maximum of three essential oils in a body massage blend, and one essential oil for the face.
- Explain why you are using each essential oil, giving its properties.
- Note the percentage blend used each time.
- Note the carrier oil(s) used and explain your choice.

Aftercare

After the massage, rouse the client gently, gradually raising the head off the couch. Offer a suitable drink, such as mineral water or a fruit tea. While you are fetching it, the client can wake up fully, and you can raise the head end of the couch to a sitting position. This is a good time to explain what to do after the massage. You can either discuss the points below with the client or write them down for the client to read.

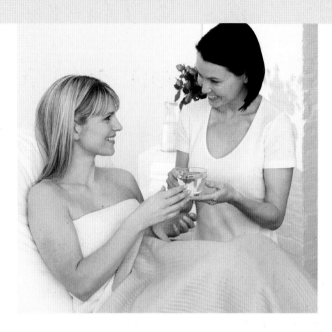

- Avoid taking a bath or shower for 6–8 hours to give the oils time to be absorbed completely. This also applies to swimming, both in a pool or in the sea.
- Avoid sunbathing or having a sunbed treatment because certain oils used in aromatherapy massage may cause irritation of the skin if the body is exposed to ultraviolet light.
- Avoid strenuous exercise because the body might sweat out the essential oils.
- Spend a restful evening, with a light meal followed by an early night.

- Don't drink any alcohol after aromatherapy but do drink lots of water.
- Don't worry if you feel slightly unwell, or develop a headache; this could be due to the effects of toxins leaving the body and it will not last long. Most clients feel very good after an aromatherapy treatment.

Response to treatment

You will also need to keep additional notes on:

- the client's reaction to the treatment (see box)
- how you felt a treatment worked, for example: did the client fall asleep, talk throughout the treatment, become emotionally upset?
- any comments you wish to make regarding the client
- the client's progress
- any referrals you make (and keep a note of any follow-up)
- any changes that occurred after the treatment, such as differences in posture or attitude
- any home treatments you recommend (see page 150) and instructions you gave
- any changes you make to the next treatment and why.

Summary

At the end of the treatment period, you should write a summary of:
- any improvements, not just physically but emotionally, mentally and in lifestyle
- anything that did not change or got worse
- final feedback from the client
- how you felt the treatment went
- general comments and conclusions.

FEEDBACK

It is a good idea to ask the client for some feedback about the experience, especially after the first session. You can either ask the following questions directly or provide a questionnaire.
- Was there any aspect of the initial consultation that you found embarrassing or confusing?
- Was there anything you liked or disliked about the treatment room?
- Were you happy about the hygiene standards?
- Was the massage couch comfortable?
- Did you feel too warm or too cold?
- Did you enjoy the scent of the oils?
- Did you like the music?
- Was the therapy uncomfortable at any time?
- Did you dislike any part of the therapy?
- Would you consult an aromatherapist in the future?

Home treatments

One of the most pleasurable ways to enjoy essential oils is in your bath, but essential oils can be used in a number of ways around the home. Take note of any precautions mentioned here and also on pages 108–9.

Bathing

Essential oils can relax and sedate or uplift and stimulate, but aromatic baths are mostly used for their stress-reducing properties. The oils work both by absorption into the skin and by inhalation as they evaporate.

To get the full benefits, make sure the room is warm. Shut the door and turn off the taps before adding the blended oil. Don't add oils neat to the bathwater: dilute 8–10 drops in 5 ml (1 teaspoon) of carrier oil. An alternative to carrier oil is to disperse the drops in 10 ml (or 2 teaspoons) of full-fat or dried milk.

Refreshing blend: to ease cold, coughs, exhaustion, and tired or over-worked muscles
2 drops pine
2 drops juniper
2 drops sweet basil

Invigorating and stimulating blend: to ease poor circulation
2 drops sweet basil
2 drops patchouli
2 drops juniper or rosemary

Revitalizing blend: to ease aches and pains, help regulate menstruation and alleviate fluid retention
2 drops grapefruit
2 drops eucalyptus
2 drops geranium

Relaxing blend: to ease stress, insomnia, anxiety and shock
2 drops Roman chamomile or neroli
3 drops lavender or 2 drops rose or 2 drops jasmine

Soothing blend: to soothe arthritis, rheumatism and headaches
3 drops lavender
2 drops Roman chamomile
1 drop juniper

CHILDREN'S BATHS

1 drop of essential oil (diluted in carrier oil or full-fat/dried milk, as above) in a baby bath is sufficient for an infant, while 2–3 drops added to half a bath of water is sufficient for a toddler.

Make sure children do not rub their eyes.

Bathing in essential oils can bring relief to children suffering from chickenpox or other irritating infections (see Chapter Seven, page 221).

Comforting blend: to soothe constipation, indigestion and stress
3 drops petitgrain
2 drops sweet orange
2 drops lavender

Relieving blend: to soothe psoriasis, dermatitis, eczema, shingles, cystitis and stress
2 drops bergamot
1 drop eucalyptus
2 drops tea tree

To relieve depression or high blood pressure
3 drops lavender
2 drops bergamot
1 drop ylang ylang

Showering

Mix the essential oils into 10 ml (2 teaspoons) of carrier oil first and massage into the skin before getting under the spray. Do not apply to the feet because of the danger of slipping.

Foot or hand bath

These provide relief for rheumatism and arthritis. Add 5 drops of diluted essential oils to a basin of warm water, then soak the hands or feet for about 10–15 minutes. Oils can be chosen for their smell alone, or for specific properties: lavender and pine to refresh tired feet; ginger to boost circulation; cypress to help reduce perspiration.

Shampoos

Add 2–3 drops to your shampoo or to 100 ml (3–4 fl oz) of water for the last rinse. Be careful not to get it into the eyes.

Saunas

Adding 2–3 drops of essential oils such as eucalyptus, tea tree or pine to at least 600 ml (1 pint) of water and throwing it on the hot stones is particularly good for relieving nasal congestion or as an air disinfectant and antiseptic.

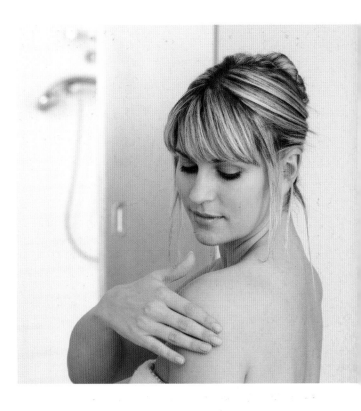

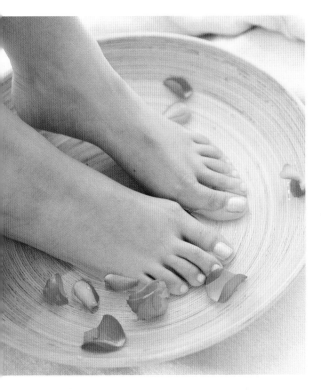

Compresses

Compresses help reduce fever, inflammation and pain, improve circulation and relieve tiredness/headache and fluid/lymphatic congestion. They are ideal for oversensitive areas of the body or where pressure cannot be applied because of stiffness or congestion. Always use cloths made of natural fibres and use only enough water to soak the compress.

Hot compresses relieve muscular pain and help with arthritic conditions. Add a few drops of essential oils to a small bowl of very hot water and, wearing rubber gloves, dip in a folded cotton cloth or flannel. Squeeze out any excess water and place the cloth carefully (checking the heat) over the affected area. Cover with foil or plastic wrap and a towel to keep in the heat. Remove after about 15 minutes and gently manipulate the joint to relieve the pain.

Cold compresses are a good first aid treatment for sprains and swellings and to soothe inflammation; applied to the feet they can reduce fever. Follow the same procedure as for a hot compress but use 100 ml (3–4 fl oz) of cold water and six ice cubes. Do not allow a cold compress to dry out.

You can also apply hot and cold compresses alternately to improve the circulation in injuries such as sprained ligaments and bruises.

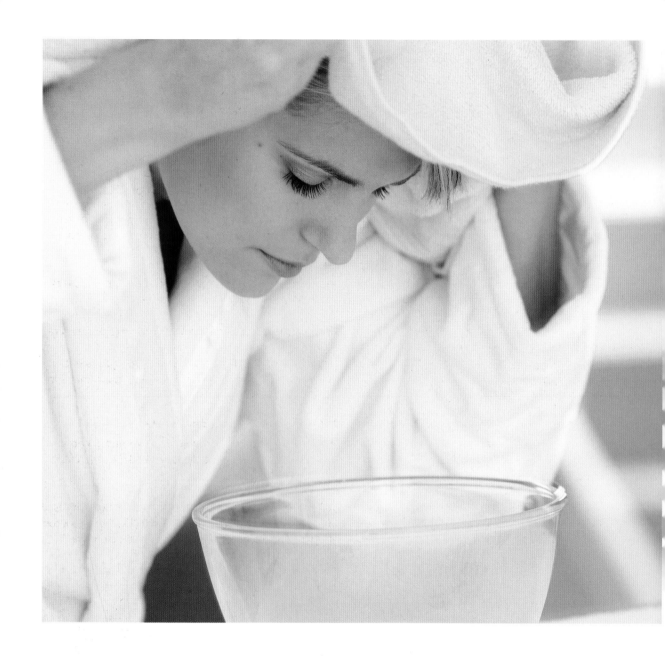

Inhalation and facial steaming

Place a bowl of hot (not boiling) water on a table and add 6–8 drops of essential oils. Slowly breathe in the vapours. To turn this into a facial steam, add just 3–5 drops to the water, drape a towel over your head and lower your head over the bowl. Close your eyes, so the fumes don't irritate or burn them. Inhale for one minute then rest, repeating this several times. Do this two or three times a day to relieve congestion and other respiratory symptoms.

An alternative method is to put a few drops of tea tree or ravensara (see tea tree in the Directory of essential oils, page 88), on a tissue and inhale occasionally.

Caution: Asthmatics should be careful when using this method, because the intensity of the essential oils may be overpowering and provoke an attack.

Creams and lotions

Essential oils can be incorporated into cleansers, toners and moisturizers. Choose a base that is unperfumed and made of pure, natural materials (suppliers of essential oil sell plain base creams). Calamine lotion can also be used as a base, as can zinc oxide cream; both are widely available from pharmacies. Check that the essential oil you have chosen is safe to use in this way.

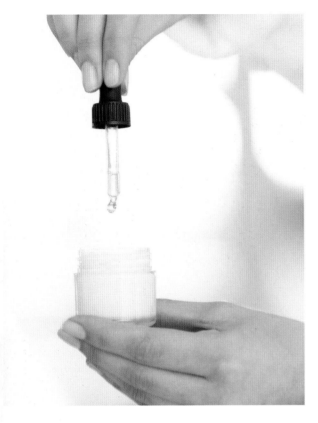

Room vaporizers and diffusers

Warmed essential oils releasing their aromas into a room can:

- relieve respiratory conditions and headache
- aid sleep and relaxation
- combat the spread of infectious bugs in offices
- counteract unpleasant odours.

Vaporizers and diffusers work either by candles or electrical elements or as a ring designed to rest on a light bulb. Add 4–6 drops of oils to 1 tablespoon (15 ml) of water in the bowl of the vaporizer (ideally purified water so that no chemicals are released during heating). Make sure the water never dries up, because the oils that remain may burn and produce undesirable odours. It is best not to let the oils burn for longer than two hours, as by this time the lighter molecules will have vapourized, leaving the heavier molecules, which evaporate at a slower rate.

Caution: Never leave vaporizers with candles unattended: essential oils are extremely volatile and can ignite at high temperatures or if exposed to a naked flame. Don't leave any vaporizer burning in a room where there are children.

Insect repellent

Certain essential oils are powerful natural insecticides. Add a few drops of lemongrass, tea tree and thyme to a damp cloth and wipe the insides of wardrobes and around window frames. For outdoors, dilute 8 drops of tea tree and 8 drops of thyme in 100 ml (3–4 fl oz) of water in a clean spray bottle and then spritz the air.

For insect bites and stings

Essential oils with antiseptic and anti-inflammatory properties help reduce swelling, itchiness and inflammation. Try lavender neat, or Roman or German chamomile, peppermint or basil in a 1 per cent solution.

To counteract jet lag

After a long-haul flight, try the following blends in 10 ml (2 teaspoons) of carrier oil:

- for swollen feet: 2 drops grapefruit, l drop cypress and l drop juniper
- to stay awake: 1 drop lavender and 2 drops rosemary
- to sleep: l drop geranium, 1 drop sweet marjoram and 2 drops lavender.

To counteract travel sickness

Put a few drops of peppermint, ginger or melissa on a tissue and inhale occasionally before and during travel.

Room spray

Make a therapeutic air freshener by mixing a few drops of your favourite essential oil with 100 ml (3–4 fl oz) of water in a pump-action spray bottle. Shake well before use.

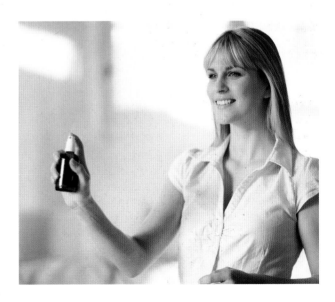

Seated massage

It is possible to conduct a 15-minute seated massage without removing the client's clothing, in which case no massage oil is used. As an on-site massage, this may take place in an office or other working environment, so you will need to adapt what is available: a chair in front of a desk or table, preferably a high one, will suffice. Take pillows or towels to act as supports. This sequence can also be used for a pregnant woman who would be uncomfortable lying face down.

Setting the scene

The client should be sitting in a chair in front of the desk or table. Make sure that he or she is sitting correctly, with a straight back, and use the pillows or towels to enhance comfort and relaxation.

For an on-site massage, establish a relaxed atmosphere by placing a burner with a destressing blend of essential oils near the client so that they can inhale the aroma. If convenient, play some music of the client's choice during the treatment. At the end of the massage, offer your client a glass of water or herbal tea.

There was a time when a therapist visiting an office or clinic to give a massage was unheard of but with today's high-pressure lifestyles many companies encourage this treatment for their staff. Obviously some busy people would prefer an aromatherapy massage in a salon after work but long working hours often mean this may not be possible. With so much time spent sitting in front of computer screens one of the most effective ways to obtain relief to the neck and shoulder muscles is to have a seated massage.

Be aware that women may prefer not to have the head massaged due to hair rearrangement but men really enjoy a head, neck and shoulder massage.

The most popular time for seated massage seems to be during the lunch break and before the client has actually eaten. There are also a few shoulder exercises which can be recommended after the massage has been completed.

Massage sequence

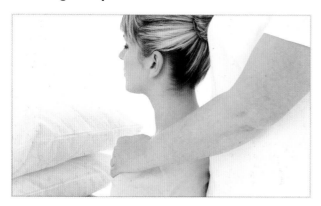

1 Stand behind the chair, place your hands flat on the client's shoulders and ask him or her to breathe deeply. On an out breath, pull the shoulders gently back, pushing them into the back of the chair. Repeat three times.

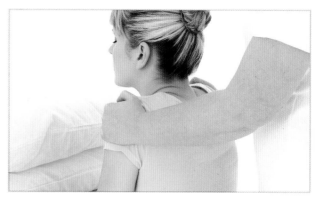

2 To improve shoulder mobility, rotate the shoulders forwards and backwards and upwards and downwards. This will rotate the whole ball-and-socket joint.

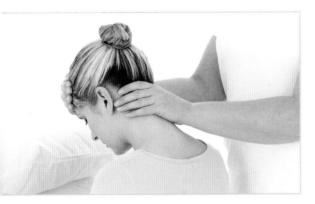

3 Place one hand on the forehead and, with the other hand, tip the head slowly forwards and backwards. Repeat movement three times.

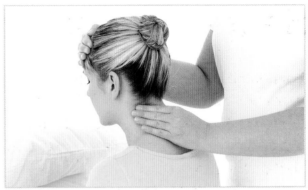

4 Keeping one hand on the forehead, work your other hand up the back of the neck on either side of the spine from the seventh cervical vertebra to the base of the cranium.

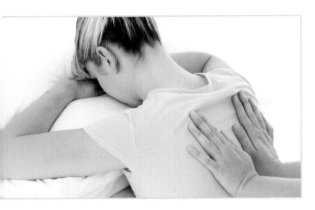

5 Now ask the client to lean forwards and rest on the pillows on the desk and relax. Effleurage up the back with both hands.

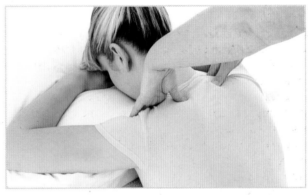

6 With your thumb, make circular movements along the trapezius muscle, starting from the seventh cervical vertebra and sliding back and upwards to the cranium. Use fairly deep pressure. Repeat three times.

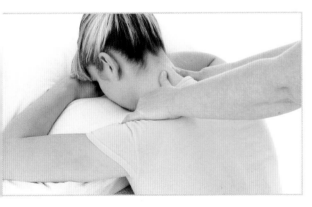

7 Circle with the thumbs down the neck muscle to the fifth cervical vertebra and push deeply upwards with the hand. Repeat three times.

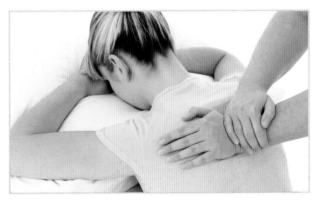

8 Deep knead along either side of the spine with the heel of the left hand, supporting the wrist with the right hand and pushing deeply upwards with each application. Repeat three times on each side of the spine.

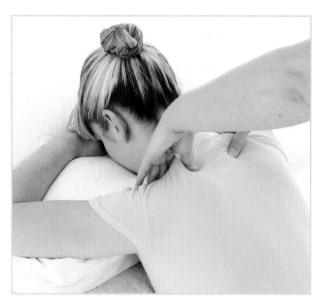

9 Work on the trapezius muscles by kneading and lifting, paying attention to the pressure points (see page 114 and using friction movements according to the amount of tension detected. Do not work too long as it could cause pain.

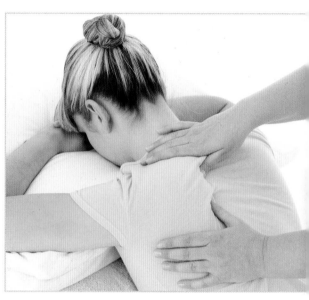

10 Work on the scapula in a similar way.

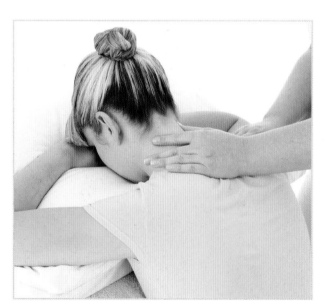

11 Work again on the neck with thumb and forefinger up to the cranium to release tension (see Step 6). Repeat three times.

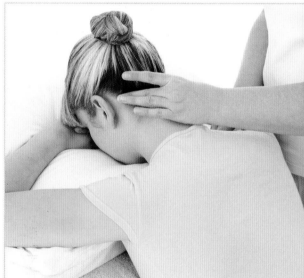

12 To loosen the scalp, work along the base of the cranium, from the mastoid process (just behind the ear) to the occipital vertebra, applying careful pressure to the points where the muscles are attached, which can be quite painful.

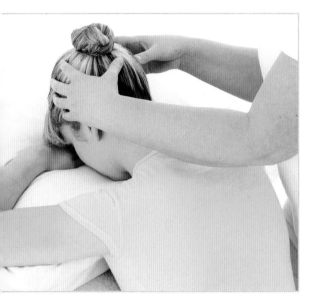

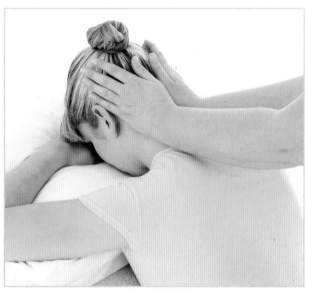

13 Now massage the whole cranium with your thumbs and fingers, making sure that the skin of the scalp is loosened from the underlying bone and that there is movement.

14 Effleurage downwards from the top of the head towards the back and shake off any negative energy.

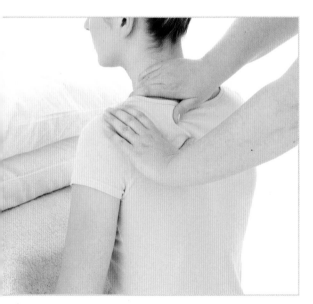

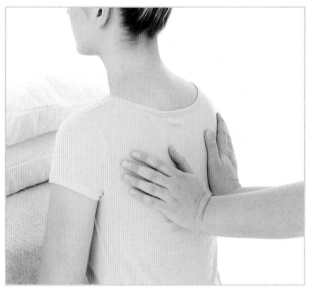

15 Ask the client to sit up slowly and resume work on the back. Work on the trapezius muscles again, using rolling movements and palmar kneading. Then pull the shoulders gently back (see Step 1).

16 Finally, stroke down the back and shake off to release the negative energy.

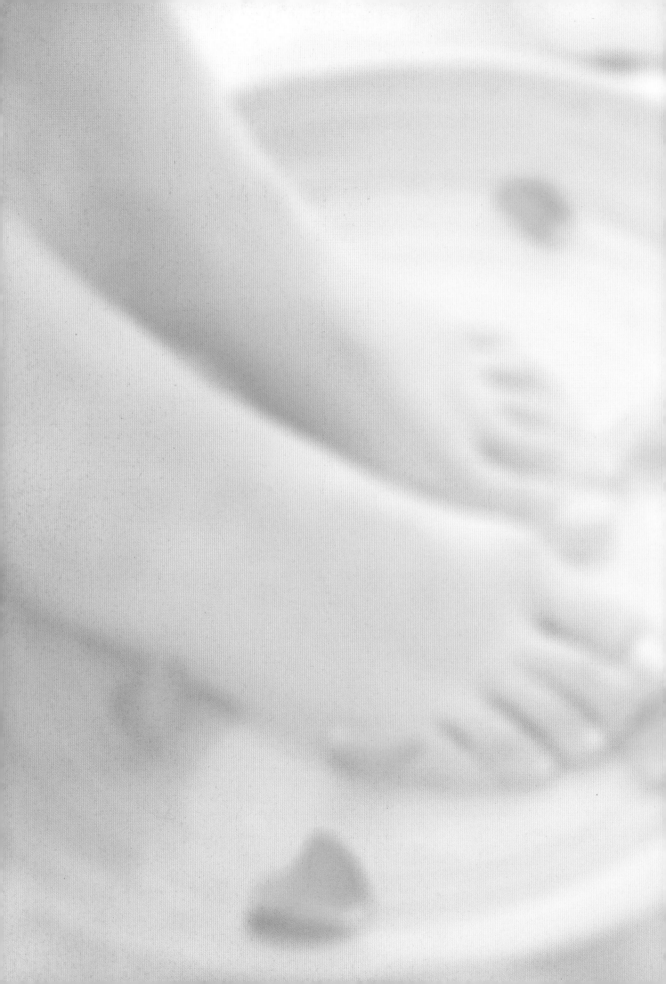

Body systems

To ensure safe and effective treatment, aromatherapists must have sufficient knowledge of anatomy: how the body is structured and what it's made of – and physiology: how the body works. The body systems, though studied as separate units, are interrelated. When one part of the body shows an imbalance, it is a reflection of disharmony within the whole. Aromatherapists are taught to think of the whole mind and body, taking a holistic approach to their work.

Cells and tissues 160

Skin 164

The respiratory system 170

The circulatory system 174

The lymphatic system 180

The nervous system 184

The digestive system 190

The urinary system 194

The endocrine system 196

The reproductive system 200

The musculoskeletal system 206

Cells and tissues

A cell is the fundamental unit of all living organisms and is the simplest form of life. Each of us begins life as a single cell that divides and multiplies. Cells group together to form specialized tissues, for example, blood, muscle and bone. Tissues in turn group together to form organs such as the liver or skin, each contributing a specific role to maintaining the body as a whole.

Cells

Cells consist of the elements of carbon, hydrogen, nitrogen plus some other trace elements, but take many forms in the body. Cells can do many things, some of which are associated with their structure or location.

Cell structure

A cell consists of plasma membrane enclosing a fluid in which float a number of small structures, called organelles. At the centre of the cell is a nucleus, enclosed within its own membrane.

Nucleus

Every cell in the body, with the exception of mature red blood cells, has a nucleus. The nucleus is the largest organelle; it acts like the brain of the cell and is essential for reproduction. The information required by the cell is stored in DNA, which carries the genetic materials for replication. The DNA strands are found in long coiled structures known as chromosomes. Each human cell normally has 23 pairs of chromosomes.

The nucleus is contained within a semi-permeable membrane with tiny pores through which some substances can pass between it and the cytoplasm.

Cell membrane and cytoplasm

A cell's fine semi-permeable outer membrane maintains the shape of the cell and acts as a protection for the contents. It also deals with the exchange of nutrients and waste materials passing in and out of the cell. The outer surface of the membrane is covered in cilia, tiny hair-like projections that help move materials outside the cells.

Inside the membrane, the gel-like, semi-transparent cytoplasm contains a variety of different organelles, each with its own function (see box). Many chemical reactions occur in this part of the cell.

ORGANELLES

Centrioles contained within a dense region of cytoplasm called centrosome and associated with cell division.

Ribosomes tiny organelles made up of RNA and protein whose function is to manufacture proteins for use both inside and outside the cell.

Endoplasmic reticulum a series of membranes connected to the manufacture and transport of enzymes and other materials out of the cell. Also detoxifies harmful agents.

Mitochondria sausage-shaped structures that act as the power house of the cell, because they provide the energy needed from food molecules.

Lysomes small oval cells or sacs producing a variety of enzymes that deal with harmful substances and destroy any part of the cell that is worn out or damaged.

Golgi body/apparatus attached to the flattened membranous sacs within the cytoplasm; transports the protein manufactured in the cell and later transports it out of the cell or stores it.

Cell functions

As well as forming organisms that perform many different functions, cells also act in a number of ways at an individual level. For example, they respond to stimuli, such as heat – a reaction known as irritability. They also absorb and secrete substances through their semi-permeable membrane, in a process called cell respiration.

Cell The basic unit of all living organisms can reproduce itself exactly. Each cell is bounded by a cell membrane of lipids and proteins that controls the passage of substances in and out of the cell.

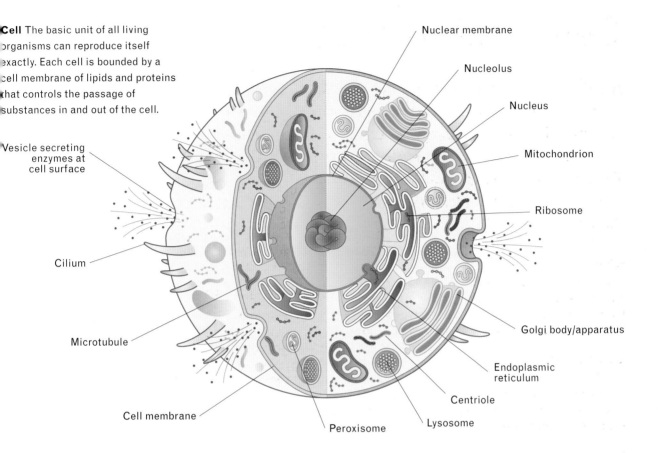

One of the vital substances cells absorb is oxygen from the blood. Oxygen allows other materials manufactured or absorbed in the cell to be broken down to provide energy. All the biochemical reactions that occur in cells create the body's metabolism. The process can be broken down into:

- anabolism: the synthesis of substances, which is energy-consuming
- catabolism: the breaking down of processes, which is energy-releasing.

Metabolic rate is the speed at which these reactions happen, and is influenced by age, exercise, body and environmental temperature, thyroid hormone, the sympathetic nervous system and drugs. Basal metabolism is the least amount of reactions that can occur to keep the body alive. As a point of interest the anabolic process is more evident between 4 am and 10 am and the catabolic process between 4 pm and 10 pm.

What a cell does is reproduced on a larger scale throughout the body and throughout life. If the cell cannot perform its usual functions it results in disease and illness.

Cell division

Cells also reproduce constantly, by dividing into two. The nucleus divides and is followed by the division of the cytoplasm to form two identical 'daughter' cells. This ongoing process is called mitosis, and cells in the human body continue to do this throughout life, new cells replacing old ones that fail and die and are reabsorbed or shed. The average lifespan of a cell varies – red blood cells, for example, last about 120 days, but hair and skin cells are replaced much more often.

Meiosis is a special process of cell division that occurs in the reproductive cells. As an ovum grows to maturity in the ovaries and spermatozoa multiply in the testes, the chromosomes do not replicate as they do in mitosis. Instead, each of the 23 pairs of chromosomes separates and one from each pair moves to opposite poles of the 'parent' cell, so that when it divides, each of the 'daughter' cells has only 23 chromosomes. Fertilizing an ovum with a sperm produces a zygote with, once more, the full complement of 46 chromosomes, half from the father and half from the mother – which means the child inherits some characteristics, such as colour of hair, eyes and height, from each parent.

Tissue

Tissues consist of a large number of similar cells and are classified according to size, shape and function. The many variants come in two basic forms: epithelial tissue and connective tissue.

Epithelial tissue or epithelium

Epithelial tissue covers and protects the external and internal surfaces of the body, and lines the multitude of cavities and tubes. The lining of the uterus, the inner surfaces of blood vessels and the skin are all examples of epithelial tissue.

The cells forming epithelial tissue are closely packed together, either in a single layer (simple) or several layers (compound), and arranged in different formations according to the function of the tissue. The more active the tissue the taller the cells.

Simple epithelium

The single layer of cells usually rests on a basement membrane, which is inert connective tissue that gives the cells their nourishment.

The squamous (pavement) is like the flat stones of a pavement, forming a very smooth membrane through which substances can easily pass. Examples are lining of blood vessels, heart, lymph vessels and the alveoli of the lungs.

Cuboidal are cube-shaped cells found in areas where absorption and excretion takes place. Examples are

tubules of the kidneys, the ovaries, thyroid gland, pancreas and salivary glands.

Columnar are taller and wider cells found in the lining of some organs. Examples are linings of the small and large intestine, and the stomach gall bladder.

Ciliated are columnar cells with fine, hair-like projections called cilia, which propel in one direction the contents of the tubes they line. Examples are lining of the respiratory passages and uterine tubes.

Compound epithelium

The main function of compound epithelium is to protect the underlying structures. The cells are of different shapes and configurations, and as the cells grow towards the surface they become flattened. There is usually no basement membrane.

Stratified; found on wet or dry surfaces subject to wear and tear. On a dry surface, the top layer consists of dead cells to which the protein keratin has been added, protecting and preventing drying out of deeper cells from where they develop. Examples (non-keratinized) are the lining of the mouth, pharynx, oesophagus, conjunctiva of the eyes. Examples (keratinized) are skin, hair, nails.

Transitional; composed of several layers of pear-shaped cells, and allows for stretching, for example, as an organ expands. Examples are the lining of the uterus and the bladder.

Simple epithelium

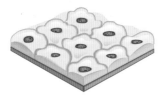

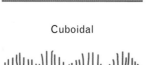

Squamous (pavement)　　　　Cuboidal

Compound epithelium

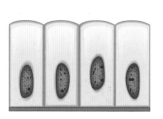

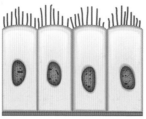

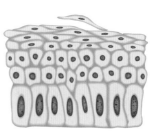

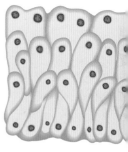

Columnar　　　　Ciliated　　　　Stratified　　　　Transitional

Connective tissue

Connective tissue connects other tissues and organs and gives support and protection to the body. The cells of connective tissue are more widely spaced than in epithelial tissue, leaving room for intercellular substance (matrix). The matrix can be semi-solid-like jelly, or dense and rigid. The cells and fibres in the matrix and certain chemicals determine the pliability or rigidity of the tissue, from the solidity of bone, through to the elasticity of tendons and the softness of fat.

Cartilage is a firm type of connective tissue, with a quite solid matrix. There are three types:

- **Hyaline cartilage:** smooth and glossy, found at joint surfaces of bone, between the ribs, part of the larynx, trachea and bronchi.
- **White fibro-cartilage:** found at the joint surfaces of the bone. It also forms, for example, pads between the vertebrae, between the bones of the knee and on the rim of the hip and shoulder socket.
- **Yellow fibro-cartilage** consists of elastic fibres running through a solid matrix. It forms, for example, the earlobes, epiglottis, middle layer of blood vessel walls.

There are also specialized forms of tissue, such as lymphoid tissue found in the lymph nodes and organs associated with the lymphatic system (see page 180). Blood is also classed as a connective tissue, but is liquid because it contains no fibres.

Areolar tissue is the most widely distributed connective tissue found in humans. It is composed of fibrocytes, which allow for elasticity and are found in almost every part of the body.

Adipose tissue is composed of specialized cells for the storage of energy in the form of fat (adipocytes). Adipose

MEMBRANES

Membranes are made from thin layers of epithelial cells. They cover organs and surfaces, reducing friction and secreting specific juices. There are three basic types:

- Mucous membrane coats and protects the lining of the alimentary, respiratory and genito-urinary tracts.
- Synovial membrane is found in bursae (protective sacs lining joint cavities), surrounding tendons that could be injured by rubbing against bone.
- Serous membrane is found in the thoracic cavity, pleura surrounding the lungs, pericardium surrounding the heart and the peritoneum surrounding the abdominal organs.

tissue insulates the body and protects organs as well as producing certain hormones. It also contains many small blood vessels.

The white fibrous connective tissue is made up mainly of closely packed bundles of collagen fibres. This makes it very strong and it is found in tendons (attaching muscle to bone) and ligaments (binding bones together). The cells of this type of tissue produce both collagen and elastin, which respectively give strength and elasticity to the tissue.

Yellow elastic tissue is composed of bundles of elastin and can be found in areas where stretching of various organs requires help to return them to their original shape and size. The fibres can stretch up to one and a half times their length before relaxing, when they snap back to their original length.

Connective tissue

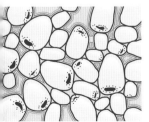

Areolar tissue

Adipose tissue

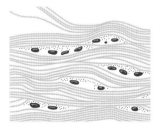

White fibrous tissue

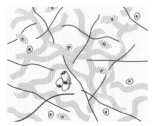

Yellow elastic fibrocartilage

The skin

The skin is the largest organ of the body, and an important one for aromatherapists to study as it is one of the principal ways essential oils are absorbed. The health of the body in general is often reflected in the state of the skin.

The structure of the skin

The skin forms the protective covering over the entire surface of the body. The colour varies according to race, individual variation, the season, location of the body and age. It also varies in thickness on different parts of the body and is thinnest on the lips and eyelids.

Examine skin under a magnifying glass and it appears to be covered by a pattern of criss-crossing lines. Fine hairs and barely visible pores, which are the outlets for the sweat glands, can also be seen. There are also ostia, tiny openings through which the sebaceous glands secrete sebum.

The skin is composed of two layers: the epidermis and the dermis. As the skin constantly regenerates itself, cells reproduce at the deepest level of the epidermis and work their way through to the surface until they die and are shed, a process taking about six weeks.

Layers of the skin The skin is a complex organ composed of two levels: the epidermis and the dermis. The hypodermis is not part of the skin, but connects the skin to the muscle and bone underneath and provides it with nerves and blood vessels.

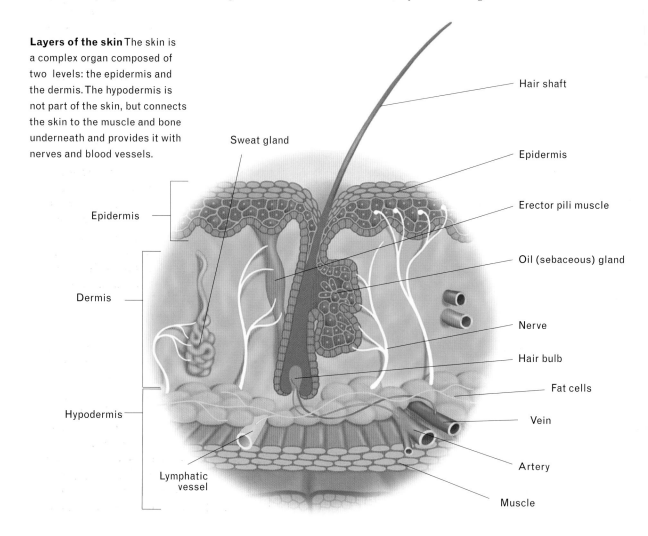

Epidermis

Dermis

Hypodermis

Sweat gland

Lymphatic vessel

Hair shaft

Epidermis

Erector pili muscle

Oil (sebaceous) gland

Nerve

Hair bulb

Fat cells

Vein

Artery

Muscle

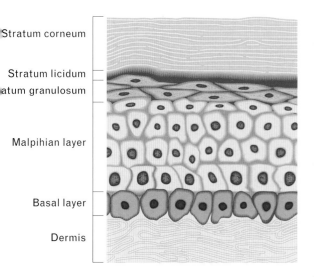

Stratum corneum

Stratum licidum

atum granulosum

Malpihian layer

Basal layer

Dermis

The dermis

Also called the cutis or 'true skin', the dermis contains blood vessels, lymph vessels, nerves, sweat, sebaceous glands and hair follicles, and is thicker in men than women. Its key functions are to provide support, strength and elasticity. The dermis is divided into a superficial papillary level and a deeper reticular level.

The papillary layer lies directly beneath the epidermis and its tissues contain some fine collagen and elastin fibres embedded in a rich matrix. Into the papillae reach capillary loops and tactile (touch) nerve endings.

The reticular layer contains dense, coarse fibres, some of which branch down into the underlying layers, binding the two together. Blood vessels are loosely entwined with fibres to allow for dilation and constriction.

The dermis contains various types of fibrous tissue that give it its texture and strength:

- collagen, produced by cells called fibroblasts, is a hard white, inelastic protein fibre found in bundles that lie parallel to the skin's surface. Collagen gives strength to the skin.
- elastin, also produced by fibroblasts, is a yellow protein fibre that allows the skin to stretch and snap back. It forms a network of branching fibres.

Reticular fibres are made by the protein collagen and form a branching network which has a supporting function.

The dermis has an abundant supply of blood vessels forming a fine network of capillaries supplying sweat glands, sebaceous glands, hair follicles and the dermis itself. This network also supplies nutrients and oxygen to the epidermis, which has no blood supply. (See page 174, for how gases and nutrients circulate in the bloodstream.)

Lymph vessels also form a network throughout the dermis and the deeper layers of the epidermis. They generally accompany the course of veins.

The subcutaneous layer/hypodermis

Also called the hypodermis or sub-cutis, this is not part of the skin, but a layer of fatty tissue containing the same collagen and elastin fibres as the dermis. Through it run the arteries and veins that supply the skin. This layer gives us our contours, acts as a protective cushion for the outer skin and is an energy store, and its depth depends on age, sex and health. Its fat cells help to insulate the body by reducing heat loss. Areolar and adipose tissue (see page 163) act as shock absorbers, supporting more delicate tissues such as blood vessels and nerve endings. Below the subcutaneous layer lies the subdermal muscle layer.

he epidermis

he top layer of the skin is composed of stratified pithelium. It is thickest on the palms of the hands and bles of the feet. There are no blood vessels or nerve ndings in the epidermis, but its deeper layers are athed in interstitial fluid that is drained away as lymph.

Basal or germinative layer A single layer of constantly dividing cells lying between the dermis and the epidemis. Special cells in this layer, called melanocytes, produce melanin, the substance responsible for skin pigmentation. When the skin is exposed to the sun, melanin production increases.

Malpighian layer (prickle layer) So-called because the cells in this layer have short, prickly looking projections for making contact with neighbouring cells. These cells are very active; the cytoplasm is denser and filled with different substances (cholesterol, amino-acids).

Stratum granulosum The nuclei of these flat, granular cells are reaching the end of their life and have become egg-shaped. Granules of keratohyaline appear in the cytoplasm, a fatty substance that permeates and softens the skin's keratin.

Stratum licidum A layer of homogenous, transparent cells. It is at this level of the epidermis that cellular death actually occurs.

Stratum corneum (horny layer) Composed of flat, thin, non-nucleated, dead cells. These are constantly being rubbed off (exfoliated). The horny layer is a highly efficient protective shield, and one of its most important roles is to prevent evaporation of moisture from the tissues.

Functions of the skin

As well as providing a waterproof covering for the body, the skin has several other useful functions.

Protection

The skin protects the body's deeper and more delicate structures, and acts as a barrier against the invasion of microbes and harmful agents. In this it is helped by its slightly acidic nature. The mix of sweat and sebum on the surface of the skin (see opposite) form what is known as the acid mantle, which inhibits the growth of organisms on the skin. The skin's production of melanin (see page 165) is also a protective, helping shield the body from the sun's dangerous ultraviolet rays.

Absorption and elimination

The skin's ability to absorb some microscopic substances while repelling others is significant to aromatherapy. How it does this and the effects are described in Chapter Two (see page 34). The skin also acts as a mini excretory system, eliminating waste and toxins through perspiration.

Sensation

Sensory nerve endings relay information to the brain about environment affecting the skin, such as touch, pressure, heat and cold. They trigger reflex actions to unpleasant or painful stimuli, protecting the body from further injury.

THE PH OF THE SKIN

The pH scale measures acidity or alkalinity, and ranges from 0–14, with 7 being neutral. The higher the number the more alkaline the substance. The skin has a pH between 4.5 and 6, making it a little acidic.

Regulation of body temperature

The skin controls our surface body temperature and maintains our internal body heat, a balance sometimes referred to as homeostasis (see also page 195). It achieves this through perspiration from the sweat glands, and the expansion and contraction of blood vessels in the dermis (vasodilation and vasoconstriction). Any increase in body temperature will cause the capillaries near the skin's surface to dilate, allowing more blood to circulate nearer to the surface, where heat will be lost by radiation and convection. This is what gives pale skins a flushed look when hot. Increased amounts of sweat also provide a cooling effect as it evaporates from the surface of the skin. A decrease in body temperature will trigger the opposite effects.

Vitamin D production

There is a fatty substance in the skin (modified cholesterol molecules) that the ultraviolet light from the sun converts into vitamin D. This circulates in the blood and is used, with calcium and phosphorus, in the formation and maintenance of bone. Any vitamin D in excess of immediate requirements is stored in the liver. A lack of Vitamin D in children can result in rickets, a softening of the bones which can lead to fractures and deformity. A similar condition in adults is known as Osteomalacia.

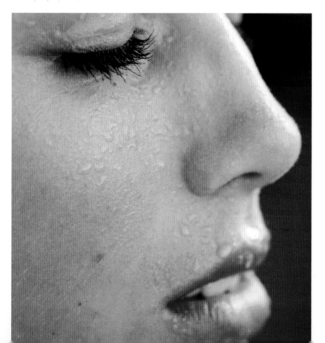

Perspiration from the sweat glands is part of the body's way of controlling its surface temperature. The evaporation of sweat from the surface of the skin produces a cooling effect.

Hair and skin glands

Embedded in the skin are a number of structures that affect how it functions.

Hair

Hair grows from a sac-like depression of epidermal cells called a follicle. At its base is a cluster of cells called the bulb, and as these cells multiply they are pushed upwards away from their source of nutrition, die and are converted to keratin. They emerge from the skin as a hair.

Hair grows all over the body, with the exception of the palms of the hands and the soles of the feet. It protects the skin, helps conserve warmth and assists our sense of touch. Hair colour depends on melanin: white hair is the result of the replacement of melanin by tiny air bubbles.

Attached at an angle to the base of each hair follicle is a small smooth muscle, called the Erector pili. As its name implies, it makes the hair stand erect in response to either cold or fear.

Sweat glands

These are widely distributed but are most numerous in the palms of the hands, the soles of the feet, the armpits and groin. There are two types of sweat glands: eccrine (the majority, which open directly on to the surface of the skin) and apocrine. These open into hair follicles and are only found in the genital and underarm regions. They do not become active until puberty and produce a fatty secretion which, if decomposed by surface microbes, causes an unpleasant odour.

Sweat glands are stimulated by sympathetic nerves in response to raised body temperature and fear but the most important function is in the regulation of body temperature (see opposite). The amount of sweat produced is governed by the hypothalamus part of the endocrine system (see page 196).

Sebaceous glands

These secretory epithelial cells derive from the same tissue as hair follicles. They produce sebum, an oily substance containing fats and cholesterol that flows into hair follicles and keeps hair soft and shiny. They are most numerous on the scalp and face, and some open on to the chest and back. Sebum provides some waterproofing and acts as a bactericidal and fungicidal agent. It also prevents drying and cracking of skin, especially on exposure to heat and sunshine. The secretion of sebum is stimulated by the release of certain hormones.

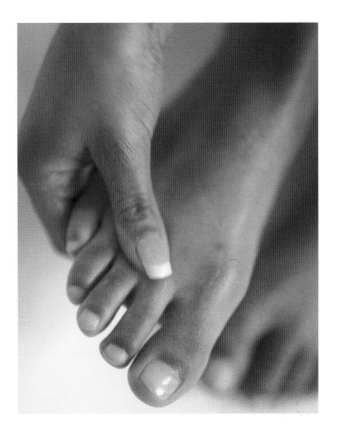

Nails on the hands and feet are made of the same cells as the epidermis and the hair and can benefit from the use of essential oils. Protein and vitamin A are particularly important in maintaining healthy nails.

Nails

Nails are constructed from the same cells as epidermis and hair, and consist of a hard, horny type of keratinized dead cell. Each nail grows out from the nail bed in the germinative zone of the epidermis, and the root is covered by the hemispherical cuticle, or lanula. Fingernails grow more quickly than toenails and growth is quicker when the environmental temperature is high. The nail forms a protective covering which supports the blood vessels and nerves at the ends of the fingers and toes. The nails also help transfer the sensation of touch along the nerves beneath them.

How aromatherapy can help

Skin problems are often symptoms of an underlying problem, and as aromatherapy is a holistic approach, you need to take this into account. Aromatherapy can help skin complaints but results can be slow.

Conditions helped by aromatherapy include:

- Dry skin: the following oils are helpful: geranium, neroli, German chamomile, ylang ylang, rose and palmarosa.
- Oily skin: Try lemon, geranium, petitgrain, cedarwood and sandalwood.
- Athlete's foot: can be treated with tea tree in a footbath or neat on a lint pad.

Essential oils which are made up of small organic molecules can diffuse through the skin by entering the hair follicles and the ducts of the sweat glands to the capillaries and circulation. The rate of diffusion depends on the surface area, the thickness (viscosity) of the carrier oil used and the evaporation (volatility) rate of the essential oils.

Aromatherapy massage will increase the absorption rate and, as the essential oils are antisepti and some anti-bacterial and anti-fungal ,such as Tea tree and Ravensara, they can help the skin's protective function.

Essential oils can also help the ageing process – oils such as Frankincense and Neroli are said to help the skin cells to regenerate and are known as cytophylactic.

It is known that Geranium can also regulate the sebum secretion of both oily and dry skins.

CASE STUDY 1 **ECZEMA**

Brenda's two children (Morgan, 6, and Sophie, 8) had atopic inherited eczema, characterized by itchiness with inflammation on the elbows and backs of the knees. Morgan also had itchy eyelids, which scratching had made very sore. Stress seemed to be the emotional factor for Sophie, who became very tired and tearful, especially after school, and could not sleep because of the itchiness. The children had been to the doctor, who had taken them off dairy products and arranged allergy tests.

CHOICE OF OILS
Roman chamomile and geranium are good anti-inflammatories, lavender is a general soothant and de-stresser, and it, sweet marjoram and sandalwood make a good night-time combination to help sleeplessness.

BLEND 1: FOR ITCHY EYELIDS
8 ml carrot oil
4 ml wheatgerm oil
This blend of carrier oils was chosen for its soothing properties, to be gently rubbed on to eyelids.

BLEND 2: FOR ITCHY SKIN AND STRESS
10 ml of the above carrier oils
1 drop Roman chamomile
1 drop lavender
1 drop geranium
3 drops = 1½ per cent blend to be used twice a day for two weeks

BLEND 3: TO AID SLEEP
2 drops sweet marjoram
1 drop sandalwood
2 drops lavender
Diffused into the bedroom for two hours to help relaxation.

TREATMENT
Morgan and Sophie attended the clinic twice a week for two weeks, but most of the treatment was carried out at home.

AFTERCARE
As these are children, the aromatherapy blend was discontinued after two weeks, but they continued to use the carrier mix to improve skin texture. A spray of equal amounts of Roman chamomile and *Rosa damascena* hydrolat proved effective and could be used as often as required, as hydrolats are more suitable for children. (See page 41 for a description of hydrolats).

OUTCOME
By changing to a more healthy lifestyle based around a balanced diet with lots of fresh fruit and vegetables, adequate intake of water, less stress and occasionally using the aromatherapy blend, Brenda has found that she was able to keep her children's eczema at bay, although it was pointed out that the condition may return.

CASE STUDY 2: **ACNE**

George, 17, was suffering from bad acne: his skin was very inflamed and had many blackheads, papules and pustules. A course of antibiotics from his doctor had helped, but the acne returned once the course was completed. George was very depressed about his skin, and felt that examinations and a stressful home life contributed to his condition.

CHOICE OF OILS

Several good essential oils can help clear the infection, reduce the amount of sebum produced, minimize scarring and promote the growth of new skin tissue. Especially effective are niaoli, tea tree and lemon, which are highly antiseptic. Bergamot and petitgrain are also astringent, and lavender is soothing and healing. Geranium, as a balancing oil for mind and body, balances the secretion of sebum.

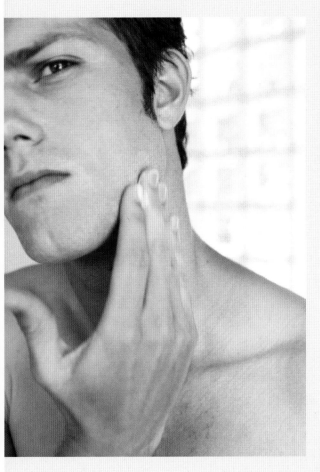

BLEND

10 ml jojoba carrier oil (good for controlling accumulation of excessive sebum and preventing build-up)
2 drops lavender
1 drop geranium
2 drops bergamot
5 drops = 2½ per cent blend

TREATMENT

Massaging the pustulated area will aggravate the condition, so a compress was put on to the inflamed areas, and the remaining blend applied to skin areas not badly affected and to prevent the acne spreading further. Tea tree was applied directly on the pustules with cotton buds, as an antiseptic and to work on the sebum directly. (Care must be taken with the use of tea tree and it is better applied directly than in a blend.) This was continued until the pustules dried up. Later, other essential oils such as juniper, grapefruit and rosemary were introduced to eliminate the toxins.

AFTERCARE

George was warned not to squeeze his blackheads and spots, and given advice on diet and exercise. He was asked to avoid processed foods containing saturated fats and refined sugars, and foods high in iodine such as sushi (seaweed wraps) and shellfish, but to include zinc and vitamin A in his diet. A good 15-minute walk in the fresh air at regular intervals throughout the day was advised (but not running or jogging, as sweating can aggravate the condition). To relieve stress, a warm bath with a blend of lavender and Roman chamomile was recommended at night.

OUTCOME

George attended the clinic for treatment at least twice a week and after about a month there was a definite improvement, and this meant he began to feel better about himself. The treatment, together with a gentle cleansing routine, cleared the condition after eight weeks.

Skin conditions such as acne can be improved and often cleared using aromatherapy.

The respiratory system

It is the lungs and associated air passages that maintain the exchange of oxygen and carbon dioxide that keeps us alive. The respiratory system is also involved in detecting smell, in speech and in regulating pH.

The upper respiratory tract

The body depends on receiving a constant supply of oxygen to all its cells, which use it to release energy and produce carbon dioxide as a waste product, in a process known as cell respiration.

The intake of oxygen begins with the nose. As we inhale, the nostrils filter, moisten and warm incoming air thanks to an epithileal lining with tiny cilia (hairs) that trap bacteria and dust. The epithelium secretes mucus containing a sticky protective fluid to prevent dust and bacteria entering the throat and lungs.

Once air has passed through the nose it moves on to the naso-pharynx, the upper part of the nasal cavity behind the nose, which is lined with mucous membranes. The pharynx serves as an air and food passage; it cannot be used for both purposes at the same time, otherwise choking would result.

The larynx is a short funnel-shaped passage connecting the pharynx to the trachea and contains the vocal cords: air passing over the vocal cords produces the voice. At the top of the larynx there is a flap of tissue called the epiglottis, which closes to stop food entering the trachea (windpipe) during the process of swallowing. The trachea, which carries air between the larynx and the lungs, consists of a tube surrounded by C-shaped rings of cartilage that act to keep it open. The trachea passes down through the thorax and connects with the bronchi, which pass into the lungs.

The lungs

The bronchi lead to and carry air into each lung. The right bronchus is wider and more vertical than the left. Both are further divided into a network of narrower passages called bronchioles, which divide into ever smaller branchioles within the lungs.

There are two lungs, the left one being smaller than the right as it shares chest space with the heart. They are cone-shaped spongy organs, each surrounded by a specialized membrane called the pleura. The pleura consists of two layers moistened by a special fluid resembling lymph, which acts as a lubricant enabling the two surfaces to glide smoothly over each other during respiration.

The lungs are pink coloured because of the large number of blood vessels inside them. The ever-branching branchioles, which form a vast network, end in millions of tiny air sacs called alveoli, which are arranged in lobules and resemble bunches of grapes. They are surrounded by an equally vast network of tiny blood vessels, called pulmonary capillaries. The barrier between the air in the alveoli and the blood in the capillaries is so thin that oxygen and carbon dioxide can pass across it.

Interchange of gases in and out of lungs

During inhalation, oxygen is taken in through the nose and mouth. It flows along the trachea and bronchial tubes to the alveoli of the lungs, where it diffuses through the thin film of moisture lining the alveoli. The air, rich with oxygen, comes into contact with the blood in the capillary network surrounding the alveoli. The oxygen diffuses across a permeable membrane wall surrounding the alveoli to be taken up by the red blood cells. This oxygen-rich blood is carried to the heart, then pumped to cells throughout the body. Carbon dioxide, collected by the respiring cells around the body, passes in the opposite direction by diffusing from the capillary walls into the alveoli; it is passed through the bronchi and trachea, and exhaled through the nose and mouth.

Muscles that aid respiration

Two sets of muscles lie between the ribs, known as the internal and external intercostal muscles. Together they are responsible for raising and lowering the chest during inspiration (breathing in) and expiration (breathing out).

The diaphragm is a dome-shaped sheet of muscle that separates the thorax (chest cavity) from the abdomen. It has three openings to allow for the passage of the oesophagus, the aorta and the vena cava.

The mechanism of respiration involves the intercostal muscles contracting, moving the ribcage upwards and

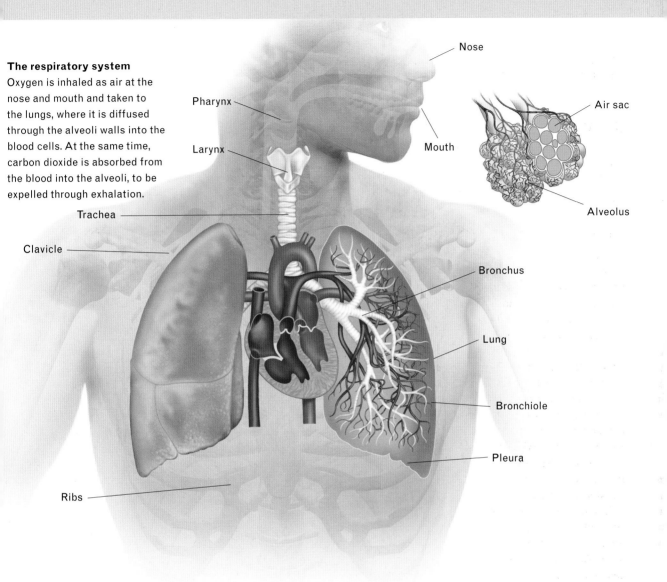

The respiratory system
Oxygen is inhaled as air at the nose and mouth and taken to the lungs, where it is diffused through the alveoli walls into the blood cells. At the same time, carbon dioxide is absorbed from the blood into the alveoli, to be expelled through exhalation.

Nose

Pharynx

Larynx

Mouth

Air sac

Alveolus

Trachea

Clavicle

Bronchus

Lung

Bronchiole

Pleura

Ribs

outwards, and the diaphragm contracting downwards, to a more flattened position. This causes the space inside the thorax to increase in volume and so decrease the pressure inside it. During expiration the intercostal muscles relax, the diaphragm returns to its dome shape on relaxation and the ribcage returns to the normal position. This has the effect of reducing the volume within the thorax, increasing the air pressure in the lungs and forcing out air.

Regulating breathing

Control of respiration is partly voluntary but mainly involuntary, and is achieved through both chemical and neurological means. Voluntary control is exerted during activities such as speaking and singing. Involuntary respiration is controlled by nerve cells in the brain's medulla oblongata, in what is known as the respiratory

centre. It is further controlled by chemoreceptors in the walls of the aorta and carotid arteries.

Other functions of the respiratory system

As explained, air passing over the vocal cords in the larynx is what allows us to speak. This is why we cannot talk when we are gasping for breath – for instance from running too fast – and why breath control is so important to singers. Of great importance to aromatherapy is the respiratory system's role in olfaction, or how we sense different smells. This is explained in greater detail in Chapter Two (see page 32). The respiratory system is also one way in which the body regulates the blood's pH, or acid–alkaline balance. Carbon dioxide is slightly acidic, and so a build-up of carbon dioxide in the body's system, usually due to a lung or breathing disorder, can cause respiratory acidosis.

Disorders of the respiratory system

Viral infections such as common cold, influenza and tonsillitis affect the respiratory systems, and diseases or disorders that interfere with normal breathing will have an effect on the entire body.

Asthma

There are two types of bronchial asthma: extrinsic (allergic or atopic) and intrinsic. In both types the mucous membrane and muscle layers of the bronchi become thickened and the mucous glands enlarge. During an attack, spasmodic contraction of bronchial muscle and excessive secretion of mucous constrict and reduce the airways. Inspiration is normal but expiration is only partial. The duration of attacks can vary from a few minutes to hours.

Allergic reactions

These include hay fever, a condition of hypersensitivity that develops as a reaction to foreign antigens such as pollen and dust mites, sensitizing the airways.

Acute sinusitis

The sinuses are cavities within the bones of the front of the face, which become painful if the mucous membrane lining them becomes inflamed or congested. This is often caused by the spread of microbes from the nose and pharynx.

Bronchitis

Bronchitis is a bacterial infection usually preceded by a cold or influenza. It can be acute or chronic; chronic bronchitis being a progressive inflammatory disease caused by several factors, including smoking or atmospheric pollutants.

Emphysema

This chronic obstructive pulmonary disease results in an irreversible distention of the respiratory bronchioles, alveolar ducts and alveoli.

Tonsillitis

Viruses and bacteria are common causes of inflammation of the tonsils and walls of the pharynx.

CASE STUDY 1: **EMPHYSEMA**

Sonia, aged 80, had a heart and lung problem from smoking heavily when she was younger. Her breathing was so difficult that she needed help from a nebulizer and oxygen.

CHOICE OF OILS

Frankincense deepens the breath, eucalyptus helps clear the upper respiratory tract and benzoin is a good expectorant. Other suitable oils would include ginger, Scots pine and petitgrain.

BLEND

Carrier oil of 10 ml calendula and 10 ml refined avocado
2 drops eucalyptus
2 drops frankincense
2 drops benzoin
6 drops = 3 per cent blend (age appropriate)

TREATMENT

The blend was gently massaged into her chest and back every day.

AFTERCARE

Vaporizing oils in the bedroom for a short while (no longer than an hour) was also beneficial. Choices included Scots pine and thyme.

OUTCOME

The blend of oils helped to relieve her breathing and enabled Sonia to sleep at night.

CASE STUDY 2: **SINUSITIS**

Ava, 30, from Singapore, suffered regularly from sinusitis, which is quite a common complaint in the Far East due to climatic conditions. Delicate bone structure is also a contributing factor. Working and sleeping in air-conditioned buildings was not helping the condition.

BLEND
10 ml of carrier oil
2 drops eucalyptus radiata
2 drops Scots pine
2 drops frankincense
6 drops = 3 per cent blend

TREATMENT
A few aromatherapy massages with some of the same blend mixed into a small amount of hydrosol, on the chest area and back. A gentle face massage emphasizing the sinus acupressure pressure points below the cheek bones using a 1 per cent dilution of frankincense and sandalwood was also most helpful for the pain.

AFTERCARE
It was suggested Ava infusing one or two essential oils in the bedroom at night, and try burning a small amount of Scots pine in the office if her colleagues were agreeable, as the smell would be pleasant.

OUTCOME
This seemed to relieve the problem considerably for Ava.

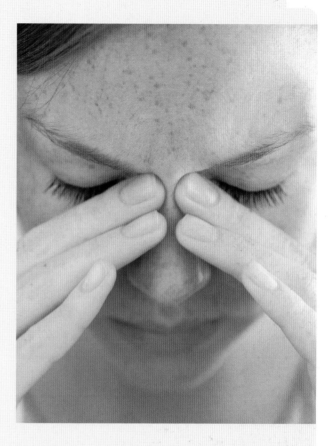

Sinusitis is an inflammation of the sinuses, which can cause pain in the nose, cheeks, teeth and head. Essential oils can help with the pain and an aromatherapy massage can help relieve some of the pressure that contributes to the pain.

How aromatherapy may help

Unlike herbal remedies, essential oils lack demulcent properties, whose action soothes irritated and inflamed mucous membranes. However, they are extremely helpful for a number of common respiratory problems. The principal actions of essential oils having an affinity with the respiratory system are antispasmodics and expectorants.
Antispasmodics These relax spasms in the bronchial tubes. For problems such as asthma and dry coughs, try Roman chamomile, cypress and sweet thyme.
Expectorants These promote the removal of mucus and phlegm. For catarrhal problems such as sinusitis and coughs, try eucalyptus globulus, eucalyptus radiata, Scots pine, benzoin and frankincense.
Antiseptic and antiviral Essential oils such as bergamot, pine, lavender, eucalyptus and tea tree will help infections of the respiratory tract.
Immunostimulants Essential oils can strengthen and support the immune response in two ways; by stimulating the immune system or by directly inhibiting the micro-organisms responsible. There are a number of essential oils that help by acting against a wide variety of viruses and bacteria, such as eucalyptus, lemon, rosemary, thyme and tea tree.

The circulatory system

Blood circulating throughout the body's immensely long and complex network of arteries, veins and capillaries ensures that every cell receives supplies of food, oxygen and other nutrients essential to life. Enabling all this is the heart, which works ceaselessly to pump blood to the furthest parts of the body.

The structure of the heart

The heart is an organ about the size of a fist that lies in the thorax above the diaphragm and between the lungs. The heart is a muscle composed of three distinct layers:
Pericardium: the outer layer is a smooth, membranous covering, which is formed of an outer fibrous layer and an inner, serous coat. Between these layers a serous fluid is secreted that reduces friction as the beating heart moves.
Myocardium: the middle layer of the heart is formed of a specialized, involuntary muscular tissue. This cardiac muscle is exceptionally strong as the fibres are bonded together in branches and it has to be able to contract rhythmically throughout life.
Endocardium: the inner lining of the myocardium layer is a very thin membrane consisting of flattened epithelial cells. It is continuous with the lining of the blood vessels.

The heart is divided into a right and left side by a partition called a septum and each side is further divided into a thin-walled atrium above and a thick-walled ventricle below. The top two chambers of the heart (the left and right atria) take in blood from the body from the large veins and pump it to the bottom chambers. The lower chambers, the left and right ventricles, pump blood to the body's organs and tissues.

When cardiac muscle contracts it squeezes blood out of the heart and into arteries that carry it to all parts of the body. When cardiac muscle relaxes the heart fills with blood from the veins. This mechanism of contraction and relaxation is the heartbeat.

Blood flow through the heart

Blood is supplied to the heart by the two coronary arteries (right and left), which originate from the base of the aorta, and a series of valves regulates the flow of blood through the heart. Between the right atrium and the right ventricle is the tricuspid valve, and between the left atrium and the left ventricle is the bicuspid or mitral valve. The aortic valve regulates the flow from the right ventricle to the pulmonary artery. These valves open and close when the pressure changes within the chambers. Mis-functioning of any of these valves causes arrhythmia, or irregular heartbeat, and if either of the coronary arteries is unable to supply sufficient blood to the heart a heart attack occurs.

Deoxygenated blood returns from the body and flows to the right atrium of the heart via the largest veins of the body, the superior and inferior vena cavae. When this is full, it empties through the tricuspid valve into the right ventricle from where it is then forced through the pulmonary artery, which carries the deoxygenated blood to the lungs. Here a gaseous exchange takes place, the blood passing carbon dioxide into the lungs and absorbing oxygen from them (see Respiratory System,

BLOOD PRESSURE

Blood pressure is the amount of pressure exerted on the arteries by blood as it flows through them. It is measured in millimetres of mercury (mmHg) and given as two figures: the diastoic followed by the systolic. Readings can vary quite considerably in the same person at different times of day or in different conditions. As an approximate guide, readings in the range of 90/60 to about 125/80 can be considered normal, and your blood pressure is considered high if the systolic is 140 or above or the diastolic is 90 or above.

Blood flow through the heart
Oxygenated blood from the lungs arrives in the left atrium of the heart via two pulmonary veins, passing to the aorta and then on to the rest of the body. The venae cavae deposit deoxygenated blood in the right atrium, from where it is pumped via the pulmonary artery to the lungs.

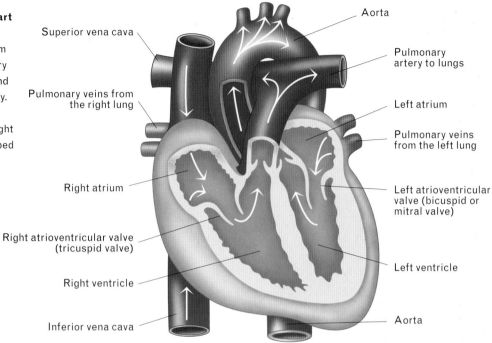

Superior vena cava

Pulmonary veins from the right lung

Right atrium

Right atrioventricular valve (tricuspid valve)

Right ventricle

Inferior vena cava

Aorta

Pulmonary artery to lungs

Left atrium

Pulmonary veins from the left lung

Left atrioventricular valve (bicuspid or mitral valve)

Left ventricle

Aorta

page 170). The oxygenated blood returns to the heart via the pulmonary veins, which empty the blood into the left atrium. It passes through the bicuspid valve and into the left ventricle, then is forced into the largest artery of the body, the aorta, which carries the oxygenated blood to the rest of the body.

The cardiac cycle

The function of the heart is to maintain a constant circulation of blood throughout the body. It acts as a pump, beating about 60–70 times a minute at rest but speeding up during exercise. The contraction and relaxation of the heart, known as the cardiac cycle, is divided into two phases: **diastole**, when blood is passing from the veins into the atria then into the ventricles and the heart muscle is relaxed; and **systole**, when the ventricles contract and the valves in the heart are pushed closed, causing the pressure in the arteries to increase. This gives the pulse.

Blood

All tissues in the body receive a blood supply, even the bone. It is the fluid in which all materials are transported to and from individual cells in the body and could be termed the main transport system of the body.

Blood is made up of plasma, a watery fluid containing billions of red blood cells (erythrocytes), white cells (leucocytes) and cell fragments (platelets).

Erythrocytes (red blood cells) are biconcave discs made from cytoplasm surrounded by an elastic membrane and make up more than 90 per cent of the blood. They are formed in red bone marrow and contain haemoglobin, which is a protein containing iron (which gives blood its red colour) and has a natural affinity with oxygen. The function of red blood cells is to transport oxygen to the cells and carry carbon dioxide away from the cells.

Leucocytes (white blood cells) are the largest of all the blood cells and appear white due to their lack of haemoglobin. Their main function is to fight infection and protect the body against viruses, toxins and bacteria. There are different types of leucocytes and they have different functions within the body.

- **Granulocytes** form approximately 75 per cent of the total number of white cells. They capture bacteria and digest them slowly, a process known as phagocytosis.
- **Lymphocytes** form roughly 23 per cent of the total number of white cells. They are formed in lymph nodes and produce antibodies that kill foreign proteins.
- **Monocytes** form approximately 2 per cent of white cells. They can ingest foreign proteins in the blood.

Platelets (thrombocytes) are formed in the red bone marrow and they play an important part in the clotting process of blood. Damaged tissues initiate the release of chemicals that attract platelets, these stick together and trigger the formation of a blood clot.

Plasma is a slightly alkaline, yellowish fluid in which the blood cells float and it consists of 96 per cent water together with important compounds such as proteins (albumen, fibrinogen, globulin); antibodies and soluble salts (sodium chloride, potassium chloride, calcium phosphate); food substances (amino acids, glucose, fatty acids, glycerol); waste products (urea, carbon dioxide) and hormones.

Blood vessels

The blood vessels that transport blood around the body all take the form of thin hollow tubes, but they differ slightly in size and structure, according to their function.
Arteries carry blood away from the heart and have thick muscular and elastic walls to withstand the pressure of the blood flowing through them. Arteries do not contain valves except at the base of the pulmonary artery. They carry oxygenated blood (with the exception of the pulmonary artery to the lungs). Arteries give rise to small blood vessels called arterioles, which deliver blood to the capillaries.
Veins carry blood toward the heart. They have thinner muscular walls than arteries, since the blood in them is under low pressure, and contain valves to prevent the back-flow of blood. Veins carry deoxygenated blood (with the exception of the pulmonary veins from the lungs). They form finer blood vessels called venules, which continue from capillaries.
Capillaries are the smallest vessels and link arterioles and venules, completing the circular system. The wall of a capillary vessel is just a single layer of cells thick, so it allows matter to diffusion through it to and from tissues.

Systems within the circulatory system

Pulmonary circulation is related to respiration and is the system between the heart and the lungs, where a high concentration of blood oxygen is restored and the concentration of carbon dioxide in the blood is lowered.

The systemic (or general) circulation is the largest and its function is to bring nutrients and oxygen to all the systems of the body and carry waste materials away from the tissues for elimination.

The portal circulation is within the systemic circulation, and describes the circulatory system that collects blood from the digestive organs and delivers it to the liver for processing via the hepatic portal vein. The portal system allows blood with concentrations of glucose, fat and protein to have these substances processed before it enters the great systemic circulation.

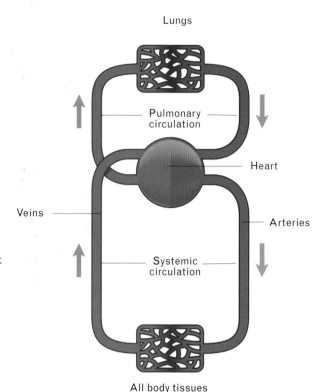

Systemic circulation Blood flows from the heart to every cell in the body via an extensive network of veins, arteries and capillaries. This simplified diagram shows how oxygenated blood flows from the lungs to the body and deoxygenated blood flows from the body back to the heart to be reoxygenated.

THE FUNCTIONS OF BLOOD

- Transport of oxygen from the lungs to the body tissues
- Transport of carbon dioxide from the body tissues to the lungs
- Transport of excretory products
- Transport of digested food
- Distribution of heat
- Distribution of hormones
- Clotting (to prevent loss of blood from a wound)

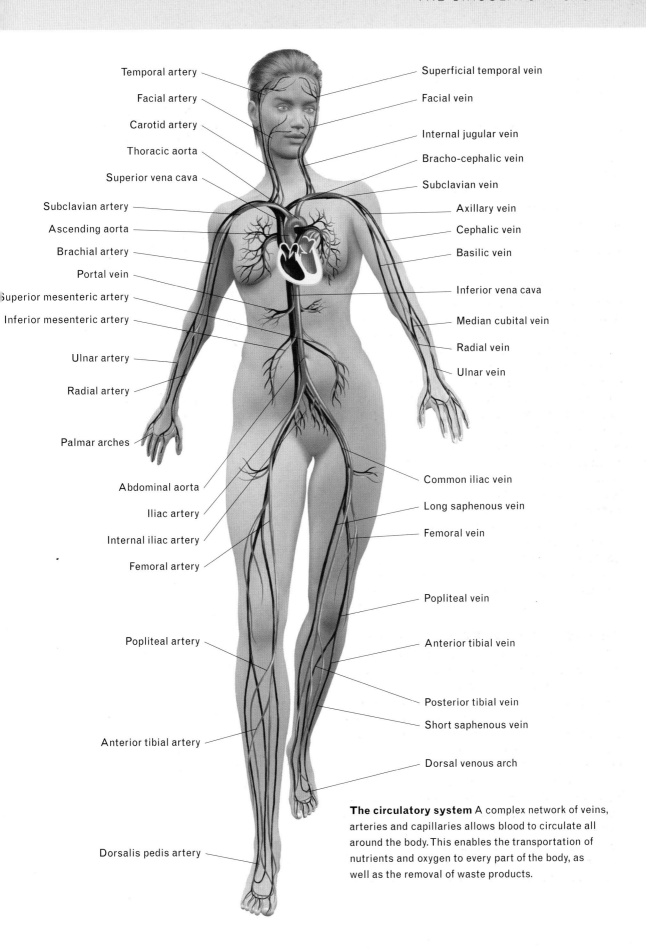

Temporal artery

Facial artery

Carotid artery

Thoracic aorta

Superior vena cava

Subclavian artery

Ascending aorta

Brachial artery

Portal vein

Superior mesenteric artery

Inferior mesenteric artery

Ulnar artery

Radial artery

Palmar arches

Abdominal aorta

Iliac artery

Internal iliac artery

Femoral artery

Popliteal artery

Anterior tibial artery

Dorsalis pedis artery

Superficial temporal vein

Facial vein

Internal jugular vein

Bracho-cephalic vein

Subclavian vein

Axillary vein

Cephalic vein

Basilic vein

Inferior vena cava

Median cubital vein

Radial vein

Ulnar vein

Common iliac vein

Long saphenous vein

Femoral vein

Popliteal vein

Anterior tibial vein

Posterior tibial vein

Short saphenous vein

Dorsal venous arch

The circulatory system A complex network of veins, arteries and capillaries allows blood to circulate all around the body. This enables the transportation of nutrients and oxygen to every part of the body, as well as the removal of waste products.

Disorders of the circulatory system

Aromatherapists will come across many of the following disorders and there are some excellent essential oils that may help.

Heart disease

Congenital and other heart conditions, high and low blood pressure, arrhythmia and embolisms are all symptoms that the heart is not functioning as it should. With medical referral, some adaptation of massage methods and care with the choice of essential oils, a treatment may be given.

Varicose veins

A varicosed vein is so dilated that the valves do not close to prevent backward flow of blood, so it loses elasticity and strength. The walls of the vessels become swollen and bulge out, becoming visible through the skin. Varicose veins are mostly seen in the legs and rupture easily if injured. Aromatherapists must take care not to put pressure on the veins themselves but may gently apply a suitable essential oil blend.

Hypertension

Blood pressure varies from individual to individual (see page 174), but may be considered high if it is sustained at a higher than generally accepted normal maximum level for a particular age group. It may be brought on by emotional stress or poor diet.

Anaemia

This is caused by a condition where the haemoglobin level in the blood is very low. The main symptoms are excessive fatigue, breathlessness, pale skin and poor resistance to infection.

Palpatations

This varies from person to person but is mostly shown by a fast irregular heartbeat. Palpitations may be associated with emotion, stress, stimulants or exercise.

CASE STUDY 2: **HYPERTENSION**

Simon, a high-powered businessman aged 50, had symptoms of extreme tiredness yet could not sleep. He was overweight, with a high flushed colour.

CHOICE OF OILS

Ylang ylang and sweet marjoram help with high blood pressure, and lavender and chamomile make a good combination as a sedative.

BLEND FOR THE BODY

20 ml carrier oil (due to his size): 10 ml grapeseed and 10 ml avocado for penetrative powers
2 drops Roman chamomile
4 drops lavender
1 drop ylang ylang
2 drops sweet marjoram
9 drops = 2¼ per cent blend

BLEND FOR THE FACE

A small amount (further diluted) of the first three essential oils (sweet marjoram is not suitable for use on the face).

TREATMENT

His high blood pressure benefited from a gentle aromatherapy treatment to help him to relax. After an hour's massage he fell into a deep sleep.

OUTCOME

That night he slept round until 9 am the next morning. He became a convert to aromatherapy and after a few similar treatments started to feel he could properly unwind from his stressful work life.

CASE STUDY 1: **HIGH STRESS LEVELS**

Gina, a 54-year-old with an executive job as an adviser for a successful TV programme, had a stressful life which gave her very little time for herself and she was exhausted from the long hours and her blood pressure was high.

CHOICE OF OILS

There is a wide choice of oils to aid relaxation and de-stress, so the ones used on Gina were those that she found most pleasant. Grapefruit is great as a detox, geranium is always useful as a balancing oil, and ylang ylang was included to lower her blood pressure. An alternative for her face could be neroli, which is uplifting.

BLEND FOR THE BODY

10 ml carrier oil, made up as 5 ml sweet almond for her dry skin, 3 ml avocado for penetrative powers and 2 ml evening primrose for her age
2 drops grapefruit
1 drop geranium
1 drop ylang ylang
4 drops = 2 per cent blend

BLEND FOR THE FACE

7 ml calendula carrier for her mature skin
1 drop rose otto
1 drop frankincense

TREATMENT

Regular body and facial treatments whenever she could manage were the most helpful way of getting her to relax.

OUTCOME

Gina benefited from regular weekly treatments and has always said how much better she felt, expecially the next day during work.

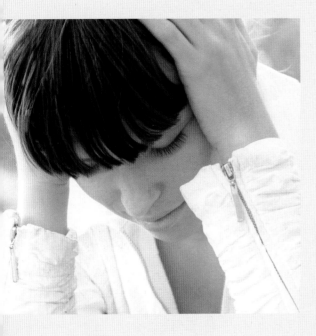

Stress, exhaustion and tension can cause numerous conditions, such as headaches, high blood pressure and skin problems, all of which can be helped by aromatherapy.

Stroke

This is caused by the blocking of blood flow to the brain or the bursting of a blood vessel and is usually associated with high blood pressure. It can vary in severity and may result in permanent or temporary paralysis if severe.

How aromatherapy may help

When circulatory problems arise, there is often a need to deal with fluid retention. Regular massage helps the body to eliminate excess fluid and toxic wastes, irrespective of which essential oils are applied. In addition, there are essential oils with properties that can help specific circulatory problems.

Hypertensives are oils that raise the blood pressure and stimulate the circulation. Oils include black pepper, rosemary and spike lavender.
Hypotensives are oils that lower the blood pressure. Oils include ylang ylang, true lavender and sweet marjoram.
Tonics and astringents are oils that strengthen and tone the whole system, which is especially helpful for varicose veins. Oils include cypress, lemon, and juniper.
Rubifacients are oils that warm and stimulate the circulation locally, causing the capillaries to dilate and thereby increasing the blood flow. Oils include black pepper, eucalyptus and ginger.

The lymphatic system

Alongside the blood's circulatory system is another fluid circulatory network that works closely with it, acting as a cleaning process and also guarding the body against infection: the lymphatic system.

What is lympth?

Lymph is a clear, straw-coloured liquid that is a derivative of blood plasma (see page 175). It has a similar composition to plasma, but with a lower concentration of plasma proteins. When plasma passes out of the capillaries of the circulatory system it forms what is called intercellular fluid. Excess intercellular fluid drains from the body's tissues into lymphatic capillaries, where it becomes known as lymph. It then flows through the lymph system's vessels and nodes and is ultimately returned to the bloodstream.

Lymph contains white cells, mainly lymphocytes, together with waste products that the system is dealing with at any particular time, such as dead cells and any micro-organisms.

The lymphatic network

The lymphatic system consists of lymphatic capillaries, lymphatic vessels, lymph nodes and lymph ducts.

Lymphatic capillaries

These commence in the tissue spaces of the body as minute, elastic blind-ended tubes, similar to blood capillaries in structure although they are wider and less regular in shape. They consist of a single layer of epithelial tissue, which makes it possible for tissue fluid to enter them. They are also more permeable than blood capillaries, allowing for larger substances to pass through their walls. Molecular substances in the tissue fluids to large to pass into the veins can easily pass into the lymphatic system. These molecular substances are mostly proteins but notably also include foreign invaders such as bacteria: fighting infection within the body is a principal function of the lymphatic system. Capillaries called lacteal capillaries also help rid the small intestines of fat deposits that have accumulated there.

Lymphatic vessels

Lymphatic vessels are vein-like tubes composed of connective tissue lined with epithelial cells. They carry lymph through the body to the great veins in the neck: the left and right subclavian veins. About 2–4 litres (3.5–7 pints) of lymph pass into the venous system every day.

As the lymphatic system lacks a pump, lymph flow is created by other mechanisms. The major ones are the contraction of the body muscles in general movement, which tends to force the fluid along, compression from the pulsing in the arteries and the drawing action due to the change of pressures in the chest during inspiration. There are numerous one-way valves in the long vessels to make sure the lymph moves only in one direction and prevent it from flowing backwards.

Lymph nodes

Before lymph is discharged into the bloodstream it passes through at least one lymph node. There are more than a hundred of these oval structures situated in clusters around the body. Some lie just under the skin, whereas others are deeply seated. The principal clusters are found in the following places, which can be recognized as sites where 'swollen glands' arise in cases of infection:

- Head and neck. Occipital nodes are located at the back of the head; submandibular nodes in the jaw and cervical nodes around the neck (divided into deep and superficial groups). They can become enlarged if there is an upper respiratory tract infection.
- Armpits. These axillary nodes drain lymph from the upper extremities and the breasts, and can become enlarged following infection.
- Elbow. These are called supertrochlear or cuboidal nodes
- Groin. These are referred to as inguinal nodes and drain the lower extremities and the genitals.
- Back of the knee. These are called popliteal nodes.

Each lymph node receives lymph from several different lymph vessels. Lymph nodes contain infection-fighting lymphocytes, macrophages and white blood cells, and as lymph flows slowly through a node, any micro-organisms,

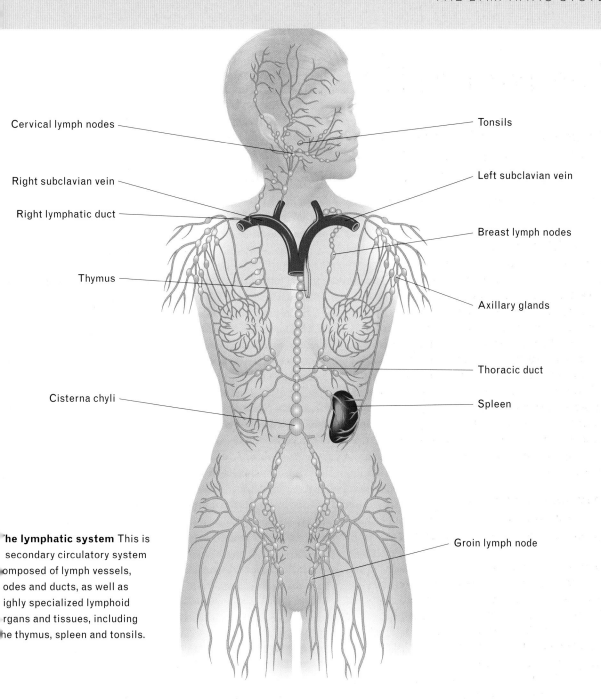

Cervical lymph nodes

Tonsils

Right subclavian vein

Left subclavian vein

Right lymphatic duct

Breast lymph nodes

Thymus

Axillary glands

Thoracic duct

Cisterna chyli

Spleen

Groin lymph node

The lymphatic system This is a secondary circulatory system composed of lymph vessels, nodes and ducts, as well as highly specialized lymphoid organs and tissues, including the thymus, spleen and tonsils.

ell debris or infective bacteria potentially harmful to the body are filtered out, so that when lymph enters the blood, it has been cleared of any foreign matter.

Once filtered, the lymph leaves the node and drains into further vessels that lead to one of two ducts.

Lymph ducts

The thoracic duct is the main collecting duct of the lymphatic system. It begins at the cisterna chyli, a specialized lymph sac found in front of the first two lumbar vertebrae. The cisterna chyli acts as a temporary storage pouch for chyle, a milky fluid rich with fat globules absorbed by lymph capillaries from the small intestines. The thoracic duct drains lymph from the left side of the head and neck, the left arm, left side of the chest area and both legs. It returns it to the bloodstream by connecting into the left subclavian vein at the base of the neck.

Lymph from a smaller proportion of the body – the right half of the head and neck, right chest area and right arm – drains into the right lymphatic duct, situated at the base of the neck, which feeds into the right subclavian vein.

The immune system

The lymphatic system fights off organisms that may present a
threat to the body's health with lymphocytes (white blood cells),
in particular phagocytes and macrophages. These are produced
in bone marrow and several supporting organs.

The spleen

The spleen is a large nodule of lymphoid tissue that is a
deep purplish-red in colour. It is situated high up at the
back of the abdomen, protected by the lower part of the
ribcage and immediately under the diaphragm, between
the stomach and the left kidney. The functions of the
spleen are:

* formation of lymphocytes
* provision of a reservoir for blood
* formation of antibodies and antitoxins
* destruction of worn-out erythrocytes (red blood cells)
* production of erythrocytes before birth.

The tonsils and adenoids

These small oval bodies are found either side of the soft
palate (palatine tonsils) and at the back of the tongue
(lingual tonsils). The pharyngeal tonsils (more commonly
known as adenoids) are located behind the nose, on the
back wall of the upper pharynx. The tonsils provide a
defence against micro-organisms that enter the mouth
and nose, and are the first line of defence from bacteria
invading the body.

The thymus

The thymus is a triangular-shaped gland made up of
lymphatic tissue located in the upper chest. It plays an
important role in the development of immunity before
birth and in newborn babies, promoting the development
and maturation of certain lymphocytes and programming
them to become T cells of the immune system (see box).
The thymus is at its most active in childhood, atrophying
after puberty.

The immune response

The body's defence mechanism, called the immune
response, is geared to ridding the body of unwanted
invaders such as disease and infection, and expelling
impurities, such as toxins, in order to keep the body healthy.

Some individual immunity is inborn, inherited and
passed down the generations – which is why some
communities or racial groups appear to have a resistance
to or vulnerability to certain infections. Acquired
immunity develops during a person's lifetime: as we
encounter various specific antigens our body learns to
recognize them and builds up a resistance. Immunity can
be acquired in a number of ways: it can be passive (from
the placenta or breast milk, for example), through direct
contact with the disease or through vaccination.

Although antibiotics have played an important role in
modern medicine in fighting bacterial infections, antiviral
drugs have not been successful. Among a number of
common conditions caused by viruses, two of the most
serious are:

* **AIDS (Acquired Immune Deficiency Syndrome)** is
  caused by the human immuno-deficiency virus (HIV),
  which attacks the body's natural immune system and
  makes it very vulnerable to other infections.
* **Hepatitis B** is a disease of the liver caused by a virus
  (HBV) which is transmitted by infected blood and tissue
  fluids. The virus is very resistant.

ANTIGENS AND ANTIBODIES

An antigen is a foreign substance that produces an
immune response. That response is called an antibody.
Each antibody is specific, initiating and stimulating the
activity of certain lymphocyte cells designed to
overpower or remove a particular antigen. Lymphocyte
cells are classified as T or B cells. B cells manufacture
specific antibodies that circulate in the blood. There are
several types of T cell, each with a different function:
'killer' cells destroy foreign cells directly, 'helper' cells
release substances that stimulate other lymphocytes
and macrophages, 'suppressor' cells suppress the
immune response and 'memory' cells remember an
antigen and can initiate a rapid response if that
antigen is met again.

CASE STUDY 1: **DETOX**

Carole, aged 44 and looking after her recently disabled husband, was suffering from general fluid retention. She felt very bloated and her legs were heavy and swollen. Although she was careful with her diet, she did tend to eat comfort food in the evenings. Her doctor had said there was no problem with her kidneys but she felt her lymphatic circulation was rather sluggish and that she needed a detox.

CHOICE OF OILS
Essential oils suitable for helping this type of problem are mainly the diuretic oils, in particular juniper, sweet fennel, rosemary and, to a lesser degree, geranium, sandalwood and patchouli. An excellent detoxifying oil is grapefruit and other useful oils are lemon, cypress and, again, sweet fennel. Palmarosa used in the face blend hydrates the skin and promotes cell regeneration.

BLEND FOR THE BODY
20ml carrier oil: 10 ml avocado (for deeper penetration) and 10 ml sweet almond (a good emollient)
5 drops grapefruit
3 drops juniper
1 drop sweet fennel
3 drops geranium
12 drops = 3 per cent blend

BLEND FOR THE FACE
5 ml sweet almond carrier oil
1 drop palmarosa

TREATMENT
Carol attended once a week for a full body aromatherapy and also used the prescribed blend of oils on her legs during the week (taking home the remainder of the 20 ml blended for her). She was advised on changes to her diet to help detox and lose weight: asparagus, fennel root and rhubarb as diuretics, with a reduction in fats. She was encouraged to take some exercise such as cycling and walking, to help circulation in her legs.

OUTCOME
After two months, Carol felt she was making good progress. She was feeling much 'lighter' and following instructions with diet and exercise. Her legs were much more shapely and she had also taken a course of manual lymphatic drainage to speed up the process. She continued with monthly maintenance treatments.

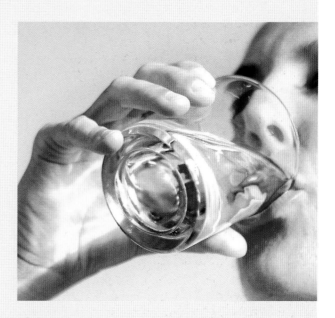

Drinking water helps to detox the body and after an aromatherapy treatment a glass of water helps to flush the oils through the body.

How aromatherapy can support the lymphatic system
When the body's immune system is weak, it is difficult to fight infection and people with low resistance can find themselves constantly assailed with coughs, colds and other ailments.
Suitable essential oils: bergamot, chamomile and thyme can help to increase the production of white blood cells to help fight infection.

If the lymphatic system's regulation of fluid in the body's tissues is compromised, an excess of fluid within the tissue spaces causes swelling (oedema). Lymphoedema, in which limbs become waterlogged, is a condition associated with post-cancer patients. Although manual lymphatic drainage is the most suitable treatment, aromatherapy massage can help generally.
Suitable essential oils: juniper, sweet fennel and sandalwood act as diuretics to help expel excess water.

The nervous system

The nervous system is the body's control centre, determining its actions and reactions, and how it adjusts to the environment. It is also responsible for all mental processes and emotional responses. The central nervous system (CNS) comprises the brain and the spinal cord, while the peripheral nervous system consists of the nerves that extend from the brain and from the spinal cord to all parts of the body.

The brain

The brain is an extremely complex mass of nervous tissue lying within the protection of the cranium. Its function is to coordinate the nerve stimuli received and carry out the correct responses. The main parts of the brain are the cerebrum, cerebellum and the brain stem, comprising the midbrain, pons varolii and medulla oblongata.

Cerebrum

The cerebrum is the largest part of the brain and is divided into two halves called cerebral hemispheres. Deep within the brain the hemispheres are connected by a mass of nerve fibres called the corpus callosum. Each hemisphere is divided into lobes, which take the names

of the bones of the cranium under which they lie: frontal, parietal, temporal and occipital. Different areas of the lobes specialize in different functions.

The superficial or outer layer of the cerebrum is composed of nerve cells, or grey matter, forming the cerebral cortex. This is concerned with all forms of conscious activity, all sensory perception, initiation and control of voluntary movements; thinking, reasoning, emotion, memory and intelligence.

Deep in the core of the brain is the diencephalons, which includes the basal nuclei, the area of grey matter thought to influence skeletal muscle tone; the thalamus, a relay and interpretation centre of all sensory impulses except olfaction; and the hypothalamus, which regulates

Lobes of the brain The frontal lobe controls personality, judgement, planning and aspects of speech and movement. The temporal lobe recognizes sound and memory. The parietal lobe deals with stimuli like temperature and pain. The occipital lobe interprets visual imagining.

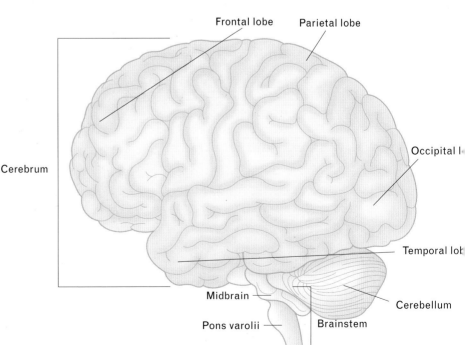

Frontal lobe   Parietal lobe

Occipital l

Cerebrum

Temporal lob

Midbrain

Cerebellum

Pons varolii

Brainstem

Medulla oblongata

the autonomic nervous system, controlling hunger, thirst, body temperature, heart and blood vessels and the limbic system.

Cerebellum

The cerebellum is a cauliflower-shaped structure located at the back of the cranium, below the cerebrum. Its function is coordination of skeletal muscles associated with voluntary motor movement and the maintenance of balance. It also coordinates the activity controlled by the autonomic nervous system. The cerebellum connects to the brain stem with three bands of neural fibres linked to the midbrain, the pons varolii and the medulla oblongata.

Brain stem

The midbrain, tucked in below the cerebrum, contains the main pathways connecting the cerebrum with the lower parts of the brain and with the spinal cord.

The pons varolii consists mainly of nerve fibres forming a bridge between the two hemispheres of the cerebrum. These act as neural relay stations and are also associated with the cranial nerves.

The medulla oblongata extends down from the pons to become the spinal cord. The vital control centres within the medulla oblongata include those for the heart, lungs and intestines. It also contains the reflex centres of vomiting, coughing, sneezing and swallowing. One of the special features of the medulla oblongata is the decussation of the pyramids, where the majority of motor nerves descending from the motor area in the cerebrum to the spinal cord cross from one side to the other. This means that the left hemisphere of the cerebrum controls the right half of the body and vice versa.

Neurons

The nervous system is made up of millions of cells known as neurons, supported by a special type of connective tissue called glial cells. Neurons perform the main functions of the brain through two properties:

- irritability: the ability to sense things and convert it to a nerve impulse
- conductivity: the ability to carry impulses around the body.

There are three types of neuron:
- sensory (or afferent) neurons transmit impulses from the periphery of the body to the spinal cord. The impulses may then pass *to* the brain or to connector neurons of the reflex arcs. Sensations transmitted include heat, cold, pain, taste, smell, sight and hearing.

- Motor (or efferent) neurons originate in the brain, spinal cord and autonomic ganglia. They conduct impulses *away* from the brain and spinal cord to effect actions. These can be voluntary (such as muscular contraction), reflexive (such as blinking), or trigger glandular secretions.
- Mixed neurons describe neurons whose sensory and motor nerves are enclosed within the same sheath of connective tissue. They are found outside the spinal cord in the body.

Each neuron has only one axon, which carries information, in the form of electrical impulses, away from the cell, but many dendrites, which receive impulses from other neurons' axons. Neurons are not anatomically connected to each other, and the point of transmission from one neuron to another is called a synapse. To bridge the synaptic gap, a transmitting neuron secretes specific chemicals, called neurotransmitters, to convey the impulse to neighbouring neurons. Millions of such connections form an almost instantaneous 'information highway'. Once the impulse has crossed the gap the neurotransmitters are neutralized by enzymes.

HOW NEURONS TRANSMIT INFORMATION

Each neuron consists of three basic parts: a cell body containing the nucleus, an axon and numerous dendrites.

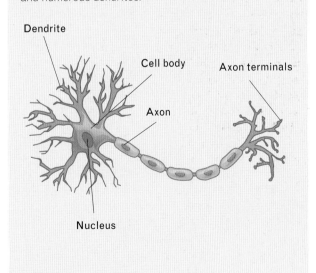

Dendrite

Cell body

Axon terminals

Axon

Nucleus

The spinal cord

The spinal cord is an extension of the brain stem, forming one continuous structure. Together the brain and spinal cord are called the central nervous system (CNS).

Just as the brain is protected by the cranium, the spinal cord is protected by the vertebrae of the spine. Both are further protected by three layers of special connective tissue collectively known as the meninges:

- The dura mater consists of two layers of strong, thick fibrous membrane, its outer part forming the periosteum.
- The arachnoid mater is a serum-bathed membrane lying close to the underside of the dura mater (called arachnoid because of its delicate, spider's web-like structure). Beneath it is the subarachnoid space, containing protective and nourishing cerebrospinal fluid.
- The pia mater is the innermost layer, a fine connective tissue richly supplied with blood vessels. It completely covering the convolutions of the brain and continues downwards to the spinal cord and beyond as the filum terminale, finally fusing with the periosteum at the coccyx.

NERVOUS REFLEXES

The spinal cord is the centre of reflex action, by which our body reacts to a sensory stimulus without involving the brain. A typical sequence is the kneejerk reaction:
- sensory receptors pick up tap on edge of knee, sensory neurons route this information via the spinal cord to relevant motor nerves in the leg
- lower leg jerks spasmodically.

The sequence is known as a reflex arc.

Many reflexes occur as a matter of course in our body, affecting our heart, blood vessels, stomach, intestines and breathing. The brain registers this activity, which is why we are aware of a kneejerk reaction or a blink, but does not control it.

When massaging it is important to be aware of this reflexive. Ganglia situated on either side of the spine correspond with the sympathetic nervous system, so pressure put on them closes the reflex action, but must be precise.

Except for the cranial nerves, the spinal cord is the nervous tissue link between the brain and the rest of the body, and also is the centre for reflex actions which provide a fast response to external or internal stimuli (see box).

The peripheral nervous system

This consists of 31 pairs of spinal nerves, 12 pairs of cranial nerves and the autonomic nervous system.

Most of the nerves of the peripheral nervous system are composed of sensory nerve fibres conveying impulses from sensory end organs *to* the brain, and motor nerve fibres conveying impulses *from* the brain through the spinal cord to, for example, skeletal muscles.

There are 12 pairs of cranial nerves originating from the nuclei in the brain, some sensory, some motor and some mixed.

The 31 pairs of spinal nerves emerge, one from either side of the vertebral canal, and each is a mixed nerve – formed by the union of a motor and a sensory nerve. They are named according to the vertebrae with which they are associated and congregate in five large groups or plexuses (see illustration).

The autonomic nervous system

The autonomic (or involuntary) nervous system controls areas of the body over which there is no conscious control. It is divided into two sections the sympathetic system and the parasympathetic system.

The sympathetic system prepares the body for dealing with emergency situations, especially to stimulate functions of the 'fight or flight' response (see Stress, page 229). Processes that are not necessary for overcoming the perceived emergency are inhibited – muscular movements of the gastro-intestinal tract and digestive secretions are slowed down, for example, or even stopped.

The parasympathetic system is primarily concerned with activities that restore and conserve body energy. It is a 'peacemaker', slowing down the effects of the sympathetic system and restoring balance (homeostasis). Impulses reduce the heart rate, reduce bronchial capacity, increase blood supply to the internal organs, increase digestive activity and adjust glandular secretions.

It must be remembered that the autonomic nervous system is not a separate nervous system. The two systems work closely together to regulate the internal workings of the body.

The nervous system is responsible for receiving and interpreting information from inside and outside the body and works closely with the endocrine system.

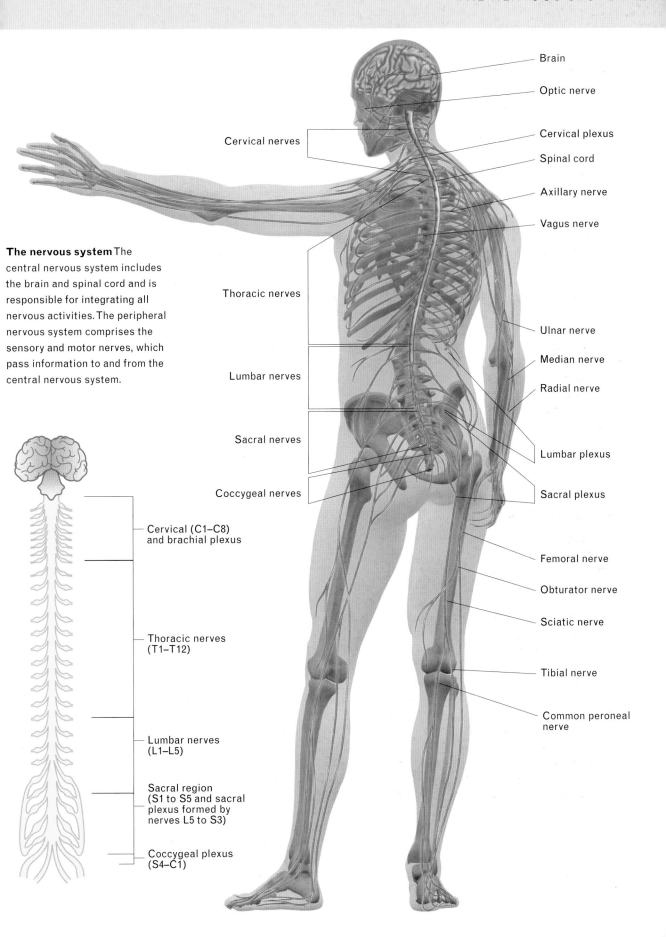

The nervous system The central nervous system includes the brain and spinal cord and is responsible for integrating all nervous activities. The peripheral nervous system comprises the sensory and motor nerves, which pass information to and from the central nervous system.

Brain

Optic nerve

Cervical plexus

Spinal cord

Axillary nerve

Vagus nerve

Ulnar nerve

Median nerve

Radial nerve

Lumbar plexus

Sacral plexus

Femoral nerve

Obturator nerve

Sciatic nerve

Tibial nerve

Common peroneal nerve

Cervical nerves

Thoracic nerves

Lumbar nerves

Sacral nerves

Coccygeal nerves

Cervical (C1–C8) and brachial plexus

Thoracic nerves (T1–T12)

Lumbar nerves (L1–L5)

Sacral region (S1 to S5 and sacral plexus formed by nerves L5 to S3)

Coccygeal plexus (S4–C1)

Disorders of the nervous system

Conditons can take many forms, as the nervous system affects not only the physical functioning of the body, but its mental and emotional state.

Constricted or damaged nerves

This can vary from carpal tunnel syndrome (pressure on the median nerve of the wrist) or sciatica to cerebral palsy (caused by damage to the CNS of the body during pregnancy or soon after the birth).

Degenerative nerve diseases

These include motor neurone disease, Parkinson's disease and multiple sclerosis.

Neurological conditions

These can range from migraines and epilepsy to Alzheimer's disease and other forms of dementia.

Anxiety, depression and psychological disturbance

These more nebulous nervous conditions are usually described as multi-factorial, as they can be the result of several causes coming together, from overwork to worry about another medical condition to a chemical imbalance in the brain. Symptoms can be equally varied, including: insomnia, an ability concentration, loss of libido, eating disorders and physical tics.

How aromatherapy can help

Many of the above conditions are medical but aromatherapy treatments can really help. A body that

---

CASE STUDY 1: **ANOREXIA NERVOSA**

Suzie, aged 15½ years, had been at boarding school from the age of 11 and suddenly decided she would become vegetarian. Every time she came home for the holidays she became more fussy about food and was getting very thin. She had also stopped menstruating. This is obviously a psychological problem that manifested itself as an eating disorder.

CHOICE OF OILS

Rose otto helps with menstruation difficulties, and is uplifting, and Suzie chose jasmine from among the oils suitable for uterine support. Basil provides a stimulant to the digestive and nervous systems, and rosemary is also a tonic to the nerves. The blend for the head and face had a rich, nourishing base, as her skin was so dry and it seemed as though some of her hair had fallen out.

BLEND FOR THE BODY

About 20 mg odourless base cream.
2 drops rose otto
1 drop basil
1 drop rosemary
4 drops = 1 per cent blend

BLEND FOR THE FACE

10 ml sweet almond
1 drop jasmine

TREATMENT

As body image is so important to those with anorexia, a luxury body massage with a rich cream for the body was appealing. Micheline Arcier recommended that stimulation to the nervous system while working on the spinal ganglia area was important and that a slow, relaxing massage was not a good way to stimulate the appetite in the hypothalamus, so the first part of the massage – pressure points on the spinal ganglia – was quite fast. Suzie really enjoyed her first massage and had a course of six treatments over the holiday period.

OUTCOME

Suzie was persuaded to try to eat a few smaller, nourishing meals. Suzie's mother arranged an appointment with the doctor, who was also very helpful with advice and pleased about the therapy. About six months later Suzie came into the clinic looking much better.

CASE STUDY 2: **ANXIETY AND TENSION HEADACHES**

Lucy, aged 39 with two school-aged children, was suffering from anxiety and tension headaches due to overwork and domestic problems. She had a fairly hectic social life connected to her husband's work and he was often late home. Sometimes she rushed out of the house without having breakfast. Her skin was playing up, she was sleeping badly, dreaming a lot and hoped that aromatherapy would help.

CHOICE OF OILS

Geranium is the oil Lucy needed to balance her skin – in fact, she needed her body balancing too, and the other oils in the blend were chosen to relax her nerves and slow down her thoughts. Basil acts as an antidepressant and helps clear the mind. According to Micheline Arcier, vetiver is the oil of tranquillity.

BLEND FOR THE BODY:

10 ml carrier oil, 5 ml jojoba and 5 ml calendula, both good emollients
1 drop basil
2 drops geranium
1 drop frankincense
1 drop neroli
5 drops = 2½ per cent blend

BLEND FOR THE FACE:

7 ml carrier oil: hazelnut, good for combination skin
1 drop geranium
1 drop petitgrain (also good for combination skin)

TREATMENT

A full body aromatherapy massage, with the following essential oils should help her. Follow-up treatments about once a month.

AFTERCARE

Once her skin had settled down, the facial blend was changed to a drop each of frankincense and rose, to help regeneration. She was advised to massage vetiver in a carrier oil in an anticlockwise motion over her solar plexus whenever she felt stressed.

OUTCOME

Lucy continued to have a massage every few weeks or whenever she felt the stress was getting to her, and she said it was so good to have time when she felt relaxed and cosseted.

---

is relaxed is better able to deal with life situations than when stressed. Learning to control the mind and balance the body with relaxation techniques is an essential part of holistic health care. The following oils may help different conditions:

Antidepressants: basil, bergamot, lavender, lemon, neroli, rose, sandalwood and ylang ylang.
Nervine tonics strengthen the nervous system, helpful in cases of nervous debility, stress or shock: clary sage, juniper, basil, rosemary and lemongrass (*Cymbopogon citratus*).
Nervine relaxants help to alleviate tension and anxiety: Roman and German Chamomile, bergamot, lavender, sweet marjoram, melissa, neroli and vetiver.
Soothing to the emotions: geranium, rosewood, jasmine.

See also Chapter Seven, which looks in more detail at treating people with a variety of stress-related conditions.

If treating someone with a medical condition, always put the client's doctor in the picture or get permission from a patient's medical team. Check whether a relaxing or stimulating massage is best for the patient. If giving treatment to someone with multiple sclerosis, for example, the session should be short (20 minutes) but brisk, as the patient needs to be stimulated to carry on through the day rather than lulled into relaxing. Use stimulating movement to the ganglia on the back and stroke the essential oils (include basil) on the legs.

Caution: Care should be taken with the use of basil and juniper, as too high a dosage could be toxic in certain cases. It is also worth mentioning that if a woman is pregnant or hoping to become pregnant it would be better not to use clary sage or jasmine.

The digestive system

The digestive system is the collective name to the alimentary canal, accessory organs such as the liver and the series of digestive processes that convert what we eat and drink into substances that keep the whole body alive and functioning.

The alimentary canal

Starting at the mouth and ending at the anus, the alimentary canal consists in essence of a long tube through which food passes. It changes its form and function several times, and includes the pharynx, oesophagus, stomach and intestines.

The mouth

The digestive process starts as soon as food is put into the mouth. The action of chewing starts to break down food and the sight and smell of food triggers the reflex action of salivating. Saliva contains a digestive enzyme, ptyalin (amylase), which is involved in the first stage of the digestion of carbohydrates.

The pharynx and oesophagus

Chewed food moves to the pharynx at the back of the mouth to be swallowed. The oral pharynx is shared by both air and food, but food then passes into the laryngeal pharynx, where muscles force it down the oesophagus. This long tube is composed of voluntary and involuntary muscle fibres, which work in a wave-like motion called peristalsis, propelling food downwards to the stomach.

Peritoneum

A closed sac, it is the largest serous membrane of the body and contains the abdominal organs of the digestive system and the pelvic organs. It produces a serus that acts as a lubricant to prevent friction with other organs.

The stomach

This is a muscular sac-like organ beneath the diaphragm. At either end of the stomach are valves, called sphincters, which control the movement of food in and out. Food enters the stomach from the oesophagus through the cardiac sphincter and then later leaves via the pyloric sphincter to enter the duodenum.

Mechanical and chemical digestion continue in the stomach. The food particles are churned down to a liquid state called chyme. Gastric juice contains the enzymes pepsin and rennin, and hydrochloric acid provides the correct medium for the digestive juices to work. Proteins are broken down to peptones. Food is held in the stomach until the chyme is ready for release into the first part of the small intestine.

The small intestine

Completion of the chemical digestion of food and subsequent absorption of nutrients takes place in the small intestine. This part of the digestive tract ends with the ileocecal valve, which prevents the backflow of waste material that has passed into the large intestine.

The walls of the small intestines have four layers, containing muscle, blood vessels, lymph vessels, nerves and a mucous membrane. The inner wall is covered with villi, tiny finger-like projections that increase the surface area for absorption and contain a network of blood and lymph vessels. Peristaltic movements mix food with intestinal and pancreatic juices as well as bile from the liver, and push the digested matter against the villi, through which nutrients are absorbed into the blood and lymph vessels. Peptones from the stomach are broken down to polypeptides and finally to amino-acids; carbohydrates are broken down to simple sugars such as glucose, and fats and oils are broken down to fatty acids and glycerol, which may be used for energy by muscles or stored.

The large intestine

Undigested food, plus roughage and unabsorbed digestive juice, pass from the small intestine into the large intestine in a liquid form. The large intestine is formed of three parts: the ascending, transverse and descending colon. The first part of the ascending colon consists of a lined pouch called the caecum, from which extends the appendix. Here sodium and water are reabsorbed and the remains, consisting of undigestible food, dead cells and bacteria, wait to be expelled out of the body through the anal canal as faeces. The anus is guarded by two sphincter muscles – the internal sphincter is under involuntary control and the external sphincter is under voluntary control.

The digestive system Ingested food is broken down in the alimentary canal to a form that can be assimilated by the body. Digestion begins in the mouth with the action of saliva on food, but most of the process takes place within the stomach and small intestine.

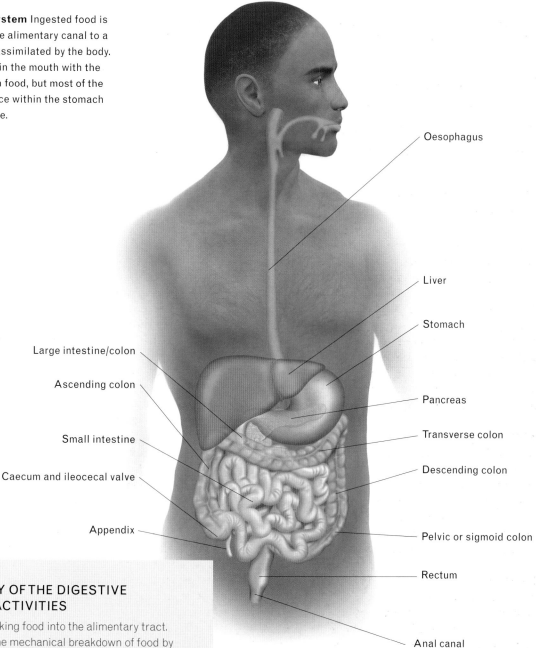

Oesophagus

Liver

Stomach

Pancreas

Large intestine/colon

Ascending colon

Transverse colon

Small intestine

Descending colon

Caecum and ileocecal valve

Appendix

Pelvic or sigmoid colon

Rectum

Anal canal

A SUMMARY OF THE DIGESTIVE SYSTEM'S ACTIVITIES

- Ingestion: taking food into the alimentary tract.
- Digestion: the mechanical breakdown of food by mastication (chewing) and the chemical breakdown by enzymes.
- Absorption: extraction of nutrients processed into usable form and passing them through the walls of the alimentary canal into the blood and lymph capillaries for transportation to where they are needed.
- Elimination: excretion of food substances that cannot be digested and absorbed.

The accessory organs

Various secretions are passed into the alimentary canal to aid digestion. Some, such as saliva and gastric juices, come from glands within the lining membrane of the canal, but others are supplied by what are known as accessory organs of digestion.

The liver

The liver is the largest internal organ in the body and is essential to our survival. It is also the largest gland in the body, weighing, in an adult human, between 1.4–1.6 kilograms (3–3½ pounds) It is situated in the upper right side of the abdominal cavity and consists of two unequal halves that can be further subdivided into four or eight lobes. Blood rich in nutrients is supplied to the liver via the hepatic portal vein from the stomach, spleen, pancreas and intestines. Arterial blood is supplied by the hepatic artery.

The liver carries out many vital functions relating to digestion, of which the main ones are:

- production of bile, which together with lipase from the pancreas commences the first stage of fat digestion
- synthesis of vitamin A from carotene
- storage of vitamins B12, A, D, E and K and iron
- regulation of amino-acids
- regulation of plasma proteins
- regulation of sugar levels
- detoxification of toxic waste and drugs, excreting them in bile or through the kidneys.

The liver is one of the few human organs that is able to naturally regenerate lost tissue. Up to 75 per cent of the liver can be removed and the remaining tissue can regenerate into a whole liver.

The gall bladder

This small, pear-shaped sac attached to the posterior surface of the liver acts as a reservoir for bile produced by the liver. As the gall bladder absorbs water from the bile it stores, what it sends out through the bile duct to the duodenum is 10 to 15 times more concentrated than liver bile. It releases this bile to help digest food containing fat and to help neutralize acid in partly digested food. The body can survive without the gall bladder and it is often surgically removed when gall stones develop.

The pancreas

This pale grey gland is situated high on the left side of the abdominal cavity, behind the stomach. It consists of a many lobules made up of small alveoli which secrete pancreatic juice containing the enzymes lipase, trypsin, chymotrypsin and amylase. Lipase converts fats into monoglycerides, diglycerides and fatty acids. Trypsin and chymotrypsin convert peptones (protein) into polypeptides. Amylase converts carbohydrates (starch) into maltose. These enzymes are released into the duodenum via the pancreatic duct. Centroacinar cells line the pancreatic ducts and secrete a solution containing bicarbonates and salts into the small intestine. The secretions of the pancreas are regulated by hormones and the automatic nervous system (see Nervous system, page 184).

The pancreas is known as a dual organ as it also has an endocrine function (see page 196).

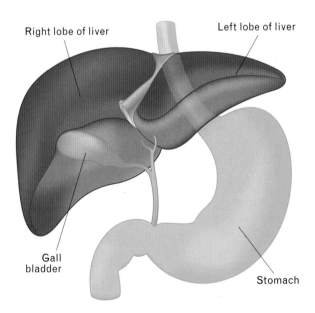

Right lobe of liver

Left lobe of liver

Gall bladder

Stomach

The liver A great detoxifier, the liver is particularly important in the digestive process. Harmful toxins that are not water-soluble are combined in the liver with natural enzymes, so they become water-soluble and can be passed to the kidneys or bowel for excretion.

Disorders of the digestive system

Most people have experienced indigestion, diarrhoea, constipation and flatulence at some time or another, but sometimes conditions resulting from dietary problems become chronic. The digestive system can also be upset by stress.

How aromatherapy may help

The antispasmodic, carminative and digestive stimulating properties of essential oils may be very helpful in treating digestive problems. Sometimes peppermint, as a carminative with antispasmodic properties, is used to treat irritable bowel syndrome, although there are other essential oils that are helpful when there is another, underlying cause.

Antispasmodics quickly relax any nervous tension that may be causing colic or other digestive spasms. They include black pepper, cardamom, German and Roman chamomile, sweet fennel, ginger, orange and clary sage.

Cholagogues increase the flow of bile and stimulate the gall bladder. Try German and Roman chamomile, lavender, peppermint, rosemary and rose.

Hepatics may help to tone and stimulate the secretions of the liver: German and Roman chamomile, cypress, grapefruit, lemon, sage and rosemary.

Carminatives relax the digestive system. Many essential oils may help, such as basil, cinnamon, sweet marjoram, black pepper and German and Roman chamomile.

CASE STUDY: **IRRITABLE BOWEL SYNDROME**

Julie, 23, was getting married and feeling very anxious about the big day, as she suffered from irritable bowel syndrome. Her symptoms were typical: abdominal pain, flatulence and alternating constipation or diarrhoea. She was becoming very worried that she might not get through the day without her symptoms spoiling the occasion.

CHOICE OF OILS
Roman chamomile helps relieve the symptoms of IBS, and the other oils were chosen to help Julie relax. As well as giving a lift to the spirits, neroli helps with muscle spasms. Peppermint is another good essential oil for IBS, but its pungent aroma doesn't make it suitable for all occasions, certainly not a wedding!

BLEND FOR THE BODY
10 ml carrier oil: 5 ml avocado oil (high degree of penetration) and 5 ml apricot kernel (nourishing and easily absorbed)
2 drops Roman chamomile
2 drops lavender
1 drop neroli
5 drops = 2½ per cent blend

BLEND FOR THE FACE
5 ml apricot kernel carrier oil
1 drop neroli

TREATMENT
Aromatherapy massage once a week. After four treatments Julie began to feel the benefits and she became much more confident about the wedding.

AFTERCARE
On her big day, she put one drop of neroli on to a small piece of cottonwool wrapped in a plastic bag and tucked it into her bra when she got dressed in the morning, leaving it there for the rest of the day.

OUTCOME
Julie had a wonderful day with no signs of her IBS. And although she was very nervous, the smell of the neroli helped calm her anxiety.

The urinary system

The urinary system regulates the composition and volume of bodily fluids, including blood, with the kidneys providing a purifying filtration system. Excess fluid and waste material is flushed out of the body as urine.

The kidneys

The kidneys are two bean-shaped organs that lie on the posterior wall of the abdomen, on either side of the spine. Each is about 12 cm (5 in) long and consists of an outer layer called a fibrous capsule, a cortex and a central medulla that contains renal pyramids.

The kidneys perform the following functions:

- filter impurities and metabolic waste from blood, preventing toxins from accumulating in the body
- regulate the amounts of body fluid and salt levels in the body
- maintain the normal pH balance of blood.

Each kidney consists of more than a million nephrons. These are tiny blood filtration units in the form of a tubule closed at one end. The closed end is indented in a tiny cup-shaped structure called a glomerular capsule. Blood

enters each kidney medulla from the renal arteries and divides to form a network of capillaries called the glomerulus. Almost encasing the glomerulus is a sac called the Bowmans capsule. Continuing from this there are various loops and collecting tubules in the nephron, which help the process of simple filtration that takes pla through the semi-permeable walls of the glomerulus an Bowmans capsule. As filtered fluid drains down the nephron, most water and nutrients such as glucose, amino acids mineral salts and vitamins are reabsorbed I the blood. What remains is urine, which consists of wate salts and protein wastes. It varies in colour according to composition and quality.

On average, a human being produces 1.5 litres of urin every 24 hours, although this can vary due to a number factors, such as taking certain medication that affects urine production. Drugs that cause the body to produce more urine are called diuretics.

The bladder and urethra

Urine is transported from the kidneys to the bladder through two very fine tubes, the ureters, which propel it along by the peristaltic contraction of their muscular walls. The urinary bladder is a pear-shaped sac that lies in the pelvic cavity, behind the pubis. The size of the bladder varies according to the amount of urine it contains. The bladder can comfortably hold up to 200–400 ml of urine for up to five hours but is capable of containing up to 800 ml. It has four layers of tissue forming a muscular wall.

The urethra is a canal that extends from the neck of the bladder to the outside of the body. The exit from the bladder is guarded by a round sphincter of muscles, which must relax before urine can be expelled from the body (a process known as micturation). The flow of urin is also helped by the contraction of the muscular wall of the bladder. The urethra is shorter in a female, where it is 3–5 cm (1½–2 inches) long, than in a male, where it is 15 cm (8 inches) long and also serves as a conducting channel for semen.

The kidneys

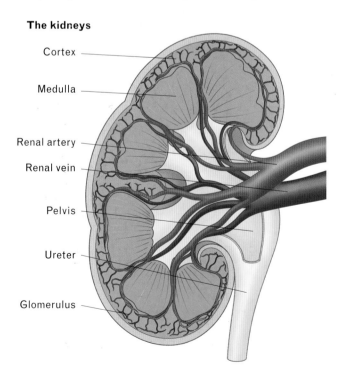

Cortex

Medulla

Renal artery

Renal vein

Pelvis

Ureter

Glomerulus

Disorders of the urinary system

The urinary system is remarkably self-regulating – even with the complete loss of one kidney – but if kidney failure does occur it has a severe effect on the entire body, because of their role in purification and homeostasis. Trouble is more likely to occur in the bladder and narrow urinary tract.

Urinary tract infection

Cystitis is an inflammation and infection of the urinary bladder wall. Sometimes towards the end of pregnancy the foetus may obstruct the flow of urine, and in the male, prostatis may cause a local infection or obstruction. Symptoms of a bacterial infection such as cystitis include fever, lower back pain, frequent urination, blood in the urine and a burning sensation on passing urine.

Kidney stones (renal calculi)

Calcareous deposits in the kidneys and bladder mostly originate in the collecting tubules or renal papillae. They then pass into the renal pelvis where they may increase in size. This condition can be extremely painful and can require surgery, or treatment by ultrasound.

Urinary incontinence

Involuntary leakage of urine is especially common in the elderly due to loss of muscle tone. Sometimes in late pregnancy the bladder can become temporarily squeezed due to the position and weight of the baby.

The urinary system

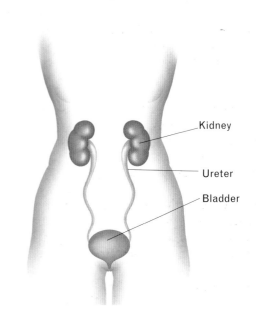

Kidney

Ureter

Bladder

HOMEOSTASIS

Homeostasis is the maintenance of a constant internal environment within the cells of the body. The water balance of the body is controlled by the collecting duct in the kidneys' nephrons, which affects the amount of water reabsorbed into the body. The brain detects how much water there is in the body and, if insufficient will release from the pituitary gland an anti-diuretic hormone (ADH) that increases the permeability of the collecting duct. If the hormone has opened the pores in the collecting duct, causing the water to be re-absorbed, the urine will be concentrated; if it is absent, all the water leaves the kidney in the urine, which is very dilute.

How aromatherapy can help

Essential oils are not usually recommended for anyone with kidney problems, as this is a medical condition, but essential oils can bring relief from urinary tract infection. Sit in a warm bath containing 4 drops of tea tree and 4 drops of bergamot diluted in at least 30 ml of carrier oil. This can also be used as a wash but because of the delicate mucous membranes, a very low dilution should be used – between 0.05 per cent and 1 per cent. Swab the opening of the urethra at frequent intervals. Sandalwood may also be used in a massage blend over the lower abdomen as it is known to be a good urinary tract antiseptic.

Some good diuretic essential oils for fluid retention are: juniper berry, sweet fennel and, to a lesser degree, sandalwood, geranium and patchouli. Some people use these for slimming purposes and cellulite problems.

The endocrine system

Many of the most important functions of the body are controlled by the endocrine system, which consists of glands that secrete various hormones into the bloodstream. Hormones act as 'chemical messengers', targeting and regulating specific cells and tissues to alter their activity and keep the body's systems in balance.

Pituitary gland

The pituitary gland and the hypothalamus act as a unit, regulating most of the other endocrine glands. The hypothalamus is not itself an endocrine gland, but part of the brain. However, it has a direct controlling effect on the pituitary gland and an indirect effect on many others – the pituitary is often referred to as the 'master gland' (or 'leader of the orchestra') and the hypothalamus as the 'conductor of the orchestra'.

The pituitary gland is the size of a pea and lies below the hypothalamus to which it is attached by a stalk. It has three lobes. The anterior lobe is linked to the hypothalamus by blood vessels, the posterior lobe is linked to the hypothalamus by nerves and between these two is a thin strip of tissue called the intermediate lobe; hormones are found in this part only during pregnancy. (One of these is the melanocyte-stimulating hormone (MSH), which triggers the production of melanin in the basal cell layer of the skin during pregnancy.)

Disorders of the pituitary gland cause hormonal imbalances that can lead to, for example, gigantism or stunted growth.

The principal trophic hormones secreted by the pituitary's anterior lobe are:

Growth (somatotrophic) hormone promotes growth of the skeleton, muscles, connective tissue and various organs. It also inhibits secretion of gastric juice and is stimulated by exercise, anxiety, sleep and hypoglycaemia (low blood sugar).
Thyroid-stimulating hormone (TSH) stimulates growth and activity of the thyroid gland. There is a circadian rhythm to the release of TSH – it is highest between 9pm and 6am and lowest between 4pm and 7pm.
Adrenocorticotrophic hormone (ACTH) stimulates the flow of blood to the adrenal cortex, increases the concentration of cholesterol and steroids within the gland

THE HORMONAL CHAIN OF COMMAND

Endocrine glands do not release hormones into the bloodstream continuously. Instead, they build up a store of hormones and release them in short bursts when triggered by hormone 'messengers'. The hypothalamus, which monitors hormone levels in the blood, produces 'releasing hormones' through the blood vessels that link it to the pituitary gland. The pituitary then releases 'trophic hormones', which convey to the relevant endocrine gland when and how much of a particular hormone to secrete. The whole system is controlled by a negative feedback mechanism.

and increases the output of steroid hormones, especially cortisol. ACTH levels are highest at about 8am and fall to their lowest at about midnight. This rhythm is maintained throughout life and is associated with the sleep pattern, and adjustment can take several days, which leads to problems such as jet-lag.
Gonadotrophic (sex) hormones control the development and growth of the ovaries and testes (see Reproductive System, page 200).

The pituitary gland also secretes two non-trophic hormones, which are manufactured in the hypothalamus but stored in the posterior lobe:

Oxytocin stimulates the uterus during labour and the breasts to produce milk after the delivery of the baby.
Anti-diuretic hormone (ADH) increases water reabsorption in the renal tubes of the kidneys and indirectly controls blood pressure.

The endocrine system The endocrine glands and tissues produce hormones, the 'chemical messengers', and release them into the bloodstream. Endocrine glands and tissues include the pituitary, thyroid, parathyroid and adrenal glands, as well as the ovaries, the testes, part of the pancreas and the placenta.

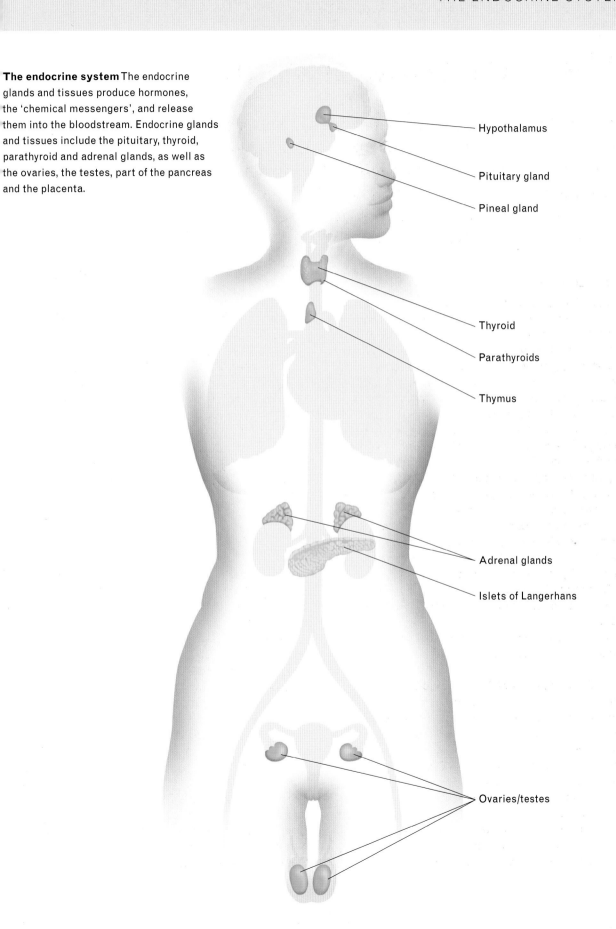

Hypothalamus

Pituitary gland

Pineal gland

Thyroid

Parathyroids

Thymus

Adrenal glands

Islets of Langerhans

Ovaries/testes

Thyroid gland

The thyroid is found in the neck in front of the larynx and trachea. It consists of two lobes, roughly cone-shaped. The thyroid takes up most of the iodine ingested in food, to manufacture the hormones triidothyronine (T3) and thyroxine (T4). After secretion, these hormones combine with colloid and are stored in the follicles as thyroglobulin. T3 and T4 both regulate growth and development, as well as influence mental, physical and metabolic activities. The thyroid gland also secretes the hormone calcitonin, which controls the level of calcium in the blood. The body will increase demand for more thyroid hormones at various time, such as during the menstrual cycle, pregnancy and puberty.

Hypersecretion by the thyroid is associated with Graves disease, which shows itself as restlessness, sweating, weight loss and an increased metabolic rate. It may also produce a goitre. Hyposecretion reduces the metabolic rate, characterized by weight increase, dry skin and brittle hair. Left untreated, physical and mental activity also slows.

Parathyroid glands

Discovered in 1880, these were the last major organ to be identified in the human body. These small glands usually sit on the posterior of the thyroid gland but in rare cases can be found within the thyroid gland. This allows the nervous and muscular systems to function properly. They secrete the hormone parathormone, which helps regulate the calcium level of the blood and tissue fluid, working together with the thyroid gland. Usually there are four parathyroid glands but there can be up to eight. When the parathyroid glands detect low calcium levels in the blood they release the parathyroid hormone. This is a protein which stimulates the body to release more calcium and also to increase calcium absorbption.

Overactivity, or hypersecretion, of this gland causes a calcium imbalance, which leads to softening of the bones and may cause tumours. The condition can be treated by surgically removing the parathyroid glands. Underactivity, or hyposecretion, can result in tetany, a spasmodic contraction of the muscles. Depending on the severity of the condition it can be treated with calcium supplements or by the introduction of intravenous calcium.

Adrenal glands

The adrenal glands are two triangular-shaped glands, one situated on top of each kidney. The glands are composed of two main parts that differ both anatomically and physiologically; the outer cortex and the inner medulla. The cortex is essential to life but the medulla is not.

The adrenal cortex produces three groups of hormones:

- glucocorticoids (cortisol and hydrocortisone) have widespread effects on the body systems, promoting the formation and storage of glycogen, raising the blood glucose level and promoting sodium and water reabsorption from the kidneys' tubules. These hormones also help the body cope with stress and have an anti-inflammatory action.
- Mineralocorticoids (aldosterone) act on the kidney tubules, retaining salts in the body, excreting potassium and maintaining the water and electrolyte balance.
- Sex corticoids control the development of the secondary sex characteristics and the function of the reproductive organs, but after puberty are believed to have little significance compared to the effects produced by the gonads (see above).

The adrenal medulla is completely surrounded by the cortex and its functions are closely allied to those of the sympathetic part of the autonomic nervous system. The principal hormones it secretes are adrenaline and noradrenaline, which are released at times of emergency and/or stress associated with conditions needed for 'fight and flight' (see Stress, page 230).

Hypersecretion by the adrenal glands is associated with Cushings syndrome, which involves weight gain, reddening of face and neck, excess growth of facial and body hair, kidney failure and raised blood pressure. Hyposecretion is associated with Addison's disease, with symptoms including weight loss, low blood sugar, brown pigmentation around joints and muscular weakness. It is treatable by replacement hormone therapy.

The islets of Langerhans

Discovered in 1869 by the German anatomist Paul Langerhans, the cells that make up the islets of Langerhans are found in clusters irregularly distributed throughout the pancreas. In a healthy adult human pancreas there are about one million islets. The hormone they secrete, insulin, lowers the level of sugar in the blood by helping the body cells to take it up and use or store it as glycogen. Without this regulatory function, diabetes develops, and the blood's sugar levels have to be adjusted through careful dietary habits or insulin injections, to avoid either hyperglycemia or hypoglycemia. There are two types of diabetes mellitis: insulin-dependent diabetes (early onset) and non-insulin dependent diabetes (late onset), which usually occurs later in life.

The pancreas This gland is composed of cell clusters (acini) that secrete pancreatic juice containing a number of enzymes concerned in digestion. It also has an important role in the endocrine system, producing hormones such as insulin.

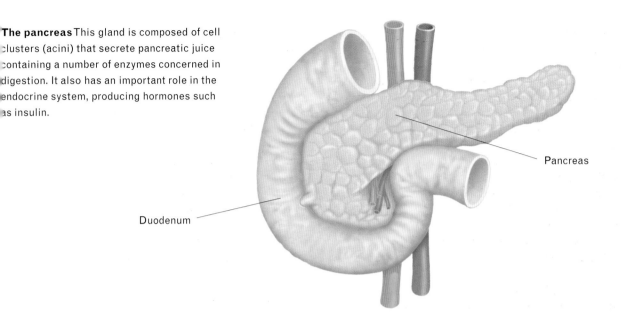

Pancreas

Duodenum

The pineal gland

Referred to as the 'third eye' in some therapies, the pineal gland is a small body, shaped like a pine cone and the size of a pea. It is situated between the two hemispheres of the brain, towards the centre, and connected to the brain by a short stalk containing nerves, many of which terminate in the hypothalamus. It releases variable amounts of the hormone melatonin, relating to the 'body clock'. During the night, when it is dark, melatonin is released in high levels, leading to drowsiness, while during the day levels are kept low. Photosensitive cells in the retina detect light and, through a series of signals, pass the information to the pineal gland. The production of melatonin is linked to hibernation in animals.

Adults have a smaller pineal gland than children, as it shrinks at puberty. There is a marked reduction in the production of melatonin when puberty starts and melatonin is thought to inhibit sexual development.

Sensitivity to light levels can lead to seasonal affective disorder (SAD), also known as winter depression.

The sex glands

The female ovaries and the male testes produce their own hormones that control the development of the secondary sex characteristics at puberty and in women affect the process of reproduction (see page 200). Typically, male testes secrete primarily androgens, including testosterone. Female ovaries make oestrogen and progesterone in varying amounts.

Hormonal imbalances can lead to conditions such as breast development in men and hirsutism (male pattern hair growth) or amenorrhea (the absence or stopping of menstruation) in women. Low oestrogen and progesterone levels can lead to polycystic ovary syndrome, which has been linked with problems conceiving. Excess oestrogen can cause endometriosis, a condition where tissue that normally lines the uterus grows outside it.

How aromatherapy can help

Some essential oils contain plant hormones known as phytohormones, which are similar in action to our own and act within the body in a similar manner, reinforcing or replacing the human hormones.

The action of some essential oils is oestrogenic (there are no essential oils with progesterone-like activity). The oestrogenic activity in sweet fennel, for example, is due to the anethole content, which is a methyl ether of oestradiol. Essential oils should be considered as one of the primary ingredients in the treatment of some disorders of the reproductive system such as the menopause (see page 204).

Geranium is another essential oil to be considered, as it is known to balance all systems, especially the skin, and directly affects the adrenal cortex. Aromatherapists should look for symptoms of stress, such as fatigue and anxiety, which can cause a hormonal imbalance. Other essential oils that can be helpful are rose and lavender, and exotics such as neroli, sandalwood and jasmine, which are all very feminine oils.

The reproductive system

The reproductive system is unique among the body systems, in that it is not vital to the survival of an individual, but is essential to the continuation of the human race.

Similarities between the sexes

The male and female organs differ in appearance and physiologically, although anatomically they develop in a similar way, and many characteristics are found in both sexes. The penis, for example, has its equivalent in the clitoris, which contains erectile tissue. The male testes are the anatomical equivalent of the female ovaries and develop similarly in the abdomen before descending into the scrotum around the time of birth.

Sex hormones are often thought of as strictly male or female, but they are in fact mostly common to both sexes, but vary in proportion and effect. Puberty is the age at which the internal reproductive organs in both sexes reach maturity. An increase in the gonadotrophic hormones FSH (follicle-stimulating hormone) and LH (luteinizing hormone) triggers the development of secondary sexual characteristics, such as the growth of breasts in girls and deepening of the voice in boys. FSH stimulates the development and ripening of the Graafian follicle, which secretes the hormone oestrogen in women; in men it stimulates the testes to produce sperm. LH helps to prepare the uterus for the fertilized ovum in a woman and in a man it acts on the testes to produce testosterone.

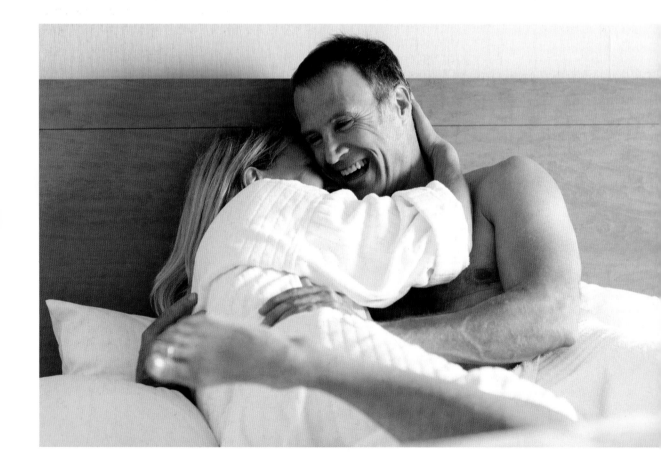

The female reproductive system

The female reproductive system consists of both internal and external organs. Its function is to produce sex hormones and egg cells, which, if fertilized, are supported and protected until birth.

The genital organs

The external genitalia, known collectively as the vulva, consists of the lip-like folds at the entrance of the vagina (labia major and minor); the clitoris, which is attached by a ligament to the symphysis pubis; the hymen, which is a thin layer of mucous membrane; and the greater vestivular glands, which lie on either side near the vaginal opening and secrete lubricatory mucus.

- The internal organs lie in the pelvic cavity and consist of the ovaries, the Fallopian tubes, the uterus and the vagina.
- The ovaries are small oval organs on either side of the uterus, where the ova (egg cells) develop. The immature eggs lie dormant in the ovary until they are stimulated by a sudden surge in the hormone FSH at the time of puberty.

- The thin Fallopian tubes, which connect the ovaries to the uterus, have tiny finger-like projections at their tip, to help sweep an egg into the tube for fertilization, then on to the uterus.
- The uterus is a small, hollow, pear-shaped organ situated in the pelvic cavity behind the bladder and in front of the rectum. It has thick muscular walls, and a central cavity capable of expanding to accommodate a foetus. The inner lining, called the endometrium, is a form of mucous membrane, part of which is shed each month during menstruation. During pregnancy, the walls of the uterus relax to accommodate the growing foetus. The muscular canal of the vagina leads from the vaginal opening to the cervix and during childbirth can stretch to allow a baby to pass through. The vagina provides an acid environment to help in the prevention of microbe growth that might infect the internal organs.

The female reproductive system Once the egg has been released from an ovary, it is drawn into the Fallopian tube. Slight contractions of the tube and the movement of tiny cilia move the egg towards the uterus. It can survive in the Fallopian tube for 24 hours and, if it is not fertilized, it will be reabsorbed by the body.

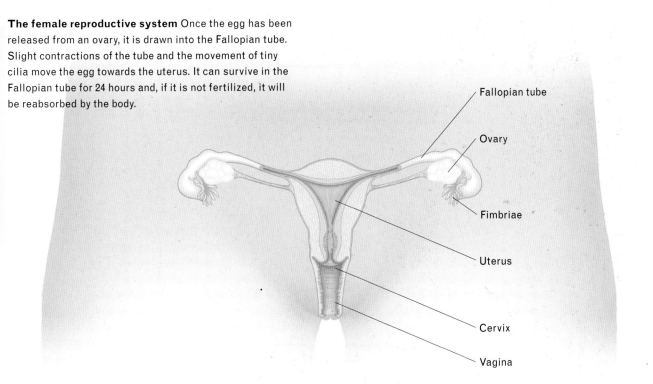

Fallopian tube

Ovary

Fimbriae

Uterus

Cervix

Vagina

The menstrual cycle

From puberty until the menopause, the reproductive system follows a cycle, usually lasting between 26 and 30 days, stimulated by hormonal changes.

The hypothalamus secretes LH-RH (luteinizing hormone-releasing hormone), which triggers the anterior pituitary to release FSH. This stimulates growth of egg follicles in the ovary and the secretion of oestrogen, leading to ovulation. The rising oestrogen levels produce a surge of luteinizing hormone (LH), which causes the release of the mature egg from the follicle.

If the egg is not fertilized, levels of both oestrogen and progesterone fall, the lining of the uterus breaks down and is shed, leading to menstruation. If fertilization occurs, the empty follicle continues to make oestrogen and progesterone, and menstruation stops for the duration of pregnancy.

Pregnancy

The nine months during which a foetus develops in the uterus is divided into three trimesters and during this time a variety of hormonal changes specific to pregnancy occur:

- HCG (human chorionic gonadotrophin), which is secreted by a layer of embryonic cells that surround the developing embryo, helps establish the pregnancy
- HPL (human placental lactogen) helps with energy and the enlargement of breasts and milk glands
- MSH (melanocyte stimulating hormone) stimulates the production of melanin. This alters the colouring of the areola of the breast, and is thought to be responsible

BREASTS

Female breasts are composed of fatty, fibrous and glandular tissue. They develop at puberty under the influence of the hormones oestrogen and progesterone. Fatty tissue covers the entire surface of the breast while fibrous tissue, in conjunction with the pectoral muscles lying directly underneath on the chest wall, provides support.

The main times of change for breasts are puberty and pregnancy. The mature breast consists of about 15–20 lobes of glandular tissue. Each lobule is made up from tiny little sacs called alveoli, which collectively form lactiferous (milk) ducts. These converge towards the nipple, where they form a lactiferous sinus whose function is to act as reservoir for milk in the event of lactation. Each nipple is surrounded by a ring of pale pink tissue called the areola, and contains about 20 minute openings from the ducts, too small to be seen.

for chloasma or 'pregnancy mask', the darkened skin sometimes seen on the face, which disappears after the birth of the baby
- Oestrogen and progesterone, working with the pituitary gland, stimulate development of the mammary glands and inhibit uterine contractions until the birth.

Menopause

Menopause is usually defined as the absence of menstrual periods for a 12-month period, accompanied by low levels of the hormone oestrogen. It usually occurs between the late 40s and early to mid 50s, and marks the end of a woman's reproductive years.

When the ovaries no longer produce an egg every month, the body's oestrogen supply diminishes and the menstrual cycle becomes irregular, eventually ceasing altogether. Side effects can include uncomfortable symptoms such as vaginal dryness, hot flushes, headaches, fatigue and sometimes uncharacteristic emotional behaviour. The glandular tissue in the breasts shrinks and low oestrogen can result in loss of bone density, leading to oesteoporosis, and thinning and dryness of the skin and hair. Menopausal women are often treated with hormone replacement therapy (HRT) to help alleviate these side effects.

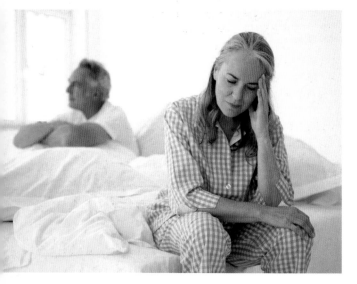

Disorders of the female reproductive system

Problems relating to the reproductive organs or the way they function can be caused by physical characteristics and by hormonal imbalances, which in turn can be influenced by such seemingly unrelated factors as diet and stress.

Amenorrhoea

The absence or stopping of the menstrual cycle at an age when regular menstruation is usual may be associated with deficiency of various hormones, depression or mental stress. Becoming underweight through anorexia or an extreme exercise regime can also cause periods to cease.

Dysmenorrhoea

Heavy, difficult and painful menstruation is thought to result from the muscle of the uterus going into spasm and congestion of the uterus, which give cramping lower abdominal pains. It can also be linked with endometriosis and, in a one-off episode, miscarriage.

Pre-menstrual syndrome (PMS)

Many women experience symptoms prior to the onset of menstruation, such as fluid retention, tender breasts and irritability are experienced. These can vary greatly from person to person, from the mildly uncomfortable to the debilitating.

Endometriosis

This is a chronic gynaecological disorder affecting women of menstrual age. It is a pelvic inflammation of the endometrium (uterus lining), resulting in lower abdominal pain and abnormal menstrual bleeding. Endometriosis occurs when stray fragments of the endometrium get into the pelvic cavity and attack different pelvic organs, causing pain during ovulation, urination and sexual intercourse. Other symptoms include fatigue and depression. Endometriosis is often linked with infertility.

Fibroids

These non-cancerous nodules develop in the muscular wall of the uterus. They are not always a problem – many women have them without knowing it – but they can causing intermittent pain and affect the menstrual cycle and fertility. Fibroids may be removed surgically or a hysterectomy may be necessary.

Polycystic ovary syndrome (PCOS)

PCOS is a hormonal disorder, in which multiple cysts develop from ovarian follicles that fail to mature into eggs. It is associated with infertility.

How aromatherapy may help

Aromatherapy can assist with many problems associated with the reproductive system. Essential oils are particularly helpful with menstrual problems and the menopause.

Antispasmodic essential oils are especially good for menstrual cramp: sweet marjoram, lavender, Roman chamomile and clary sage.

Emmenagogue: some essential oils can help promote menstruation, especially in the case of amenorrhoea and these include: sweet fennel, clary sage, juniper, jasmine and peppermint.

Uterine tonics are helpful essential oils that have a toning and strengthening effect on the uterus. They include jasmine, frankincense, rose and clary sage.

Antibacterial, antiseptic and antifungal essential oils help conditions such as thrush (*Candida albicans*). They can be added to natural yoghurt as a douche.
100 ml whole milk natural yogurt:
5 drops German chamomile
5 drops lavender
5 drops tea tree
Stir well and apply on a tampon.

See also Aromatherapy during pregnancy and childbirth (pages 214–217).

Caution: Clary sage should not be used on someone wanting to become pregnant, as it is a strong emmenagogue.

CASE STUDY 1: **ENDOMETRIOSIS**

Margaret, 43, experienced constant dragging abdominal pain, which even made her feel physically sick. She was also suffering from insomnia, which made her tired and irritable with mood swings and depression. Her doctor had suggested a hysterectomy, but she was not keen to have an operation or to go on hormone-based drugs, which could mean side effects such as weight gain and facial hair.

CHOICE OF OILS

The chosen oils all work on the uterus. In addition, rose otto is good for the emotions, Juniper helps regulate the menstrual cycle, and bergamot is an immune stimulant and uplifting oil.

BLEND

15 ml carrier oil:10 ml sweet almond and 5 ml evening primrose oil
2 drops rose otto
2 drops clary sage
3 drops lavender
2 drops cypress
9 drops = 3 per cent blend

TREATMENT

Aromatherapy massage once a week for eight weeks helped boost Margaret's immune system and energy levels; she then came once a month for a 'top up'.

AFTERCARE

Margaret also used the blend at home daily for three weeks. She was already trying to help herself with a good diet and by exercising in the gym when she felt well enough.

OUTCOME

Margaret felt better after the first treatment. Although her endometriosis hadn't gone she was experiencing much less pain and found she had increased energy levels.

CASE STUDY 2: **MENOPAUSE**

Felicity, 49, had typical menopausal symptoms of irregular menstruation, hot flushes and tremendous fatigue. They were making her feel very depressed as she normally had lots of energy. She had a very busy life and was finding it hard to cope.

CHOICE OF OILS

There are many good essential oils for menopausal problems, including bergamot, geranium (a good balancing oil that influences the endocrine system), cypress, sweet fennel, neroli, rose and ylang ylang. Clary sage helps with hot flushes, and juniper helps regulate menstruation and also fluid retention. Felicity chose ylang ylang in her blend, but neroli is another pleasant fragrance with a good uplifting effect.

BLEND

15 ml carrier oil: 5 ml borage, 5 ml evening primrose (both containing a good level of GLA) and 5 ml apricot kernel (for skin)
3 drops clary sage
3 drops geranium
1 drop juniper
2 drops ylang ylang
9 drops = 3 per cent blend

TREATMENT

Felicity tried to make time for a weekly massage, with two in the first week to start her off; she was given the remainder of the blend to take home with her to treat herself.

AFTERCARE

She was advised to eat more foods that provide the nutrients her body needed at this time of her life: more seeds, bananas and carrots, and to supplement her diet with starflower capsules, ginsing and vitamin B complex. She was also advised to avoid eating too many refined foods with artificial additives, which could aggravate her symptoms.

OUTCOME

Felicity continued with the weekly massage over a few months and then, feeling much better, arranged to have a massage once a month. Her menopausal symptoms were definitely improving, especially the hot flushes.

The male reproductive system

The male reproductive system is designed to produce sperm and deposit them inside a woman's vagina during sexual intercourse.

The genital organs

The male genitalia consists of the penis, the testes and associated glands and interconnecting tubes.

The penis has a root and a body and is composed mainly of erectile tissue rich in blood vessels, and its function is to convey urine and semen. The penis is supplied by automatic and somatic nerves. Stimulation leads to engorgement with blood and erection.

The testes develop in the abdomen and just before birth descend into the scrotum, a pouch of deeply pigmented skin, fibrous and connective tissue and smooth muscle. They have two functions: the production of testosterone, the androgen responsible for stimulating the development of the male sexual characteristics, and the production of sperm.

Sperm are produced in the testicles, and on maturation move via the vas deferens to the seminal vesicles, which produce seminal fluid. During sexual intercourse, the seminal fluid containing sperm is expelled along the penis's urethra, a process triggered by the hormones FSH and LH.

The prostate gland lies in the pelvic cavity in front of the rectum. It secretes a lubricating fluid that is added to semen.

Disorders of the male reproductive system

Males can suffer from physical distortions or inflammations such as inflammation of the glans and foreskin of the penis (balanitis) or constriction of the blood vessels to the testes (testicular torsion). Because the urethra functions as a conduit for both sperm and urine, any urinary disorder can affect sexual performance. Difficulties such as penile erection can also be psychological or emotional in cause (see Stress, page 229).

There is no period comparable to the menopause, but fertility and sexual ability tend to decline gradually with age. The prostate gland often becomes enlarged as men get older, and can cause difficulty in passing urine. Changes in the androgen/oestrogen balance may be significant to the relative frequency of prostatic tumours in men over 50 years.

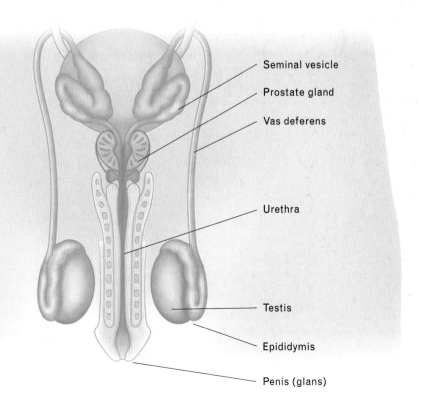

The male reproductive system
Male sperm production begins at puberty and continues until very late in life, although it starts to slow down in late middle age. Of the hundreds of million sperm in any one ejaculation, only a couple of thousand survive the journey into the uterus and on to the Fallopian tube.

Seminal vesicle

Prostate gland

Vas deferens

Urethra

Testis

Epididymis

Penis (glans)

The musculoskeletal system

The body's skeletal framework forms a protective shield for the vital organs and, in conjunction with associated muscles and joints, allows flexible movement. The extensive muscular system also contributes to other bodily functions such as breathing and digesting.

Bone structure

Bone is the hardest type of connective tissue in the body and when fully developed is composed of 25 per cent water, 30 per cent fibrous material and 45 per cent minerals. Altogether 206 bones make up the skeleton, and despite being incredibly light they are capable of bearing great weight.

Bone tissue is made from special cells called osteoblasts and takes several different forms:

Compact bone is formed of densely packed, multi-layered parallel tubes. At the centre of each is a minute hole, a Haversian canal, which provides a conduit for blood vessels and nerves. This formation makes this type of bone strong and rigid.

Cancellous bone appears spongy, as its Haversian canals spread out into a multi-branched network that contains red bone marrow.

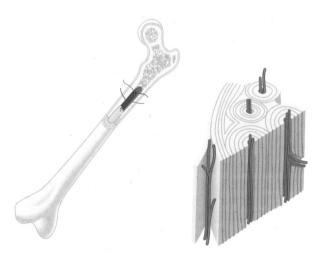

Bone section of compact bone These cross-sections show the densely packed parallel tubes that form compact bone. The Haversioan canal at the centre of each tube carries blood vessels and nerves.

Periosteum is a tough, fibrous sheeting that sheathes bone. Its inner layer produces new cells for bone growth, while the outer layer has a rich, vascular supply. Periosteum is replaced by hyaline cartilage on the articular surfaces of synovial joints and by dura mater on the inner surface of the cranial bones (see Nervous system, page 184).

Five types of bones

- **Long bones** are the strongest, such as the femur. They have a diaphysis (or shaft) and two epiphyses (extremities). The diaphysis is composed of compact bone with a central medullary canal containing fatty and yellow bone marrow. The epiphysis consists of an outer covering of compact bone with cancellous bone inside.
- **Short bones** are small ones, such as the metatarsals found in wrists and ankles.
- **Flat bones** comprise two thin layers of compact bone with cancellous bone inside. The frontal and parietal bones of the cranium are examples.
- **Irregular bones** are a mass of cancellous bone covered by a thin layer of compact bone overlaid with periosteum, such as the vertebrae.
- **Sesamoid bones** are rounded masses of bone tissue, such as the patella (knee cap).

Ossification

A bone grows by the process of ossification, which begins before birth in the embryo and is not complete until about 25 years of age. Long bones develop from cartilage and flat bones develop from a non-cartilaginous connective tissue. The osteoblasts secrete osteoid, which gradually replaces the original cartilage and membrane at, for example, either end of a long bone. The osteoid then calcifies to form new bone.

When a bone fractures, the broken ends are knitted by deposition of new bone. This healing can be delayed by many factors, including old age and infection.

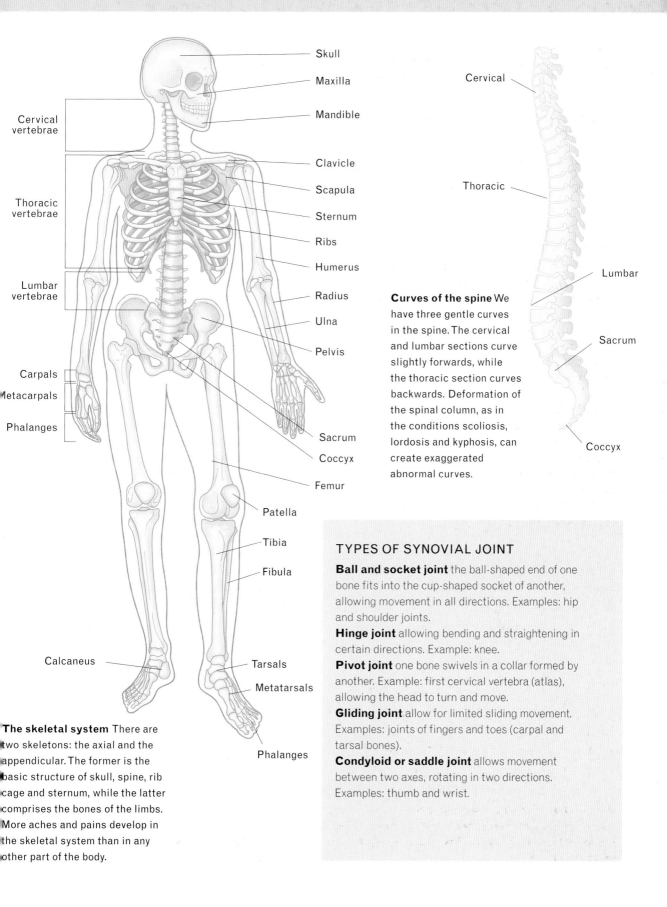

Skull

Maxilla

Mandible

Cervical vertebrae

Clavicle

Scapula

Sternum

Ribs

Thoracic vertebrae

Humerus

Radius

Ulna

Lumbar vertebrae

Pelvis

Carpals

Metacarpals

Phalanges

Sacrum

Coccyx

Femur

Patella

Tibia

Fibula

Calcaneus

Tarsals

Metatarsals

Phalanges

Cervical

Thoracic

Lumbar

Sacrum

Coccyx

Curves of the spine We have three gentle curves in the spine. The cervical and lumbar sections curve slightly forwards, while the thoracic section curves backwards. Deformation of the spinal column, as in the conditions scoliosis, lordosis and kyphosis, can create exaggerated abnormal curves.

The skeletal system There are two skeletons: the axial and the appendicular. The former is the basic structure of skull, spine, rib cage and sternum, while the latter comprises the bones of the limbs. More aches and pains develop in the skeletal system than in any other part of the body.

TYPES OF SYNOVIAL JOINT

Ball and socket joint the ball-shaped end of one bone fits into the cup-shaped socket of another, allowing movement in all directions. Examples: hip and shoulder joints.

Hinge joint allowing bending and straightening in certain directions. Example: knee.

Pivot joint one bone swivels in a collar formed by another. Example: first cervical vertebra (atlas), allowing the head to turn and move.

Gliding joint allow for limited sliding movement. Examples: joints of fingers and toes (carpal and tarsal bones).

Condyloid or saddle joint allows movement between two axes, rotating in two directions. Examples: thumb and wrist.

The functioning skeleton

The bones of the skeleton can be divided into two groups:

- The axial skeleton consists of the skull, vertebral column, ribs and sternum. These form the central core and protect the body's soft organs.
- The appendicular skeleton consists of the shoulder girdle with the bones of the upper limbs and the pelvic girdle with the bones of the lower limbs. They play a key role in movement.

The spine is the central axis from which the rest of the skeleton 'hangs'. It consists of 24 separate movable vertebrae, the sacrum (five fused bones) and the coccyx (four fused bones) giving a total of 33 bones in all.

Intervertebral discs act as shock absorbers and the cartilagineous joints they form contribute to the flexibility of the spine as a whole and protect the brain stem. Each vertebra is covered with hyaline cartilage and the neural arch, with its articulating surfaces, encloses a large ring of bone that contains the spinal cord (see Nervous system, page XX). Through and out the sides of the vertebrae run nerve fibres, blood vessels and lymph vessels.

Articulation

Bones are linked to each other by ligaments and flexible joints:

- tendons are tough, fibrous and non-elastic: they connect muscles to bones.
- ligaments are strong, fibrous and do not stretch: they connect bones together.
- Many bones of the skeleton act as levers that are worked by muscles pulling on them. All these movements require a system of joints and muscle attachments.

There are three main classifications of joint: cartilaginous, fibrous and synovial. Cartilaginous joints are slightly movable and held together by strong ligaments, such as the sacro-iliac joint. Fibrous joints are fixed, and do not allow any form of movement – for example, between the bones that make up the cranium. Synovial joints move freely. They are enclosed in a fibrous capsule lined by a synovial membrane that secretes synovial fluid to prevent friction. There are six types of sinovial joint, each with a different degree of mobility. The greater the mobility, the greater the risk of injury.

CASE STUDY: **UPPER BACK PAIN**

Amy, 24, suffered from a chronically very uncomfortable and painful neck and back, which she explained had started in her early teens after many years at dancing school. Despite some physiotherapy, which helped initially, the condition had gradually worsened due to her job sitting at a computer, and enquired about an aromatherapy treatment to help her relax and ease her discomfort.

CHOICE OF OILS
Roman chamomile and lavender act as an analgesic, sweet marjoram, ginger and its relation plai are all good for the muscle tension caused by the misalignment of the spine.

BLEND FOR THE BODY
10 ml macadamia carrier oil (a good skin lubricant and easily absorbed because of the time of day it is used)
1 drop Roman chamomile
2 drops lavender
1 drop sweet marjoram
6 drops = 3 per cent blend

BLEND FOR THE FACE
5 ml apricot kernel carrier oil
1 drop neroli

TREATMENT
Amy attended the clinic at least once a week for a full aromatherapy treatment, coming at the end of the day when she was at her stiffest after a day at work.

AFTERCARE
Amy was advised to try to spend a relaxing evening after her massage, to allow the oils to work on her whole system and to take a short break from her computer every hour. A walk at lunchtime would also help her loosen up. In the evenings Amy was recommended to take a warm lavender bath.

OUTCOME
After a few weeks there was definitely a huge improvement. She returned regularly for a back massage as a maintenance treatment to help her relax.

Disorders of the skeleton

The posture and symmetry of the entire body take their lead from the spine and poor posture or strain will have an effect throughout the body. Many problems with bones and joints become apparent in later years, as a result of cumulative use.

Osteoarthritis

This wearing away or degeneration of joints can be caused by age and general wear and tear, beginning in the joint cartilage as the cells that replace worn cartilage stop functioning. Injury or overuse may speed up the process. The effects are that the cartilage loses its smooth surface and friction in the joint increases. The bone underneath then becomes thickened and bony projections form. The joint becomes inflamed, painful and creaks as it moves. Joints particularly affected are those that take the greatest stress, such as the hips, knees, lower spine and big toes.

Rheumatoid arthritis

This rheumatoid disease involves the connective tissues of the body. The cause is unknown and occurs in about 3 per cent of people, appearing at any age. The first signs are tiredness, malaise, aches and pains and stiff joints in the morning. The synovial membrane swells and thickens and may produce excess synovial fluid. In time the cartilage lining in the joints may be destroyed and the underlying bones damaged. Eventually the bones may fuse together, making the joint rigid.

Osteoporosis

Thinning of bone is a result of inadequate replacement of the collagen framework in which calcium salts are deposited, so that the calcium is lost. The basic cause is a hormone deficiency, although poor nutrition and absorption of nutrients, prolonged inactivity and other diseases such as rheumatoid arthritis can all contribute. Symptoms include porous and brittle bones that fracture easily, even due to slight injury. It is common in women after the menopause.

How aromatherapy can help

Although essential oils cannot heal bone disorders they can help to alleviate the discomfort of arthritic and rheumatic conditions.

Anti-inflammatories As well as helping to reduce pain and inflammation in arthritic joints, certain essential oils also help to reduce swelling around injuries: chamomile (German and Roman) and lavender.

Anti-rheumatics Many essential oils have the reputation of relieving and preventing rheumatic problems, such as coriander and juniper.

Depuratives These help to detoxify the system of metabolic wastes, for example, juniper, lemon, grapefruit and rose otto.

Rubefacients By stimulating the periphery circulation, such essential oils increase blood supply to the affected area which, in turn, relieves congestion and inflammation, for example black pepper, ginger and rosemary (but take care with individuals with high blood pressure).

These problems are particularly prevalent among the elderly – see also page 234.

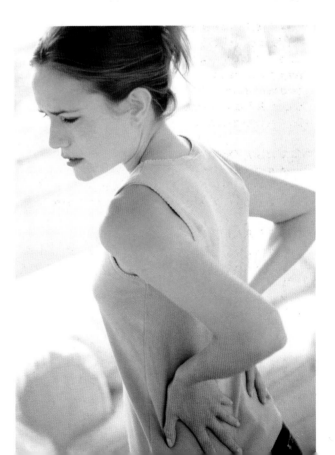

Muscles

The muscular system comprises over 600 specialized muscles, many primarily concerned with movement and body coordination. There is a relationship between muscle and bone as both contribute to movement.

Muscle structure

Muscular tissue is 75 per cent water and 20 per cent solid (most importantly the protein myosin) and 5 per cent mineral salts, glycogen and fat. About one-fifth of the bodyweight is muscle.

There are three types of muscle in the body:

Skeletal muscle is primarily attached to bone and forms the flesh of the limbs and trunk. It consists of fibres of variable length, each containing numerous thread-like structures called myofibrils. These are in alternate light and dark bands. Muscle fibres are bound together in bundles called fasciculi and surrounded by a sheath. Skeletal muscle is also called striated muscle (because of

its appearance) or voluntary muscle, because it is under our conscious control. Skeletal muscles tire rather quickly and need regular exercise.

Smooth muscle contracts or relaxes in response to nerve impulses, stretching or hormones, but it is not under voluntary control, hence its alternative name of involuntary muscle. It is found, for example, in the walls of the stomach, bowel, uterus and in blood vessels. Smooth muscles are spindle-shaped, have no striations and are bound together by connective tissue. They are designed for slow contraction over a long period, and do not tire easily. One special feature is that it can stretch and shorten and still maintain their contractile function.

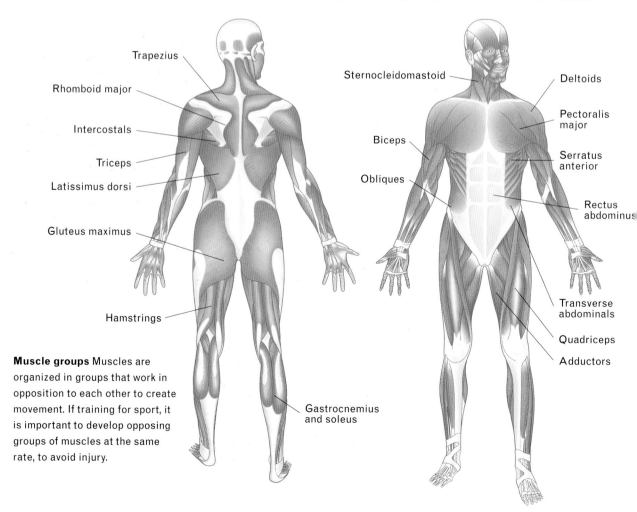

Trapezius

Rhomboid major

Intercostals

Triceps

Latissimus dorsi

Gluteus maximus

Hamstrings

Muscle groups Muscles are organized in groups that work in opposition to each other to create movement. If training for sport, it is important to develop opposing groups of muscles at the same rate, to avoid injury.

Gastrocnemius and soleus

Sternocleidomastoid

Deltoids

Pectoralis major

Biceps

Serratus anterior

Obliques

Rectus abdominus

Transverse abdominals

Quadriceps

Adductors

CASE STUDY: **MUSCULAR PAIN**

Alan, aged 44, was recovering from prostate cancer and the hospital team had put him on to an exercise programme. However, this had resulted in neck and shoulder pains. He had visited the physiotherapy department then decided to try an aromatherapy treatment to see if it would help.

CHOICE OF OILS

Alan was interested in trying some unusual combinations. Plai and lavender are analgesics that work well together, and plai may also have anti-inflammatory properties. Sandalwood relaxes and is a good masculine fragrance.

THE BLEND

10 ml carrier oil: 5ml jojoba (to help with the deeper work) and 5 ml refined avocado (for its penetrative properties)
2 drops plai
2 drops lavender
1 drop sandalwood
5 drops = 2½ per cent blend (could be increased to 3 per cent later on)

TREATMENT

Once a week, Alan received an hour's treatment on his back and upper chest. The session commenced with Swedish-style massage as the muscles were so tight, followed by the aromatherapy massage routine, which included pressure point massage, concentrating on the trapezius and deltoid muscles and concluding with some head pressure points and deep massage of the cranium.

OUTCOME

After only four treatments the physiotherapist said that whatever Alan was receiving had made such an improvement he need not visit her any more! He was delighted and continued for a further three weeks.

Cardiac muscle is a specialized type of involuntary muscle tissue found only in the walls of the heart. It contracts automatically throughout life in a rhythmic pattern, with the rate controlled by the nerves and hormones (for example, contractions can be sped up by adrenaline). Cardiac muscle is the strongest type in the body.

Muscle function

The muscular system has three main functions: movement, maintaining posture and production of heat. Even during rest a muscle is partially contracted.

When a muscle contracts it uses energy derived mainly from glucose supplied via the blood. The blood also carries oxygen, which the muscle uses to burn up the glucose. During normal activity the glucose is broken down to form water and carbon dioxide, which are removed from the muscle. However, during heavy exercise glucose is respired anaerobically, which produces lactic acid. This can accumulate, affecting elasticity and resulting in fatigue.

For a muscle to cause movement it must be held in place firmly at one end and be free to move at the other end. Muscles work in opposition to one another to create movement. The warmer a muscle is the more it relaxes and so the easier it works, with less risk of injury. Cold muscles are stiff, and may pull or tear. Good muscle tone appears firm, while poorly toned muscles appear flabby and soft to the touch.

How aromatherapy can help

Essential oils can help to reduce pain and stiffness, muscle spasm, cramp and strains. They may also alleviate symptoms of more severe muscular problems, such as muscular dystrophy (a progressive degenerative disease), fibrositis (inflammation of fibrous tissues in the muscle) and whiplash.

Aromatherpists need to understand the full benefits of the aromatherapy massage and the nervous system that regulates the activity of different muscles. When massaging the back it will be noted that tissue becomes tight and congested – this is caused by tension and fatigue. With the use of essential oils the area will become warmer and the tissues softer so that the person feels more relaxed and comfortable. Anti-inflammatory and analgesic oils give most relief and providing a blend for the bath is also helpful. Some of the most suitable essential oils are:

- Roman chamomile: soothing and analgesic, anti-inflammatory
- clary sage: antispasmodic
- sweet marjoram: calming and analgesic
- rosemary: good analgesic for stiff muscles
- plai: analgesic but cooling and anti-inflammatory
- lavender: analgesic, sedative and anti-inflammatory
- ginger: warming analgesic for pain
- black pepper: rubifacient and analgesic for muscle stiffness

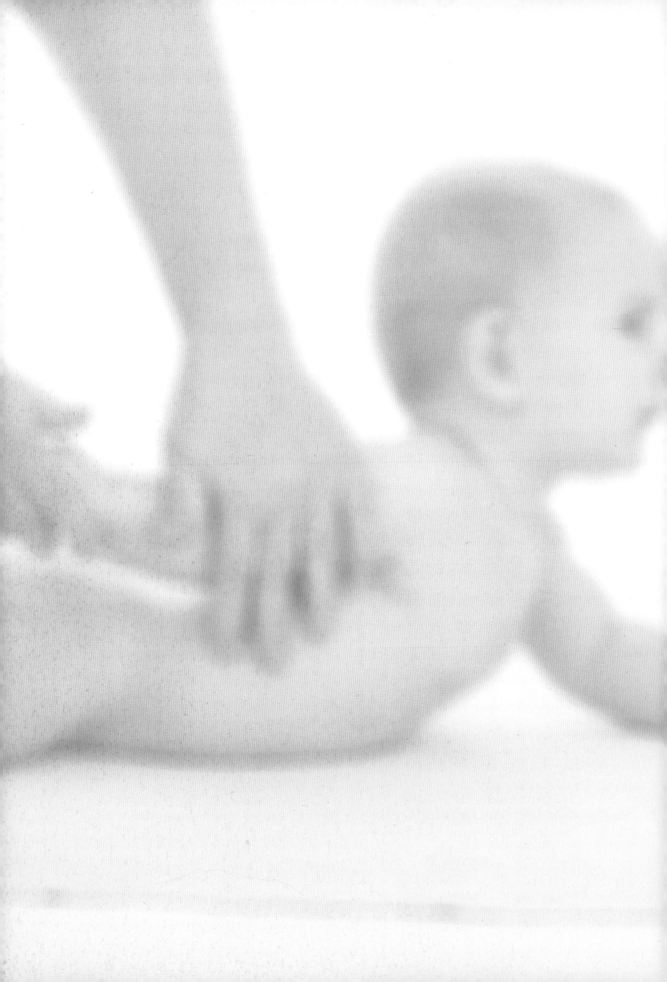

Aromatherapy for special conditions

The versatility of aromatherapy and the gentle nature of the treatment, makes it suitable for all stages of life, from babies just a few weeks old into extreme old age. It can help alleviate conditions as varied as arthritis, backache and morning sickness, ease the side-effects and anxieties of patients undergoing medical treatments and be a source of relief to overstressed bodies and troubled minds.

Aromatherapy during pregnancy and childbirth 214

Treating babies and children 220

Helping those with mental difficulties 226

Alleviating stress 229

Aromatherapy for the elderly 234

Aromatherapy and cancer 238

Aromatherapy during pregnancy and childbirth

Women today are striving to demedicalize and reduce technological intervention, and trusting their own body's abilities to give birth naturally. A holistic approach incorporating aromatherapy enables them to achieve this while balancing the body and giving relief to minor discomforts during pregnancy.

The body in pregnancy

Hormones responsible for maintaining a healthy pregnancy and development of the baby cause changes to many systems within the mother's body, affecting her both physically and emotionally.

Changes in the digestive system may cause nausea, vomiting, constipation and heartburn, while adjustments in the cardiovascular (circulatory) system may cause fluid retention (oedema) and leg cramps. A rise in blood volume raises the blood pressure but some postures the mother adopts can cause rapid lowering of blood pressure, causing dizziness and fainting.

As the baby grows it displaces the bladder, causing urinary frequency and, often, urinary tract infections. Changes in the vaginal pH can also lead to the development of thrush.

Loosening of ligaments and reduction in density of connective tissue can lead to backache and ligament pain, especially around the pelvic region.

Skin changes and worsening of pre-existing skin conditions may become apparent, and the growing pregnancy may result in stretch marks on the abdomen, breasts, thighs and buttocks.

Emotionally, women can experience episodes of tearfulness and irritability due to changing levels of hormones in the body. These exacerbate the natural anxieties, especially for a first-time mother facing unfamiliar responsibilities, probably adjusting to a new way of life after being a couple with a social life, a reduction of status and income as well as changes in body image.

In medical terms, all these may only amount to minor disorders expected during pregnancy, but can be seen to be major problems in the mother-to-be's perception.

How aromatherapy can help

Some aromatherapists may feel uneasy treating a pregnant woman, yet this is a condition to which they can bring great emotional and physical benefit. There are, however, some specific practices of which you need to be aware, and aromatherapists should undertake specialist training before offering to treat women during pregnancy and childbirth.

Essential oil usage and dosage is limited in pregnancy due to their effects on the body, which could potentially cause harm to the mother or baby, particularly in the first twelve to fourteen weeks, at the prime time of the baby's development. This is why a thorough consultation and detailed evaluation of essential oils is paramount, explaining to the mother how recommended oils will act on her body (see also page 217 for information on oils *not* to use during pregnancy or certain stages of it).

As with any client, meticulous note-taking is essential, as is ensuring the client informs her professional carers of the aromatherapy treatments she is receiving, to ensure there is collaboration between all involved, and, therefore, no fear of adverse reactions with her conventional treatments.

CARRIER OIL

For all the blends that follow, grapeseed oil would be a suitable basic carrier oil, but this can be substituted with jojoba, avocado or sweet almond if preferred. All blends are a 1 per cent dosage.

Morning sickness

This commonly occurs in the first 12 weeks of pregnancy, but it can persist for longer and may last all day in some women. The following are some suggested essential oils and their qualities, also a suggested blend but be guided by the woman as some smells may worsen her symptoms.

Petitgrain an antispasmodic, deodorizes and acts as a sedative to stomach muscles

Grapefruit a stimulant that acts as a tonic to digestive system

Lemon settles the digestive system, reducing acidity and flatulence and encouraging appetite; also helps bring down a temperature

Sweet orange similar digestion-calming properties to lemon

Ginger as lemon; also helps prevent nausea and vomiting

Suggested blend in 50 ml of a plain lotion base or grapeseed oil carrier:

- 3 drops ginger
- 3 drops lemon
- 4 drops petitigrain

Apply to inner arm, on the acupressure point just above the wrist (see page 114).

Constipation

This can occur at any time during the pregnancy. Along with advice on diet and fluid intake, any of the following is helpful:

Red mandarin for digestion and spasms

Sweet orange helps with flatulence, spasms and generally aids digestion

Grapefruit tonic, stimulant

Neroli for digestion and trapped wind

Suggested blend of a combination of two oils in a 1 per cent blend, for a very gentle clockwise massage of the lower abdomen.

Indigestion/heartburn

This becomes more common as the pregnancy grows. These essential oils and suggested blend may give relief.

Red mandarin for digestion and spasms

Sweet orange helps with flatulence, spasms and generally aids digestion

Petitgrain anti-spasmodic, deodorising

Ginger settles the digestion and aids flatulence

Sandalwood helpful for spasms and flatulence

Roman chamomile as sandalwood, and as a digestive

Lavender eases spasms and flatulence; also detoxifies

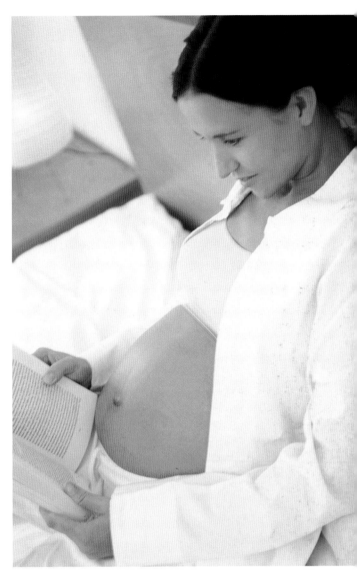

Although the use of essential oils is limited in pregnancy, careful use can be very beneficial to the expectat mother's physical and emotional well-being.

Cardamom aids spasms, flatulence and general digestive disorders

Suggested blend in 50 g plain cream base or 50 ml plain lotion base or carrier oil

- 2 drops cardamom
- 4 drops sweet orange
- 4 drops Roman chamomile

Apply this to the solar plexus area as required.

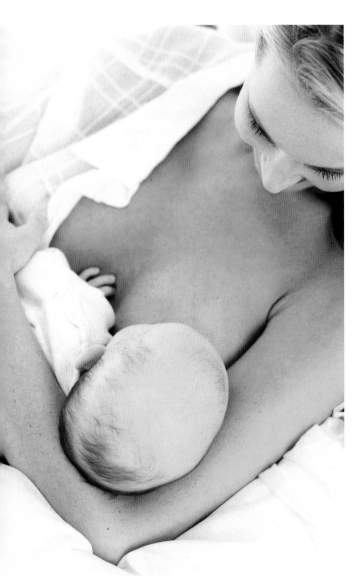

As the breasts swell during pregnancy, they are prone to stretchmarks, which also tend to occur on the thighs and especially on the abdomen.

Insomnia/stress

It is important to find the source of this problem, which could be a physical or emotional manifestation or both. The following essential oils could help with the symptoms but will not cure the root cause. You should explain this to your client and provide information on relaxation and breathing techniques as well.

Red mandarin sedative, uplifting
Sandalwood sedative
Ylang ylang anti-depressant, sedative

Lavender antidepressant, sedative, detoxicant
Roman chamomile antidepressant, sedative
Sweet marjoram sedative, restorative
Vetiver sedative; helps with nervous disorders
Valerian root strong sedative

Crisis blend in 50 g plain cream base: use for one week only then review and select another blend
- 1 drop valerian root
- 4 drops lavender
- 4 drops Roman chamomile

Apply to inner lower arm through evening and during night if required.

General blend in 50 ml plain bubblebath base
- 5 drops red mandarin
- 5 drops ylang ylang

Combine with breathing and relaxation exercises in an evening bath before bed.

Stretchmarks

Caused by stretching of the skin fibres as the pregnancy grows, these are most common on the abdomen, as it experiences the greatest growth, but can occur on the breast and thighs as well. Neroli and red mardarins are good emollient oils, and lavender acts as a counter-irritant to any deep-seated irritation.

Suggested blend in 50 g plain cream base or 50 ml grapeseed oil
- 4 drops lavender
- 3 drops neroli
- 3 drops red mandarin

Gentle abdominal, thigh or breast application

Skin rashes

Use 10 drops of Roman chamomile in a plain lotion base, or a cooled chamomile tea used as a compress is an effective soothant.

Urinary tract infection

This is common at any stage of pregnancy, so always ensure the woman has sought advice from her midwife or general practitioner first. The following essential oils are all analgesic (pain-relieving), and can assist with the distressing symptoms sometimes experienced.

Roman chamomile anti spasmodic
Niaouli a bactericide

Sandalwood anti-spasmodic, soothing and antiseptic
Eucalyptus soothing, with antiviral, bactericidal properties
Bergamot anti-spasmodic

Suggested blend a combination of these oils can be added to a warm bath with a carrier base: 4–6 drops in total of chosen essential oils. Or alternatively, in a bidet-style bath add 2–3 drops in total with a carrier base.

Essential oils to be avoided in pregnancy

Certain essential oils can cause adverse reactions in a pregnant woman. Some are only contraindicated at particular times or in particular circumstances; others should not be used at all during pregnancy. (Those listed below which do not include their Latin name are included in the Directory of Essential Oils, pages 56–109.)

Blood pressure rises naturally in pregnancy, so it is not advisable to deliberately cause a rise as this could be detrimental to the mother and baby by interfering with the blood flow to the placenta. Oils that can raise the blood pressure are:
- rosemary
- white thyme
- hyssop
- black pepper
- sage

SAFETY

Essential oils classed as abortifacient, emmenagogue or uterotonic/stimulant or any that are said to affect the uterus or hormones particularly oestrogens or progesterone should be avoided in the first 12–14 weeks of pregnancy, particularly with direct massage, especially suprapubic or sacral. Thereafter caution is advised with particular oils with some advised to be totally avoided until near term of the pregnancy.

Other areas of caution are massage in the calf area if the mother has a past history of deep vein thrombosis, vigorous massage around the heel and specific shiatsu points on the body that relate to stimulating the uterus or organs adjacent to them. Lastly, if the mother has a history of vaginal bleeding, abdominal massage is not advised.

Some essential oils have a **hormonal influence** and may interfere with oestrogen production or stimulate production of breast milk, thus confusing the natural rhythm of pregnancy and confusing the body. Such oils include:
- cypress
- basil
- cajuput (*Melaleuca leucadendron*)
- angelica (*Angelica archangelica*)
- may chang (also known as *Litsea cubeba*)
- lemongrass
- sweet fennel
- cumin (*Cuminum cyminum*)

Some essential oils described as emmenagogue should be avoided until after at least 20 weeks of pregnancy and then you should proceed cautiously if you decide to use them. These essential oils to be avoided in **early pregnancy** are:
- carrot (*Daucus carota* – see carrier oils, page 46)
- lavender
- Roman chamomile
- sweet marjoram
- peppermint
- galbanum (*Ferula galbaniflua*)

Due to their strong uterine action or because they are described as parturient (they can induce labour), essential oils to be avoided **until natural labour** (after 38 weeks) are.
- spearmint (*Mentha spicata*)
- clary sage
- melissa
- aniseed (*Pimpinella anisum*)
- nutmeg (*Myristica fragrans*)
- bay (*Laurus nobilis*)
- jasmine
- frankincense
- juniper berry
- myrrh
- rose
- dill (*Anethum graveolens*)

The following three essential oils have differing properties that can have an adverse affect **during pregnancy**:
- garlic (*Allium sativum*), which stimulates peristalsis in the digestive tract
- celery (*Apium graveolens*), which is a strong diuretic
- geranium, a hormone regulator, diuretic and anticoagulant.

Childbirth and after

Aromatherapy in labour can aid a woman's coping strategies and work in tandem with other known coping mechanisms. The main aspects of their use are to aid relief of stress and anxiety, give some relief to the discomfort of contractions and assist the efficacy of the uterus.

The stages of labour

Normal labour can occur any time from 37 to 42 weeks of pregnancy. Its start is signalled by the beginning of regular uterine contractions and the first stage runs until the cervix, the neck of the womb, becomes fully dilated. The second stage covers the journey of the baby down the birth canal and its birth. There is also a final stage, during which the placenta is expelled. This whole process can take up to 24 hours in total.

Doctors themselves aren't really sure what triggers labour. It is known that there are changes in the levels of a mother's sex hormones as progesterone drops, oestrogen rises and levels of oxytocin rise causing the womb to contract.

As the baby's glands reach maturity she, too, undergoes her own hormonal changes which contribute to sparking off labour. So it would seem that the baby is the best judge of when to put in an appearance.

Essential oil	Properties (see page 59 for unfamiliar terms)	Cautions
lavender	anti-spasmodic, sedative/calming, analgesic, uterotonic, hypotensive	Do not use at the same time as analgesics pethidine and epidural or at the same time as oxytocin/pitocin infusions (stimulate uterine contractions)
clary sage	anti-spasmodic, uterotonic, anti-depressant, euphoric, hypotensive, parturient	As above, May have a euphoric effect on others. May accelerate labour
mandarin	anti-spasmodic, sedative, analgesic, uplifting	Phototoxic
lemon	uplifting, refreshing, anti-spasmodic, hypotensive, haemostatic, immunostimulant	Do not use at the same time as analgesics pethidine and epidural. Phototoxic
peppermint	febrifuge/refreshing, expectorant, analgesic, cephalic, anti-spasmodic	Do not use if vomiting bile-stained fluid
Roman chamomile	anti-inflammatory, soothing/calming, anti-spasmodic, anti-allergenic, anti-pruritic	
frankincense	anti-inflammatory, expectorant, sedative/calming, uterotonic	Do not use at the same time as oxytocin/pitocin infusion (drug given to stimulate uterine contractions)
jasmine	anti-depressant, relaxant, uterotonic, analgesic, anti-inflammatory, sedative	As above
rose	anti-depressant, relaxant/calming, nervous sedative, anti-spasmodic, analgesic, uterotonic	As above

How aromatherapy can help

The criteria for use of aromatherapy is that the woman has completed her 37th week of pregnancy, the baby is presenting head first and there is only one baby in the uterus. Dosage is still 1 per cent at this stage. Consultation or caution is advised if:

- pain experienced is not related to labour
- if there is an underlying medical condition
- history of a previous fast labour
- waters break and there are no uterine contractions.

During labour, if massage is not required, a suitable blend could be given to the mother on a ball of cottonwool or tissue, to sniff throughout the process.

For backache and labour massage

In late pregnancy and during labour many women develop increasing pelvic discomfort and lower back pain. Application of this blend in this area can help ease this discomfort, also giving the birthing partner an active involvement in the labour process.

In 50 ml of grapeseed oil:
- 4 drops of lavender or lavandin
- 3 drops of Roman chamomile
- 3 drops of red mandarin

For reducing anxiety during labour

The essential oils used in this blend help create a euphoric state and encourage the release of the woman's own natural painkillers, Frankincense is thought to block the flow of adrenaline and substances that lead to panic attacks.

In 50 ml of plain bubblebath base:
- 4 drops of clary sage
- 6 drops of frankincense
- Add 15 ml into a warm bath after labour commences if there are no contraindications or cautions to their use.

After the birth of the baby

After the baby is born, dosage of blends can be increased to 2 per cent. A common practice in some maternity units is to offer a lavender bath (6–8 drops in a carrier added to a warm bath) to the new mother. The reasons for this are:

- it acts as an antiseptic to keep the perineal area clean
- it is analgesic and aids alleviation of soreness in the perineal area as well as muscular aches and pains
- it helps 'bring out' the bruising in the perineal area
- it helps calm and relax the mother.

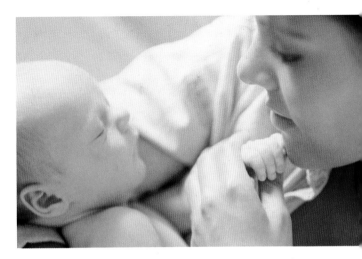

Aromatherapy can help a mother in many ways after the birth of a baby, from alleviating soreness and pain and promoting the production of breast milk to lifting the mood and balancing the emotions.

Other problems that aromatherapy can help include:

Haemorrhoids, common after pushing the baby out. Cypress can be helpful as a cream or compress.

Sore or cracked nipples caused by poor positioning when breastfeeding or if baby has a vigorous suck! Add 2–3 drops of tea tree oil to a breast-shaped bowl containing warm water, soak the nipple for five minutes after finishing a feed.

Poor breast milk supply Jasmine can promote the breast milk production, when used in a massage oil to the breasts. Make sure the nipple and surrounding breast area are free of oil before the baby feeds again.

Post natal depression This is a fairly common complaint probably due to hormonal imbalance or other stress factors. This type of depression very often necessitates something to lift the mood rather than a sedative. Suitable essential oils are bergamot, geranium, melissa and rose.

These are just some of the commonest discomforts that can follow childbirth, but you may also need to consider some essential oils that are mood- and hormone-balancers, as a new mother will pass through lots of differing stages of emotions in adjusting to her new role. Some suggested essential oils you may consider are geranium and angelica.

Treating babies and children

A baby has its first exposure to massage when it negotiates its way through the birth canal. Touch is an important aspect of life from this point on – as Dr Frederick Leboyer wrote in *Loving hands*: 'Being held, touched and caressed is like food to the baby, food as necessary as minerals, vitamins and proteins.'

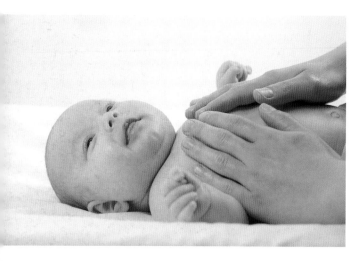

The structure of the skin

A newborn baby's skin is very delicate. It is much thinner than an adult's skin and it will take some years to develop fully and for its functions to mature.

A premature baby has little subcutaneous fat, which leads to loose skin and a wrinkly appearance. The skin has fewer layers of stratum corneum, which increases its permeability, meaning it has less of a barrier to fluid and heat loss. Also, the epidermis is not very well connected to the dermis, leaving the skin prone to blistering.

A full-term baby has a well-developed epidermis but the skin will still dry out easily. The older the baby gets, the more active the functions of the skin become. A more effectively functioning stratum corneum results in better hydrated skin.

The role of the aromatherapist

The aromatherapist plays a vital role in working with the parents/carers of babies and children, developing techniques to follow through on any treatment and strategies that can continue to be used after a visit to the therapist. These hopefully lay down a good foundation for continuing to use aromatherapy as and when required in life. Remember that you will be working as a team with any healthcare professionals, so that collaboration is always in the best interests of the child.

Babies and very young children don't have the ability to communicate verbally, so it is important to be aware that there are stages they go through when accepting new concepts and contacts. This is called the interactive sequence, and recognizing it will help you work sucessfully at the child's pace. It goes as follows:

1 resistance (not sure/hesitant)
2 tolerance
3 passive acceptance
4 enjoyment
5 cooperation
6 anticipation
7 imitation (copies massage techniques)
8 initiation (will often wish to give back)

THE BENEFITS OF AROMATHERAPY AND MASSAGE

- touch aids communication, development and growth
- aids circulation
- frees joints and aids flexibility
- cleanses the skin and removes dead cells
- aids food digestion
- boosts the immune system
- helps build a connection between the child and its carer
- essential oils can help in alleviating some distressing symptoms, which have an impact on the child and parents too.

Precautions

Don't use aromatherapy/massage:

- if the child is showing signs of distress (non-verbally telling you 'no')
- if the child has had an immunization in the previous 48 hours
- on damaged or bruised skin, or on new scar tissue
- when the child is in shock
- if the child has a heart condition
- just after a feed
- when the child is hungry
- if the child has an infected or acute skin condition
- when the child is unwell or has an infectious disease.

Specific exceptions to these are in treating eczema and chickenpox, when essential oils can provide extremely effective relief (see below).

Choosing oils

A newborn's skin is thinner and more absorbent and unable to deal with foreign substances the way an adult's can. Studies have shown, for example, that some chemical components in modern-day detergents are thought to trigger infantile eczemas and skin conditions in children. For the first six weeks of a baby's life, therefore it is recommended that even baby products are used sparingly, with plain water being used most of the time. This precaution also applies to essential oils, and their contact direct with a baby's skin should be avoided for these first few weeks.

After six weeks, the recommended dosage for babies up to one year old is 0.5 per cent (1 drop of essential oil to 10 ml of carrier oil), then for children from 1 to 8 years the recommended dosage can rise to 1 per cent.

Suggested suitable carrier oils are: sunflower, grapeseed, sweet almond, jojoba or avocado (organic if possible). Always patch test the skin first, in case of hypersensitivity. As a general rule, the younger the child the gentler the essential oil needs to be. Below are some essential oils that are particularly helpful in treating young children.

Lavender

Has a sedative calming effect and is described as a nervine, so could help with sleep problems. It is also analgesic, and anti-spasmodic so can help with muscular spasm. Other problems it can help with are psoriasis, teething and asthma. Lavender can also be used with Roman chamomile for eczema and other skin conditions.

Roman chamomile

Soothing, calming and promotes relaxation, so again can help with sleep problems. Its anti-allergenic, soothing and emollient properties help calm irritated skin such as eczema and chickenpox. It is also analgesic and anti-spasmodic and can help other common problems such as teething, colic and hayfever.

Sweet orange and mandarin

These are anti-spasmodic and settle the digestive system, so are invaluable in helping constipation and colic.

Tea tree

This immune system booster is also antiviral, antibiotic, bactericide, fungicide and can help with many conditions, particularly coughs and colds.

Frankincense

Relaxes and deepens breathing, and is calming, digestive, sedative so it can be particularly helpful with sufferers of asthma and coughs and colds.

Eucalyptus

Is cooling (febrifuge) and is also antiviral, decongestant and balsamic so can help with asthma, hayfever, coughs and cold and sinus problems.

Myrtle (*Myrtus communis*)

Is calming, sedative and a good expectorant to help with coughs and colds.

Ylang ylang

Helps to slow breathing, which is particularly helpful with panic episodes. It is also a sedative helpful with asthmatics.

Ravensara (*Ravensara aromatica*)

This is a very versatile but gentle essential oil; it is an immune system booster, a very powerful antiviral, microbiocidal, anti-infectious, anti-spasmodic and expectorant. It is useful with coughs and colds, earache, bronchiolitis and bronchitis. Particularly with chickenpox it is valuable, apply directly to each lesion with a separate cotton bud (this prevents cross infection and spread of lesions) it will help to reduce irritation and eliminate pain.

Conditions such as sleeplessness or skin irritations may be symptomatic of a quite different problem, such as a digestive disorder, so discussing any observations with health professionals involved in the child's care is an important part of the aromatherapist's role. Rest is essential for a child's growth, development and good health.

Baby massage sequence

You may not complete this whole sequence in one session the first time you do it, but be patient and build it up over each session – your baby will guide you. Always interact and keep eye contact and talk to the baby. Keep your hands well oiled.

Preparation

Before you begin, make sure the room is warm and draught-free, with subdued lighting. Prepare a soft, warm, clean surface for the baby to lie on, preferably on the floor. If the room is warm enough and the baby is happy to be completely undressed, you can take all its clothes off from the start; otherwise, begin work with the baby fully clothed and only remove nappy and lower garments when you start to massage the legs (Stage 2) and upper garments as you reach the tummy (Stage 7).

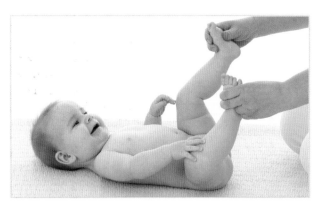

1 Start by holding baby's feet and ask for permission to begin massaging. Gently stroke the bottom of the feet and knead the tops between the thumbs and fingers. Straighten out each toe, making up rhymes or games at the same time.

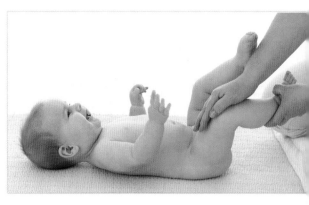

2 Replenish the oil on your hands, and gently pull baby's leg through your hand from thigh to foot, and alternate each hand (hand over hand). After a minute or so, give the leg a gentle shake. Repeat on the other leg.

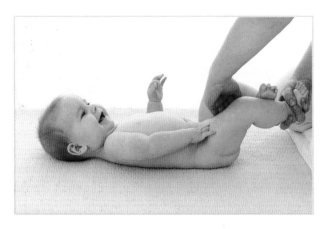

3 Hold the baby's right foot with your right hand and massage the thigh with your left hand. Repeat with opposite thigh. Do the same with the calf area of each leg.

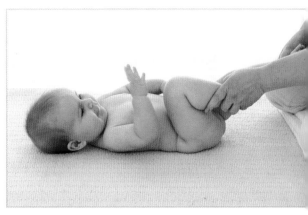

4 With baby still on its back, gently hold the legs by the ankles and, making sure the legs are relaxed, 'bicycle' them around a few times. You could sing a little song, too.

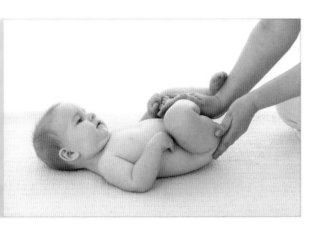

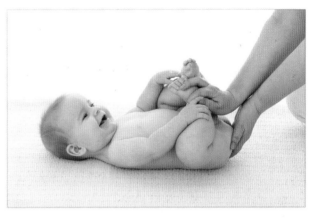

5 Using your right hand, move baby's right foot on to the abdominal area, with your left hand massage the right buttock. Repeat this on the other side.

6 Bring both legs on to the abdominal area and massage the sacral area. Do the cycling game again.

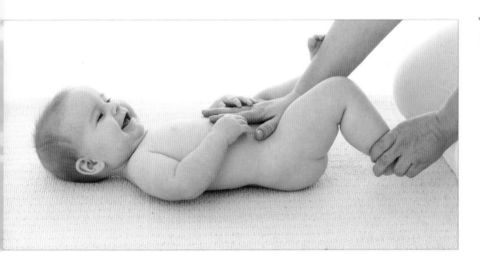

7 Put your relaxed hand on to baby's tummy and massage in a clockwise direction (towards the baby's left arm).

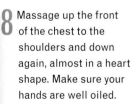

8 Massage up the front of the chest to the shoulders and down again, almost in a heart shape. Make sure your hands are well oiled.

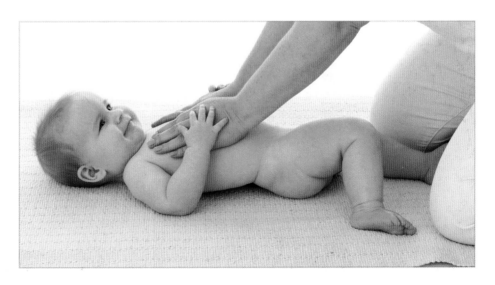

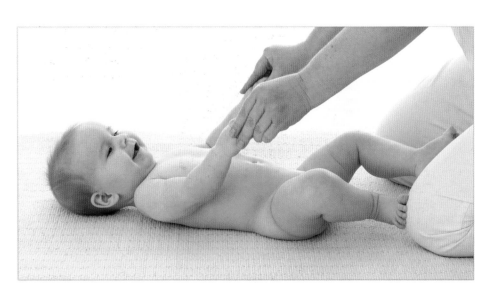

9 Repeat this movement, but continue the movements down the arms and off the hands.

10 Play a game of pat a cake (pat the hands together) and then, if baby allows, take the arms out to the side. Repeat a few times and (again if baby allows) gently each time take the arms higher to either side of the head.

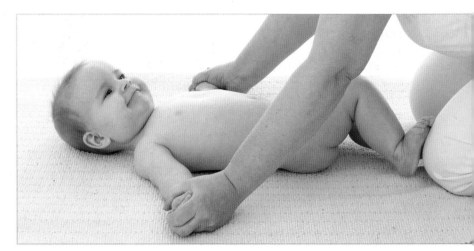

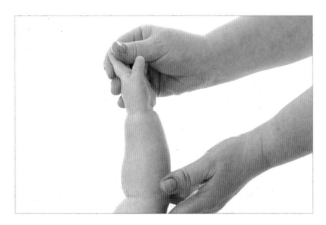

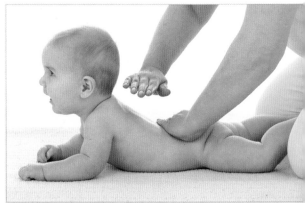

11 Massage the hands, opening out the palms and straightening the fingers.

12 If baby is happy to allow you, turn onto the tummy, massage hand over hand down the back.

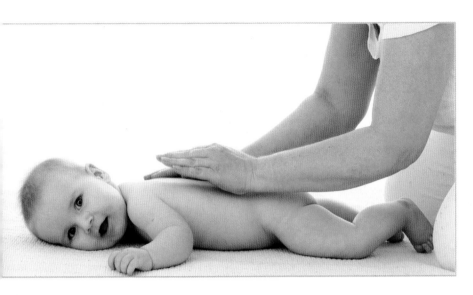

13 Cup the hands slightly and do some gentle cupping in the chest area of the back.

14 If the baby is able to rear up, bearing its weight on hands or arms, try this next movement to really open the chest and strengthen the spine. Move your well-oiled hand from the front of the chest to the side and down the baby's arm held alongside the chest. Do this a few times, and repeat with the other arm.

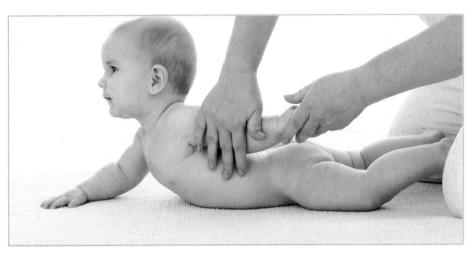

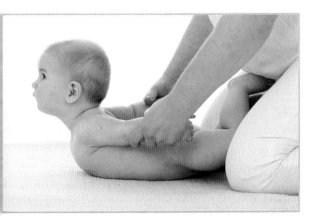

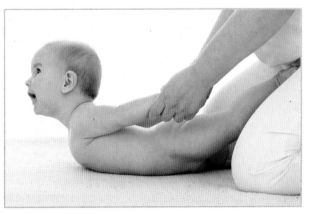

15 Now do this same movement with both arms, very gently letting the arms slide through your palms. Don't pull baby into this position.

The massage is now complete, turn the baby around for a cuddle and say thank you.

Helping those with learning difficulties

Communicating is done in many ways, and the senses of touch and smell can be powerful allies in reaching out to people whose sense of the world is different, or who have difficulty in verbal communication.

Tuning in

Start by making contact with the person in front of you. Use eye contact, talk in soothing, soft tones and use a light touch (make sure your hands are warm and dry). Be calm and ensure your body language is relaxed, with open shoulders and slow gestures. Generally have an attitude of being receptive to whatever the person is feeling – use your whole body and all your senses. This is not going to be just another massage, this is a moment of time where you can truly connect with another human being.

Introduce yourself and complete a full consultation, perhaps with the assistance of a family or staff member. Include the person as much as possible during the conversation, even if they do not or cannot speak for themselves. Ensure you know all about their conditions, so that you are prepared for an incident such as

Giving a hand massage is a good way of introducing aromatherapy to a new patient or friend. It should be accompanied by a full consultation to put the person at ease.

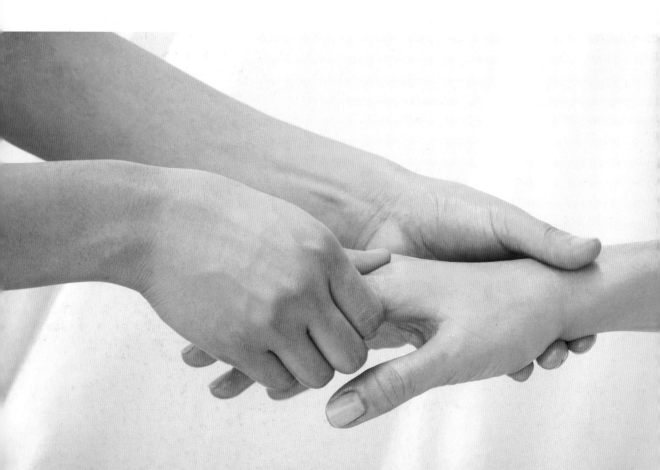

incontinence or an epileptic seizure. (In the case of epilepsy, for example, you will need to ask what signs you need to look out for – there are nine types of epilepsy and not all entail uncontrollable shaking or loss of consciousness.)

Also ask about their preferences and behaviour, and discuss the things to which they react positively and negatively (see box).

Conclude the consultation with a short hand massage in the presence of someone with whom the person feels comfortable. Make assurances that there will be more to come during your next visit and ask him to think about where he would like to be massaged: hands, feet, legs, back.

Setting the scene

Treatment should be somewhere comfortable where the session can be undisturbed: the ideal is often the person's own bedroom. The person may be able to get on to a massage couch or chair, but may be more comfortable on the bed or in an armchair. Despite the importance of comfort for the client, you need to ensure your own posture is good too – you need to be massaging for many years to come, so you need to look after yourself as much as you look after your clients. Make sure you are able to keep your back straight and do not have to bend down to a bed. Use a combination of beanbags, small plastic stools, chairs and pillows on the floor, anything to provide comfort.

Lighting is an important sensory tool to set the mood. Using bubble lamps, low lighting, coloured lights, fairy lights and so on, may all assist the person to relax both prior to and during the massage.

Music may be another source of mood enhancer. Calming music can be played just prior (and during) your visit to encourage the person to relax. It can also be used as a signal, to let the person know that he can expect a massage soon. If the person has autistic tendencies, it may be useful to use the same piece of music each time, to allow him to get used to the idea of massage to music.

Helpful pointers

- If possible, ask whether the client can have a bath or shower prior to your visit, as this will have a calming influence and also aid the absorption of oils into the skin.
- Try to find out which oils the person appears to like, but don't overwhelm with choice. Offer a maximum of three oils to smell, and allow your client to feel engaged in choosing, but not pressurized by decision-making.

CHALLENGING BEHAVIOUR

Before treating someone known to have challenging behaviour, find out the protocol that has been implemented for that individual and use it consistently. If the person becomes agitated, ask what signs you can look out for and what should be done and said in such an event.

Ensure your own safety at all times. Check that the client's behavioural history means it is safe to see that client on your own. Position yourself in the room so that you have nearest access to the door. Ensure staff or family members know where you are and that they are on hand for help should you need it.

If you sense agitation rather than acceptance or relaxation, allow some space initially by withdrawing your hands and moving back a little. Never try to force the situation by continuing with the massage. It may be necessary to leave the room. Make sure you immediately call for help as the person may harm himself, particularly if you have left bottles of oils in the room. Try to remain calm and keep your voice low and soft; raising your voice may provoke further agitation.

If the person has become agitated do not presume that it is your fault. Living constantly with some form of disability means frustrations may erupt at any time. Often the frustration is with themselves or a factor beyond anyone's control and they will lash out at you because you are closest to them – don't take it personally. Do not give up!

- Leave a small bottle in the person's home so that it can be used as an object of reference. The family or staff can then use the bottle (with some oil in it if you wish) as a visual reminder to prepare the individual for your visits.
- Never force a person to have a massage and, should they withdraw their hand or foot, then just sit back and smile and wait for them to return that hand or foot to you to continue massaging.
- You are merely there as a facilitator to relaxation. Even if you initially meet with resistance, persist with visits but perhaps try alternative methods of massage. Really tune in to the person and what you think he needs from you.
- It is worth remembering that the carers of these patients or friends also need support and some essential oils to help them.

Choosing essential oils

Use oils that are calming and grounding. Use lots of base notes such as vetiver, sandalwood, cedarwood, ylang ylang, frankincense and rose. Also try the calming oils of chamomile, juniper and lavender. Uplifting oils may be useful if the person appears low and suffers from depression. These include oils such as neroli and bergamot and melissa.

Low dilutions of 1–1½ per cent are sufficient, especially for someone on medication. Take care using oils that are stimulating, particularly on people with challenging behaviour. Epilepsy is a common additional condition, in which case, do not use rosemary, hyssop or fennel.

The reassurance of ritual

For many people with disturbed or difficult lives, the familiar is a reassuring refuge. Small rituals can help your visits to be part of a familiar pattern and reinforce the pleasurable associations. This might include following a precise order of treatment each time or incorporating a special touch such as humming or singing together.

Washing hands is necessary for reasons of hygiene, but it also provides a helpful introductory ritual. By washing both your and the clients' hands the session will start on a sensory note and starts the touch process by using something with which they are already familiar. If you only do a foot massage, use something like tea tree hydrosol and baby wipes to clean the foot prior to massage. Clients often enjoy the spray action of the hydrosol bottle and this is another small delight within that special time together.

Repetitive behaviour

Some clients you meet may rock their bodies. Sometimes you can rock to the same rhythm while massaging and this really helps you to tune in to them, and can make them feel that you are trying to get into their world and help them. On the other hand, you may aggravate the situation by mimicking them, so be very aware when you try this technique of whether you are making the person calmer or more agitated.

If you feel that the person is rocking out of agitation, you could remind them that they don't have to rock, but that this is their time to relax. This also works to aid relaxation and calmness and it is possible to feel tension easing in tight muscles.

Another common form of repetitive behaviour is humming or making sounds. Again, joining in may be a way to forge contact.

Length of treatment

Many people may not be able to tolerate more than half an hour. This is something you could build upon with time, but sessions may initially need to be kept short due to tolerance and concentration span.

Be relaxed and be yourself. It is a privilege to share time with someone who so needs you to help them relax and enjoy some pampering. If you are allowed into that private world for just a moment of time, cherish it.

Some clients may rock their bodies as you massage them. Depending on the client, they may find it comforting if you rock to the same rhythm but this can cause aggravation.

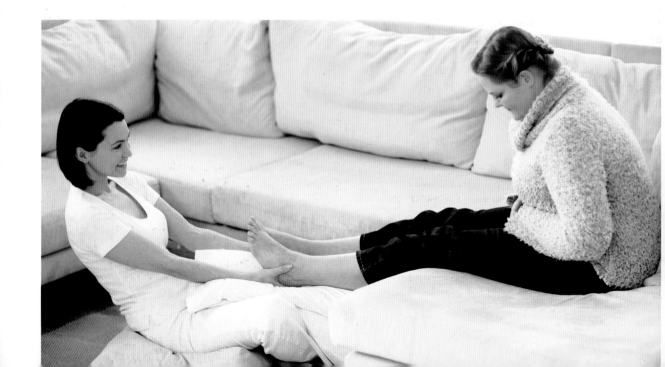

Alleviating stress

Aromatherapy has powerful effects on the chemistry and physiology of the body, but perhaps the greatest effects of all can be on the mood and the emotions. As life becomes not necessarily harder but more complex, we are expected to encompass, often single-handedly, more responsibilities in work and personal life. The result is often stress.

Recognizing stress

Stress has become part of our everyday language and doctor's surgeries are overloaded with people suffering from stress-related illnesses. But what does it really mean? To be suffering from stress is to be in a high state of tension which, if not controlled, can eventually be the beginning of a more serious physical or mental illness. At times we can all suffer from stress but is it a 'healthy' state of stress, which makes life interesting, or is it 'unhealthy' stress which makes life impossible?

Reactions under stress

Stress reactions include behavioural, emotional and physiological changes. If stress beyond a healthy level affects us only occasionally, harmony can be brought back relatively easily, but prolonged periods of stress will affect the body and the mind in many ways.

We all react differently to different stresses: stress is not so much what happens to us as the way we react to it. We cannot change the world, but we can change our attitude to it. When presented by a piece of bad news:

Person A may react by shouting, crying or getting angry (showing excess feeling), and so may become prone to high blood pressure, cardiovascular difficulties, obesity and so on.

Person B may remain calm, controlled, with stiff upper lip (showing no signs of anger or grief), but keeping everything in is more prone to infectious diseases, rheumatism and even cancer as the the perpetual assault on the nervous system affects the energy pathways.

People who fall between these extremes take bad news in their stride, do not panic, collect themselves and then let things ride for a while. These are the lucky people who know the secret of resisting stress!

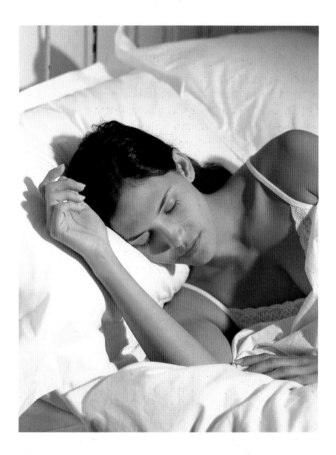

Reactions under stress vary but many people find it affects their sleeping patterns. An aromatherapy treatment before bed can help to relax the body and mind.

Women on the whole seem to cope with stress better. They are more flexible and are used to dealing with so many conflicting situations that they have become good at adapting quickly to the changing demands of the moment.

Effects on the body

When faced with a frightening or stressful situation, our body automatically rises to the challenge, equipping us to deal with whatever threatens us. Our heart rate, respiration and muscles all gear up either for fight or flight. The hormone adrenalin kickstarts additional energy reserves, blood is concentrated in the muscles where it may be needed, away from the skin, so if we are injured we do not bleed so profusely (people in physical danger are often not aware of injuries at the time). When we perceive that the danger has passed, the body then reverts to its normal state, with the excess energy having either been used up in fighting off the threat or running away from it.

In the short term the body thrives on this, even if the 'threat' is not a physical one: it helps us to think more quickly on our feet and to meet a tight deadline as well as giving us an extra push in a race or a contest.

However, when our body is on a constant state of alert, and we do not either fight or flee, the high state of tension remains, we come to ignore the distress signals and it takes longer to get back to 'square one'. The effects of stress then become cumulative, the body storing in its memory banks all that happens to it. Typical results of this are:

- stomach ulcers – a prime example of not finding the right balance, and worrying about everything.
- an altered breathing rate, preventing the body from receiving sufficient oxygen for metabolic processes. Respiration also plays an important part in the circulation of lymph fluids, and the action of the rib cage also massages the liver, which in turn affects the heart.
- lower blood sugar levels from too much adrenalin in the system, which will also have a detrimental effect on the nervous system.

Physiological signs	Emotions linked to stress	Effects on mental state	Stress addictions
heart rate increases	anxious/worried	self-critical	sweets/biscuits/cakes
blood pressure rises,	persistent thoughts	lack of clarity	sweet carbonated drinks
blood flow to muscles, lungs and brain increases	irritable	indecisive	smoking
breathing becomes fast and shallow	easily angered	poor self-esteem	tea/coffee
peripheral capillaries constrict	sense of insecurity	poor memory	alcohol
muscles tense	depressed	inconsistent	recreational drugs
red blood cells increase; white cells decrease	cry easily/feel sad	poor concentration/poor mental agility	medical drugs
adrenaline stimulated	feel alone	poor sense of direction in life	
digestive functions reduce	fearful	inability to listen accurately	
liver increases blood glucose	over/under- sensitive		

- impaired circulation: levels of fat in the blood during prolonged periods of stress will begin to 'fur up' the arteries, raising the blood pressure. And if the hormones are not able to circulate in the bloodstream efficiently our resistance to diseases and infections can be dramatically lowered.

Certain types of illnesses appear to have different emotional associations. For example, it has been observed that people suffering from cancer often seem to have difficulty expressing themselves or in letting go. There are many reported cases of cancer sufferers responding to meditation, which releases pent-up stresses. If we would listen, our body can often be telling us years before a condition develops.

The chemistry of stress
With stress the body's chemistry changes. Rapid signals stimulate the adrenal glands to produce adrenalin (see p198). Before it is possible to know what is happening the breathing changes, heart rate increases, glucose is relased into the blood and the pupils of the eyes dilate. So adrenalin prepares the body for 'fight or flight' – such as waking up and hearing a noise in the night and then there are the family rows when tempers rise and blood pressure also rises in anger. All this stress and energy is needed for emergencies. This comes from diverting energy from the body's normal maintenance and repair jobs and so the body cells are starved of certain nutrients and vitamins.

It is now known that women find it easier to talk through problems – they need to, as men produce more serotonin than women, so talking about problems increases serototin levels and that is why women alleviate stress by talking.

Therefore if your client starts to talk a lot while having her aromatherapy treatment, don't try to stop her, as it will help her to destress and off load.

How aromatherapy massage can help
Aromatherapy massage of the whole body gives a feeling of wholeness, which can give deep beneficial relaxation. It also works to rebalance the energy levels, reharmonizing painful areas that are the result of the build-up of toxins.

The pressure points on either side of the spine function like a series of little power stations to produce energy. So the massage induces a state of release of tension and you will see how hard congested tissues and muscles give way under your fingers as you work. Working on the solar plexus in an anticlockwise

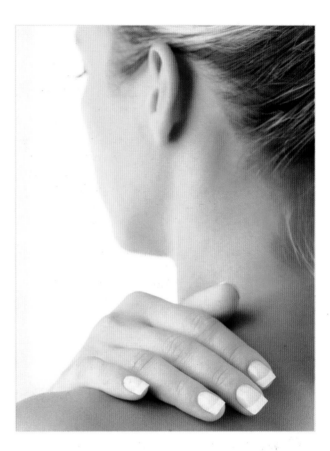

Self-massage with a blend of essential oils can give immediate relief when the shoulders and neck feel tight due to stress.

TYPICAL EFFECTS OF STRESS
- Chronic fatigue, lethargy and loss of interest in leisure activities
- Difficulty in concentrating
- Headaches, stomach disorders
- Muscular tension
- Sleep disruption
- Increased alcohol consumption
- Withdrawal from family and friends
- Irritability
- Loss of sense of humour
- Mounting pessimism
- Feelings of self-doubt

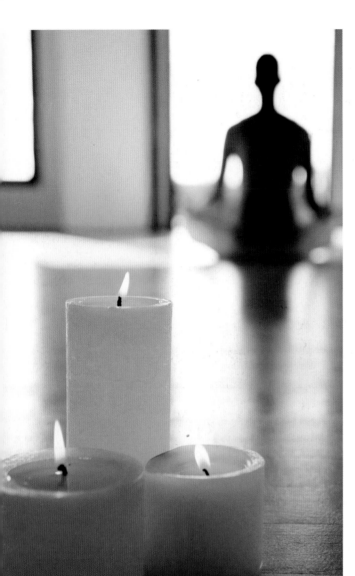

Meditation or quiet time before bed are two of the simple ways to help reduce stress levels. Low lighting and peace and quiet encourage relaxation.

direction relaxes the nerve centres and helps release inner stress. Weekly treatments are very beneficial in arresting the build-up of tensions.

How essential oils can help

Essential oils can have a profound effect, not just on the physical body but on the mental, emotional and spiritual aspects of ourselves too. Essential oils are very powerful allies in the fight against stress, and work both by scent and by absorption.

Choose essential oils for their calming and rebalancing properties, including: bergamot, geranium, chamomile, lavender, marjoram, rose, neroli, orange and petitgrain; vetiver as a bath oil, vetiver is also good for tranquillity, and don't forget pine for the immune system. The Directory of Essential Oils (page 56) gives details of others.

Consultation and advice

With clients suffering from stress, aromatherapists work on a programme to keep them relaxed and to bring them back to a more harmonious way of life. In this way we hope they will learn to cope with the specific forms of stress that affect their lives. Focusing on the individual's appraisal of stress can help the therapist work more effectively.

Consultation is very important, in order to assess, with the client, what the main stresses are. Discussion automatically releases stress, and analysing the situation together often clarifies things in a client's mind. It can also be useful to explain the lasting damage that long-term stress can do.

Aromatherapists are not trained counsellors, but it may be helpful to suggest to your client some of the following simple ways of helping to release or reduce stress levels.

- Indulge in a 'therapeutic evening' once a week, giving time to recharge the batteries: a light meal followed by an aromatic bath, a quiet time listening to music or reading, and an early night
- Regular short breaks from your work, to break the routine, if possible.
- Never to go to bed angry as it works on the subconscious level and has negative repercussions on the whole being
- Meditation
- Music or colour therapy
- Exercise such as yoga or swimming
- Getting in the habit of organizing for the following day, to avoid a sense of last-minute panic
- Sometimes simple touches, such as a herbal tea or deep breathing, can release unwanted tension.

Essential oils and emotional states

Fear	sandalwood, frankincense, cardamom
Guilt	jasmine, ylang ylang, yarrow
Anger	linden blossom, rose, German chamomile
Irritability	ylang ylang, lavender, clary sage, Roman chamomile
Depression	bergamot, mandarin, cardamon, lime
Manic depression	geranium, rose, frankincense
Anxiety	lavender, Roman chamomile, vetiver
Grief	benzoin, rose, sweet marjoram
Confusion	basil, peppermint, rosemary, lavender
Apathy	black pepper, ginger, cardamon, peppermint, lemon
Emotional breakdown	rose, sandalwood, lavender, clary sage
Trauma	neroli, frankincense, cedarwood
Regret	rose, pine, patchouli
Loneliness	benzoin, rose, linden blossom
Rejection	jasmine, grapefruit, black pepper
Argumentativeness	sweet marjoram, lavender, sandalwood, jasmine
Panic attacks	ylang ylang, neroli, frankincense
Repression	jasmine, patchouli, cardamom
Doubt	basil, frankincense, grapefruit
Indecision	lemon, grapefruit, rose
Low self-esteem	bergamot, geranium, neroli, frankincense, ylang ylang
Letting go	yarrow, patchouli, rose
Self-confidence	bergamot, geranium, frankincense, sandalwood, ylang ylang
Physical stress	lavender, chamomile, sweet marjoram, geranium
Pressure at work	neroli, basil. rosemary

Aromatherapy for the elderly

Old age can bring not only physical disabilities and weaknesses encountered with age, such as less acute sight, hearing and mobility, but can also mean having to face bereavement, loss of independence and status and faltering mental acuity. Aromatherapy can help alleviate physical discomforts and, through use of carefully selected essential oils, can lift depression and anxiety, and reduce patterns of restlessness and 'wandering' behaviour.

Osteoarthritis and rheumatoid arthritis

Degenerative joint disease can manifest itself in a number of ways. Osteoarthritis, the most common form of arthritis, is characterized by loss of cartilage and alterations of the subchondral bone. It occurs most frequently as 'wear and tear' (by the age of 65, 80 per cent of people have joints showing signs of osteoarthritis, although only 25 per cent may have symptoms), but it can also be associated with traumatic physical stress, such as surgery, fractures and injuries along joint surfaces, or the strains put on joints by obesity.

Rheumatoid arthritis typically affects the large knuckle joints of the hands as well as the wrists, elbows, knees and feet; it affects the hip joints less often than osteoarthritis does. There is evidence that, rather than relating to physical pressures, rheumatoid arthritis is an auto-immune reaction. Antibodies developing against joint tissue causes an inflammatory response as the body's adaptation to protect itself from a hostile environment. What triggers such a reaction remains largely unknown.

How aromatherapy can help

Detoxifying essential oils such as juniper, cypress, fennel and lemon are essential in helping the body eliminate toxins. They should be used in massage oils and baths.

Analgesic and anti-inflammatory oils such as German chamomile, eucalyptus, ginger, spike lavender, sweet marjoram and rosemary can be used in baths and in local massage and compresses on the affected joints. Local circulation can be stimulated by the use of rubefacient oils such as black pepper, ginger and marjoram.

Osteoarthritic joints are less likely to be inflamed, but the treatment principles using aromatherapy are similar to those that apply to rheumatoid arthritis, perhaps with more emphasis on essential oils with analgesic and rubefacient properties such as black pepper, ginger, lavender, sweet marjoram, rosemary and thyme.

Massage for the elderly must be performed very gently as they are much more vulnerable to pressure and joint injuries.

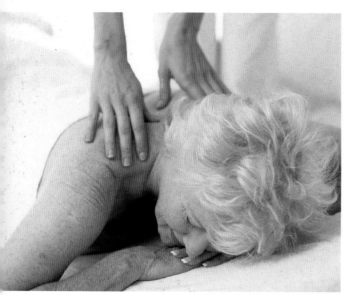

Caution: Whenever heat is applied to a painful stiff joint, it is very important to move the joint as much as possible immediately afterwards, otherwise the heat can cause congestion.

Osteoporosis

Osteoporosis is the wasting away of bone. The size of the bone remains the same but the structure becomes weaker and fragile because the balance between the breakdown of old tissue and the manufacture of replacement material becomes disrupted.

The commonest cause is ageing – all bones suffer this condition when they become old enough. The density of bones is also affected by a diet containing too little calcium or protein, by prolonged immobilization and by hormonal disorders.

Despite the high statistic of osteoporosis in the elderly (one in twelve men over the age of 50 will suffer and one woman in every four over the age of 60 will break a bone), few suffer problematic symptoms unless it occurs in the vertebrae. Severe backache and gradual compression of weakened vertebrae will cause the sufferer to become round-shouldered and shorter in stature. Women are more likely to be affected, due to hormonal changes after the menopause. Osteoporosis shows up mostly when a fall occurs and the weakened bone fractures too easily.

How aromatherapy can help

Many essential oils have analgesic (pain-relieving) properties – see Directory of Essential Oils, pages 56–109 – and one or a blend of these that appeals to the client or patient can prove very soothing.

Regular gentle exercise can help to maintain good bone density and relieve the aches and pains associated with osteoporosis in the elderly.

PREVENTION AND SELF-HELP

There is no treatment to reverse the effects of osteoporosis, but the following can help maintain good bone density:
- a mixed diet rich in calcium and protein (with calcium supplements if necessary)
- regular gentle exercise

Women (who are more prone to thinning bones than men) may benefit from HRT after the menopause. All elderly people should exercise caution to avoid falling, as broken bones will take longer to heal, and fractures will be future points of vulnerability.

WHAT IS DEMENTIA?

Dementia is a condition in which a person's ability to carry out the normal activities required in daily life becomes impaired due to a decline in memory and cognitive ability. A sufferer may also show a decline in emotional control, social behaviour, motivation and/or higher cortical functions. There are different forms of dementia, including Alzheimer's disease and vascular dementia, but in any form the changes in the brain are irreversible.

Dementia can be very frustrating and quite frightening and those afflicted often experience depression, anxiety and emotional distress, which may lead to uncharacteristically aggressive outbursts, and disturbed nights.

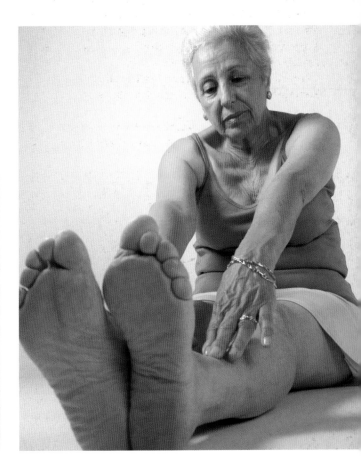

Troubled minds

While the post-retirement years can be a time of serenity after the pressures of a working life, old age can also impose its own forms of stress. Financial worries, loneliness and bereavement can be hard to bear, and those in a residential home may experience boredom with daily routine, loss of personal environment, status and identity, as well as the possible annoyances of communal living.

There is also the threat of dementia. People who have dementia may have very low moods and it is important to be alert in recognizing true depression. Dementia itself cannot be cured, but caring treatment from an empathetic aromatherapist can alleviate many of the problems that accompany it.

Depression is also seen in times of post retirement. It can be mild, moderate or severe and is usually characterized by psychological, physical and social symptoms, for example

Sometimes the simplest treatments are the best. Just holding hands with a patient, singing or humming with them or gentle stroking can be very soothing.

RECOLLECTIONS OF TIMES PAST

There have been some very good projects in various hospitals, one of which worked on the odours of essential oils. Lavender struck an obvious chord as the elderly patients thought of their gardens and of bygone times. Many recalled their grandparents' gardens and chatted happily as they remembered their childhoods. Others talked of making lavender bags and drying stems and 'forking' the flower heads into a bowl. Shoulders that were hunched at the beginning of the session had eased and the patients were fully awake, but relaxed. (The memories attached to different odours is an interesting subject: English lavender worked for the English patients – I wonder what would awaken the memories of those in other countries?)

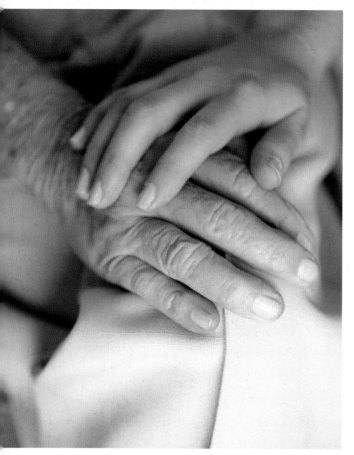

feelings of anxiety, sadness, hopelessness and reduced social activities with loss of contact with friends. The causes are varied and complex, though some triggers include distressing life events such as the death of a family member, physical illness, relationship difficulties and money problems. Many people turn to complementary therapies like aromatherapy for help.

How aromatherapy can help

For clients who would like a short massage this would be the best way to help. If appropriate, you could also provide a blend to add to the bath or for a vaporizer, so that the client could use the blend themselves between treatments. Clients or patients also seem to respond well to gentle stroking, singing/humming or even just holding a hand.

Essential oils in a room diffuser can have a good effect on anxiety – grapefruit or lemon in the morning is refreshing, while clary sage, geranium and lavender used later in the day can help to calm and balance (agitation often increases as the day progresses). Neroli and possibly jasmine are also recommended for anxiety.

Good sleep patterns can also be established, stemming from the relaxation induced by aromatherapy and the use of essential oils. Insomnia may be helped by lavender and marjoram: suggest 1–2 drops on tissues or bedclothes, in an evening bath or applied through massage or stroking.

Bergamot, lavender, neroli and rose are helpful aids to restlessness, and for the restless client who is irritable and has difficulty in sleeping, a good choice would be Roman chamomile, clary sage, lavender, sandalwood and ylang ylang. For fatigue and lethargy, try bergamot, geranium, melissa and rose.

Interestingly, a number of scientific studies have indicated that while depressed individuals have no problem identifying different odours, depression does appear to muffle the sense of smell. But whether or not clients have a reduced sense of smell, their own preferences should be taken into account when selecting oils. This will help to determine a client's changing moods and needs – usually a client's preferences will often be the right choice at that particular time.

In all cases you should take care when selecting the range of oils that the client can choose from: sedative oils may be ideal for those who are anxious, irritable or having difficulty sleeping, but are unlikely to benefit those who are feeling abnormally fatigued or lethargic. For this reason, it is important to establish precisely how depression is affecting the individual.

Rosemary is good for memory loss, but I feel that if there is a possibility of high blood pressure it is a risk. Finding out what kind of music a person likes and listening with them is relaxing and a trip down 'memory lane' in words or song provides moments of dignity and well-being for them.

Some recommended oils for physical symptoms

Before using essential oils, check on any cautions/ contraindications (see Directory of Essential Oils, page 56). If any serious medical symptoms, or if you are in doubt, consult a qualified practitioner. It is advised that only half the normal concentration of essential oils should be used when massaging the elderly, for example 1 per cent blend. Sometimes drops on a pillow or in a vapourizer/burner may be just as beneficial and preferable (it should not be forgotten though that vapourised oils will affect other people present in the room, presenting a problem in a nursing home or similar environment.

*Most widely recommended

Symptom	Recommended oils	How to use
Arthritis, swollen joints	lavender, juniper, marjoram, chamomile, cypress	Bath; compress; massage/rub affected area with massage oil and aloe vera gel
Bruises	*lavender, tea tree	Bath; compress; dab with 1–2 drops on cottonwool
Catarrh	cedarwood, eucalyptus, frankincense, mint, lavender, lemon	Inhalation; bath; compress
Poor circulation	cypress, juniper, lemon, marjoram, orange, *rosemary	Bath; massage/rub with massage oil
Constipation	*marjoram, mint, orange, tangerine, ylang ylang	Bath; massage/rub abdomen clockwise with massage oil
Convalescence	clary sage, neroli	Bath; massage; room fragrance/diffuser
Coughs/colds/flu	cedarwood, myrtle, eucalyptus, marjoram, lemon, lavender	Massage/rub throat and chest with oil; room fragrance

Aromatherapy and cancer

For most people a diagnosis of cancer is a moment of deep psychological crisis and can be the biggest and most daunting challenge they have to face. Aromatherapy, as part of complementary therapy, plays a significant role in relieving physical symptoms as well as alleviating psychological stress, bringing about profound states of relaxation and a sense of peace. Any improvement in a patient's quality of life is valuable.

Complementing medical treatments

Cancer is a very difficult disease to treat – with different outcomes – and the feeling of fear and anxiety that people experience may amplify their symptoms, not only of the side effects of their treatment but also their perception of pain and discomfort. In such situations, people need to relax in a safe and supportive environment, and in this complementary therapies play an important role. They can empower people to take control of their situation, enabling them to cope better with the unfamiliar and with the anxiety their illness provokes. For this reason an increasing number of doctors and hospitals welcome the work of a qualified aromatherapist. An important first

The diagnosis of a cancer leaves people in crisis. Aromatherapy can help with the fear, anger, denial and despair that often comes with the shock.

step, therefore, is to make contact with the oncology team or those in charge of the patient's medical treatment, and gain permission to treat.

When talking to the patient and the medical staff, ascertain which areas of the body it will be appropriate to massage. There is no scientific evidence to prove or disprove the use of massage in cases of cancer: metastatic spread does not occur just because a tumour is touched. However, it is advisable not to massage directly over tumours as the area may be painful. Once this is determined, you will know which areas need to be left out, and so decide on the massage sequence.

Use a light, gentle, non-invasive touch, and keep sessions short. After surgery, patients may not wish to undress fully or after chemotherapy women may not wish to remove their wigs. Remember that you are not treating the cancer but the person as a whole.

Caution: Avoid working on the following areas or conditions:

- directly on stoma sites, dressings and catheters
- areas affected by bony metastases
- limbs/areas affected by lymph oedema unless specifically trained
- on someone who has an infection or if someone is vomiting
- affected areas in cases of deep-vein thrombosis (DVT), phlebitis or varicose veins
- on someone who has heart disease such as unstable angina or other clinical issues
- Please note that patients may need privacy when undressing especially if they have had surgery.

Radiotherapy Avoid areas that are being treated, including entry and exit sites, for the duration of treatment and for about four to six weeks after treatment or while the skin is still sore. Encourage patients to follow the advice given by radiographers on skin care. Be aware of side effects such as digestive disturbances. Fatigue is a common side effect of treatment seldom addressed.

Chemotherapy Although there is no evidence that it is harmful to receive therapies at the same time as chemotherapy it is thought that patients should only be asking their bodies to do one thing at a time. So massage may be performed before a session of chemotherapy but not until at least 24 hours afterwards. If a patient is having continuous chemotherapy of any sort it might be advisable not to have a treatment, although some medical staff think that a drop of essential oil in a carrier applied to the forehead and shoulders could help to uplift a patient's spirits and that could not interfere with the chemotherapy at all.

Be aware of side effects of chemotherapy such as: nausea, vomiting, tiredness, lowered immunity, low blood count (platelets/white blood cells, resulting in increased susceptibility to bruising and infection), dry and peeling skin, digestive disturbances, altered sensation and loss of hair.

Choosing essential oils

Use safe, gentle oils that can be used on children and babies (see page 221), and consider using a 1–2 per cent dilution of essential oils unless otherwise indicated.

Choose oils that are soothing and uplifting, helping with a positive outlook and strengthening the immune system. Be particularly aware of smell and sensitivity – association of certain odours can cause nausea, so it is recommended that only one essential oil be used at this time and to check with the patient that it can be tolerated.

Essential oils recommended for massage may also be added to a cream or lotion if the skin is very dry: aloe vera is recommended, either direct from the plant or in cream form, but test it on the patient first. Do not apply essential oils over damaged skin.

For massage
Lavender, neroli, frankincense, sandalwood, grapefruit, mandarin/tangerine, palmarosa.

For pain
Roman chamomile, sweet marjoram, lavender, neroli. Also clary sage, but not for uterine or ovarian cancer pain. Use only 1 per cent dilution.

Before radiotherapy
Niaoli – this has been recommended in France, but not researched more widely.

For vomiting
Ginger, peppermint, rosewood have been very helpfu, as has melissa.

For fatigue
Grapefruit, neroli, lemon, mandarin.

Caution
- Do not use rosemary, sage or hyssop for cancer patients as these oils have been known to have a neurotoxic effect.
- Do not use oestrogenic-type oils on patients with hormone-related tumours such as breast, ovarian and prostate cancer, especially geranium and sweet fennel.
- Take care with photosensitive oils such as bergamot.

THE AIM OF THE AROMATHERAPIST IN RELATION TO CANCER PATIENTS
- To improve the quality of life
- To help alleviate symptoms
- To aid relaxation
- To ease away tension, stress and anxiety
- To provide comfort and security through the caring touch
- To provide an environment where the patient can talk freely one-to-one in confidence
- To give time and empathy to the patient's need, no matter how long it may take
- To use a holistic approach wherever possible to evaluate the patient's needs
- To allow patients to be at their own level of understanding, whatever it may be and not to judge the situation.
- To provide a pleasant but subtle experience combining the powerful effects of aroma and touch
- To improve the immune system
- To assist with letting go of anger and fear, accepting the facts
- Family support – to help those who are left behind with grief and loss

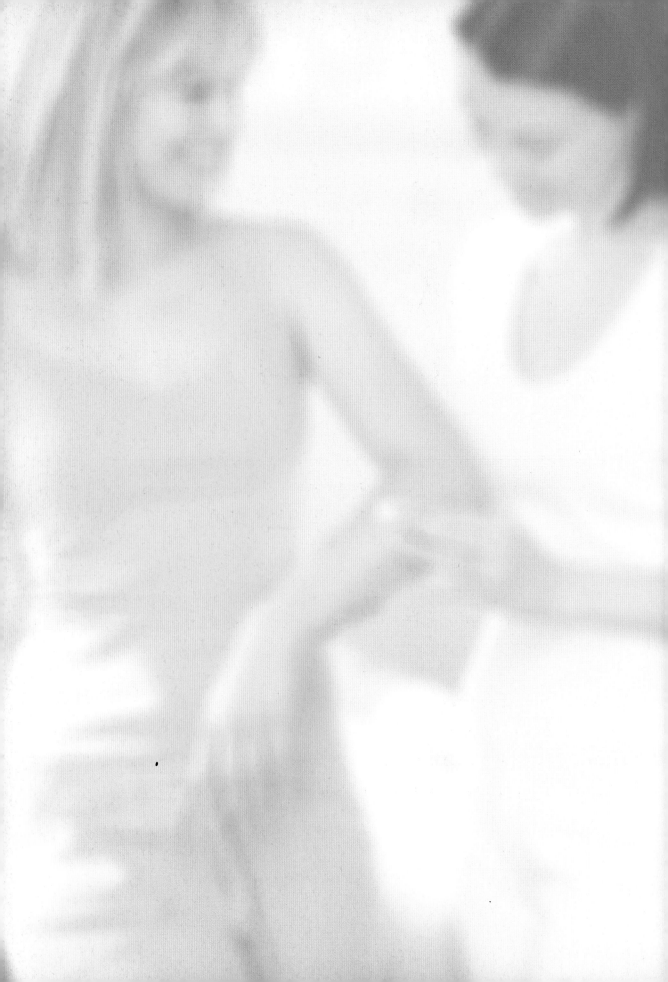

How to become a successful aromatherapist

Having completed your training and qualified as an aromatherapist you are now full of enthusiasm and wanting to get started – but how will you go about it? Gaining a diploma is a beginning, not an end, and there will now be plenty of questions to ask of yourself: about the way you wish to work, with whom and where. Running a business entails planning, budgeting, advertising, record-keeping and many other practicalities, as well as treating clients.

Going into practice 242

Setting up your own clinic 244

Advertising and promotion 246

Maintaining professional standards 248

Going into practice

There are many opportunities for a qualified aromatherapist to practise, and how and where you choose to work will depend on your personal circumstances, your personality and preferences. These may change over time and with experience.

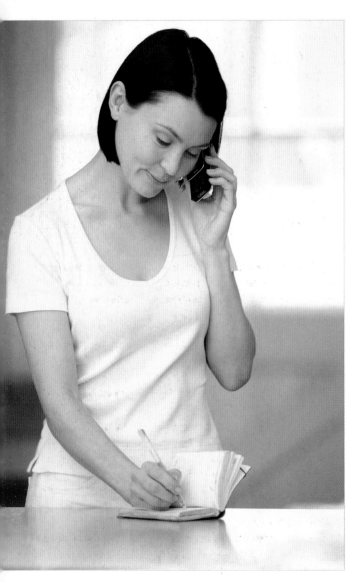

Wherever you work, a good telephone manner is important for booking in clients. An aromatherapist should be friendly, helpful and professional at all times.

The choices available

Aromatherapists work in a variety of different circumstances and settings, including:

- in a room at home
- alongside others in a group practice such as a complementary therapy clinic
- as a mobile therapist, treating clients in their own homes
- self-employed with own premises, perhaps employing others
- within a general medical practice or hospital
- in a health spa/leisure centre or beauty salon.

These are not mutually exclusive options: private practitioners may spend a day a week working in a hospital, or also offer home visits, for example.

Working in a therapy clinic

This can be a good way to start if you feel you might need support. Different clinics are set up in different ways: you might be employed or self-employed, part of a partnership or simply renting a room in shared premises. A clinic will probably have the services of a receptionist for bookings, which can be very helpful, and colleagues may be able to cover for each other in case of illness or other emergency.

When making enquiries at possible local clinics, ask about the set-up, what kind of clients they attract, and how independent you would be: for example, would you be able to advertise yourself, and to what degree would you be able to set your own hours?

Working in a hospital or doctor's surgery

This can also include hospices and homes for the elderly. It is usually preferable to have some experience before working of this type of setting, although an aromatherapist with a nursing or medical background would be more comfortable with patients from the outset. Some hospitals welcome volunteers who offer treatments, although there is still an amount of paperwork to go through before they are accepted. You would need to decide which area you are interested in and find out the name and position of the appropriate person to contact.

Setting up on your own

Aromatherapy is well suited to self-employment, but setting up your own clinic may seem quite daunting (see page 244). An alternative is to work from your own home or to visit clients in theirs.

Working from home

Quite a significant number of therapists work at home. If there is a suitable room that can be used for treatment it is not such a challenge as running a separate premises, and can often fit round your lifestyle – but it can be lonely as there is no other person to discuss any special needs of the client. Being self-employed means you will be responsible for outgoings, health and safety and taxes. You will also need to take into account:

- professional equipment, including a couch and sufficient supply of towels etc (see page 245)
- any need for special planning permission or licence to run a business from your home
- insurance
- an answerphone
- no distractions such as children or barking dogs.

Home visiting

If you plan to do home visits, you will also need to equip yourself with a portable couch, which may be quite bulky, and be well organized to ensure you have everything you need with you. You will also need to consider how far you are prepared to travel – this may depend on the area in which you live and the number of other therapists working locally – and how to charge for travelling costs and time. If possible, it is a good idea to try to book several clients in the same area, to minimize a lot of journeys to and fro.

A variation to consider is to visit people not in their own homes, but in their place of work. Providing 'on-site' massage or treatment is gaining in popularity and workers who are sitting all day in front of a computer screen, or in a call centre or at a check-out may particularly welcome you. Organizations are increasingly open to such an idea, but you may still need to work hard to sell yourself and your service to employers, and convince them of the benefits to their staff. (A step-by-step sequence for seated, or on-site massage, is shown on page 154.)

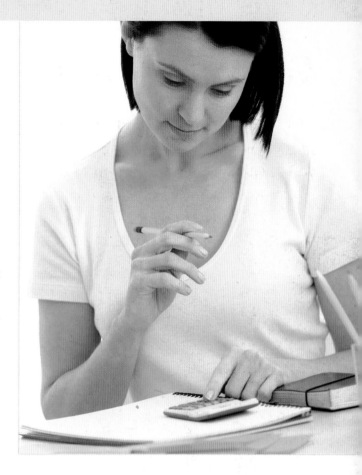

Running your own business means you will have to develop book-keeping and stock control skills. You will also be responsible for the health and safety of your clients.

Before committing to a particular course of action, first ask yourself some questions:

- Can you work anywhere, or are you tied to the home or a certain locality?
- Do you want to work full-time, or will you wish to fit your practice around other commitments, such as family or further study?
- Are you prepared to run your own business?
- Do you like the buzz of a community atmosphere or do you prefer to work alone?
- Does your main interest lie in working alongside medical professionals, or as part of the world of health and beauty? (You may not yet have sufficient experience to answer this.)

There are no right or wrong answers to these questions, but it is important that you consider honestly what is likely to suit you best before embarking on your chosen route into aromatherapy practice.

Setting up your own clinic

This can be an exciting prospect, but involves much planning and decision-making. You will, among other things, need to find yourself premises, buy equipment and advertise your services.

Researching and assessing the market

Setting up in a neighbourhood already over-supplied with aromatherapists will make it difficult to attract clients, but so will introducing aromatherapy to an area that has no experience at all of complementary therapies. Research your catchment area, find out what competition there is, what other complementary therapies are on offer and the type of clients you are likely to attract. Remember that medical centres, hospitals and offices all hold potential clients.

Once you have assured yourself of the viability of setting up an aromatherapy clinic, and perhaps inspected possible premises, draw up a business plan. Discuss your plans with a friendly bank manager and/or accountant, who should be able to advise and help. Remember to add information on your training and qualifications together with some idea of your charges or a comparison with a competitor's charges.

The right premises

Although it is important for your business that you are easy to reach, the location needs to be quiet enough for a peaceful treatment and that means eliminating all distracting noise. Check out car parking facilities and restrictions and also accessibility by public transport. Suitable premises need not be large, but the treatment room should be spacious enough to accommodate:

- a couch with enough space around it for you to move freely
- a stool or chair for yourself
- a trolley for oils, towels and accessories
- a chair for the client, and probably a table, so that you can both sit comfortably and you can take notes during a consultation.

In addition, there should be toilet facilities nearby, and also a wash basin with hot and cold water, ideally in the treatment room, for you to use during treatment.

Make a floor plan, working out carefully where the electric and plumbing points are or need to be. It is unlikely everything will be just as you require it, so get estimates for all work, including decoration, alterations and floor coverings.

Set-up costs	Running costs
adapting and decorating premises	rental of premises
furniture and equipment (see page opposite)	restocking of supplies
initial supplies (see page opposite)	insurance (of premises and professional liability)
advertising/promotion	utility bills (heating, water, lighting, telephone)
	possibly: travel cleaning and/or laundry receptionist/administrative help

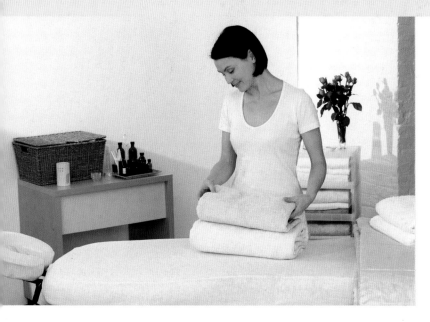

The ambience of your own clinic needs to be welcoming, professional and friendly and be fully equipped for all treatments and for all heath and safety issues that may arise.

The right ambience

The clinic should reflect the professional services you are offering. It should convey comfort and relaxation from the moment the client walks in the door. Whether you are working from home or separate premises, the following need to be right:

Colour and lighting Choose a soothing colour scheme, and avoid glaring white for the ceiling (remember the client will be looking up at the ceiling for part of the treatment). Also avoid direct overhead lighting – soft, natural or naturalistic light is preferable.

Temperature The room should be not too hot or too cold. Heating is easy to adjust, but think also about how it may need to be cooled in hot weather: open windows may let in too much noise and air-conditioning can be noisy. The room should also be well ventilated, but of course draught-free.

Sound Soothing, soft music is optional but most therapists feel it is helpful for relaxation; be aware, however, that some clients would prefer not to have background music. Soft carpeting provides a touch of luxury and helps muffle sounds but may not be practical.

Insurance

This is essential for any business and for yourself. The premises itself needs to be insured, and you will also need insurance for yourself and your clients. Being a member of a professional organization will give you access to advice on choosing not only professional indemnity insurance but other types of cover to suit your individual circumstances.

AN EQUIPMENT CHECKLIST

- massage couch – firm, comfortable with a 'face hole'
- couch stool or chair
- client chair
- trolley or small table – with drawer, if possible
- wardrobe or hooks for outdoor clothes
- small footstool, to assist clients ascending the couch
- towels and sheets
- blankets
- pillows
- paper couch roll (if used)
- essential oils
- carrier oils
- glass measuring cylinder
- glass bowls for mixing
- glass stirrers
- cottonwool
- facial tissues
- testing strips
- sanitizing agent
- cleanser and floral toner
- dark glass bottles to hold blended mixtures
- labels

Advertising and promotion

Some people enjoy the work of attracting clients, others avoid it and just hope that the custom will come to them. But for your business to get off the ground it is important to get your name known by advertising your services, however informally.

Business cards and leaflets

A printed business card may simply give your name, qualifications and contact details. You may want to give your business a name, or like to include a phrase that conveys the service you are offering – perhaps something like: 'Relax, rebalance and re-energize yourself'.

A leaflet or brochure that describes your services, perhaps including a price list, is not expensive to have printed. Have it produced in the same colours and design as your card.

Advertising

Advertising space, even in a local newspaper or magazine, can be expensive, so choose your publication carefully, to reach the most potential clients. You might also include a special offer, giving, say, 10 per cent off the first treatment. An alternative to buying space is to invite a journalist to visit your clinic for a complementary treatment which, hopefully, will lead to a free write-up.

Other, less expensive ways to advertise include placing a carefully worded card in local shops or placing flyers on car windscreens.

Networking

Invite some friends and business associates to a 'wine and snacks' evening. Hand out some brochures or price lists and suggest they might like to recommend you to others even if they do not take up your offer themselves – word of mouth is a powerful way of spreading the word about your business.

Depending on the market you are targeting you could approach leisure centres, health and golf clubs or local pharmacies, doctors' surgeries and libraries.

Spreading the word

One step up from networking is giving a talk, and there are many organizations that would be pleased to invite you, from charities and luncheon clubs to women's guilds and local social clubs. A small informal group is a good way to start, and then you can progress to larger groups as you gain confidence.

It can be daunting at first if you are not used to talking in front of an audience, but for aromatherapists there is help at hand in the form of the essential oils themselves. After a short introduction about yourself, you could say a little about the history of aromatherapy, explain what essential oils are and then encourage some audience participation. Take along with you a few popular essential oils and put a drop of an oil on some appropriately labelled strips, You can then pass these around while talking about that particular essential oil and the ways it may be used. Your audience will enjoy comparing the different aromas and it will bring alive your descriptions. Visual aids such as charts or pictures of the plants you are talking about also help make a talk interesting and memorable.

A card with headings giving the framework for your talk is a useful prompt, but never read from a script. Rehearse what you are going to say at home, with a timer, don't forget to smile, and remember to give time for a question-and-answer session at the end.

Subliminal promotion

Clients can initially be attracted by advertising, but their wish to return and to recommend you to others will depend on the impressions they take away with them. Of course your professional and empathetic treatment is key, but it is often easy to overlook little things that send out subliminal positive or negative messages: warmed, fluffy towels add a touch of pampered luxury, whereas dog-eared magazines or leaflets make a place feel run-down.

If you have a receptionist, or share one in a group practice, never forget that this person is the first point of contact your clients: a friendly smile and voice is the most important part of your business besides the actual treatment. A receptionist can also help enormously in the smooth running of the business, by:

- making and keeping track of appointment book
- taking charge of stock control (see page 245)
- ensuring the reception area is kept fresh, tidy and welcoming.

FIRST IMPRESSIONS

First impressions really count, so if the premises has
a reception area, it is important that it should appear
inviting, and present an atmosphere in which clients
feel they can relax before their treatment even begins.
Comfortable seating, a selection of magazines and fresh
flowers all contribute the right ambience. An essential
oil diffuser is a nice touch, but only if its fragrance does
not reach the treatment room, where it would interfere
with aromas of oils being used for treatment.

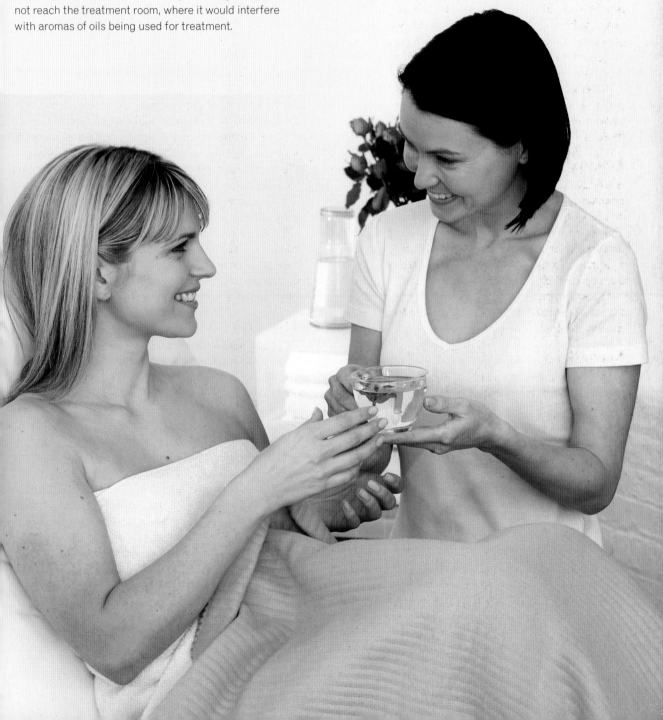

Maintaining professional standards

Professionalism should inform all areas of an aromatherapy practice, from practical niceties such as clean linen and punctuality, to a regard for a client's right to privacy and keeping your financial affairs in order.

Client records

A complete and accurate record of all consultations, including telephone calls, and treatments for each client is a must. How to do this is covered in Chapter Five (see page 110). This is a continuous process, not just paperwork to be completed on the first visit. Reaffirm past details and assess new information at each treatment. These records are a mark of professionalism; they help you make the right decisions on a treatment plan and, if necessary, are the best protection against complaints.

Show consideration and sensitivity whenever asking a client questions and ensure that the information is kept confidential – leaving record cards out and in view of others is not good practice.

Keeping accounts

Whether you are self-employed or in a partnership it is necessary to keep a detailed record of all financial transactions. You will need to keep a note of all your income and expenditures: receipts, invoices, bank statements, the appointment diary all form part of the records of your business.

Take professional advice in the early stages of setting up a business: a qualified accountant will be able to advise you on such things as tax allowances as well as prepare your annual accounts.

Routine maintenance

Supplies should be checked frequently to ensure they are in proper condition and not running low. Essential oils should be selected and ready before the client enters the room.

The facilities and equipment you use must be checked regularly to ensure they are in proper condition. Passageways must be kept clear, surfaces and linens kept clean and equipment checked against failure and safety. You are required to do all you can to eliminate the possibility of causing injury to yourself or a client.

HEALTH AND SAFETY

Ensure that your premises comply with all current health, safety and hygiene legislation – this can vary from country to country and from one year to the next.

FIRE SAFETY

- Be aware of evacuation procedures.
- Establish a policy regarding the use of open flames with candles, incense and so on.

FIRST AID

- Keep a maintained first aid kit on the premises
- Ensure the first aid kit is located in a prominent position
- Be well-trained in first aid techniques
- Keep emergency information and contact numbers posted in view near all telephones.

Professional ethics

Professional organizations set high standards which cover the way therapists conduct themselves and their relationship both with clients and with other professionals. These include both practical and ethical codes of practice.

Boundary rules between therapist and client

- Never abuse the relationship between therapist and client.
- Act in a cooperative manner with other healthcare professionals.
- Find out why a client is seeking treatment and their expectations.

- Explain the treatment and discuss any fees involved with the client before any treatment commences.
- Respect client confidentiality: never disclose client information without the prior written permission of the client, except when required to do so by law, and always ask a client's permission if you need to consult the doctor before or after giving a treatment.
- Never diagnose a medical condition and never claim to cure or give unqualified advice.
- Be aware that clients may be demanding, uncooperative, over-emotional or hypochondriac.
- Always conduct yourself in a professional manner and be courteous and respectful to a client at all times.
- Treating anyone suffering from a medical condition should be done with reference to the medical professionals involved. It is appropriate to ask clients receiving medical care to give written confirmation that they are willing to have a treatment.
- Ensure that any advertising represents the business in the most professional manner.
- Set certain work hours and let those hours be known to all your clients.
- If a client calls with an emergency problem, be flexible enough to understand and change the booking time if possible and not to charge.
- Separate your social life from your work life.

Personal safety

- When lifting equipment or clients, use proper body mechanics and lifting techniques to prevent injury.
- Know the location of the first aid kit and maintain a current first aid certification
- Wash hands before and after every treatment.
- Know the precautions and contraindications for aromatherapy and work within your scope of practice.

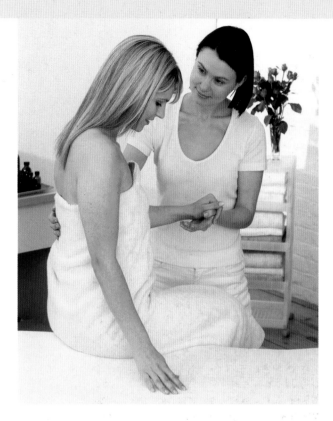

Helping the client on and off the massage couch not only ensures their safety but also shows a caring attitude.

Client safety

- Provide safe, clear entryways and passages and keep these well lit.
- Assist clients on and off the massage couch if needed.
- Check clients are not sensitive or allergic to certain products.
- Do not practise massage if you are ill or contagious.
- Avoid open wounds and sores.
- Use proper procedures in dealing with illness and injury. Refer to the proper medical authorities when such conditions arise.

Continuing professional development (CPD)

For further training and CPD points required by your professional body there are often good opportunities to build and extend your knowledge and expertise by attending seminars and conferences. There are also training congresses covering subjects such as manual lymphatic drainage, ayurvedic diagnosis, the Bowen technique and seated acupressure massage. All these combine well with aromatherapy and during these seminars and conferences there is a good opportunity to mix with other therapists, make new friends and exchange ideas.

RETAILING

Many aromatherapists are going into the market of selling essential oil blends, their own specially made cosmetics and other aromatic delights. There is a distinction drawn between selling to clients as part of their treatment and selling to the public. Products sold to the public are subject to various regulations that have become increasingly complex since labelling and legislation has come into force, and which vary from country to country.

Index

A

abdominal massage 143–4
absolutes 42
accidental swallowing of essential oils 109
Achillea millefolium (yarrow) 58, 61
acid mantle 166
acids 22
acne 16, 169
ACTH (adrenocorticotriphic hormone) 196
acupressure 114, 116
Addison's disease 198
adenoids 182
ADH (anti-diuretic hormone) 196
ADHD (attention deficit hyperactive disorder) 16
adipose tissue 113, 163
adrenal glands 198
adulterated oils 45
advertising 246
age and aromatherapy massage 121
AIDS (Acquired Immune Deficiency Syndrome) 182
alcohol 121
maceration in 43
alcohols in essential oils 22
aldehydes 22, 23
alimentary canal 190, 191
allergic reactions 172
almond 30, 47, 214
Alzheimer's disease 14, 235
amenorrhoea 203
anabolism 161
anaemia 178
anal canal 190, 191
ancient world 10, 112
androgens 199
anethol 23
aniseed oil 23
Anonaceae plant family 60
anorexia nervosa 188
anti-inflammatories 209, 234
anti-rheumatics 209
antidepressants 189

antiseptic oils 12, 14, 173
antispasmodics 173, 193, 203
antiviral oils 173
anxiety 150, 188
in childbirth 219
and tension headaches 189
Apiaceae 30
Apiaceae (Umbelliferae) plant family 60
appendicular skeleton 208
apricot kernal oil 25
Arcier, Micheline 13, 105, 116, 188
massage technique 117, 118
areolar tissue 163
arms, massaging 129
aromas, describing 51
aromatherapy massage
abdominal massage 143–4
aims of 117
arms 129
for babies 220–5
back 129
building a case history 119
buttocks 127–8
and cancer 238–9
carrier oils 46
cleansing 122
complete step-by-step treatment 122–47
opening sequences 123
polarity therapy 134
preparation 122
consultation notes 119–20
creating the right environment 118
end of treatment 147
essential oils
applying 122
dilutions of 108
measures of 54
record of 148
evaluation and aftercare 148–9
face 136–7, 136–9
feedback from clients 149

feet 145–7
focusing on the client 118
hands 142
head 124–5, 135
hips 127–7
in labour 219
legs 132–3, 145–6
backs of 132–3
the Long Journey 141
Micheline Arcier technique 117, 118
neck 124–5, 130–1, 140–1
precautions and contraindications 121
professional image 117
providing 116–18
scalp 125, 135
seated massage 115, 154–7
setting up your own clinic 244–7
shoulders 130–1
solar plexus point 133
for stress relief 231–2
talking to clients 118
aromatic rings 21
arteries 176, 177
arthritis 63, 150, 151, 209, 234
Asteraceae (Compositae) plant family 60
asthma 16, 152, 172
astringents 179
athlete's foot 168
Atlas cedarwood 21, 65
atoms 20–1
autonomic nervous system 116, 186
Avicenna 12, 112
avocado oil 25, 46, 47
axial skeleton 208
ayurvedic massage 115
ayurvedic medicine 10, 107
Aztecs 12

B

babies 220–5
aromatherapy massage for 220–5
safety guidelines and essentials oils 108
skin 220

back massage 129
back pain 208
in pregnancy and childbirth 214, 218
ball and socket joints 207
base notes 50
basic fixed oils 46
basil 23, 92, 189, 233
Bath House of the Four Winds 11
baths
children's baths 150
essential oils in 35, 150
safety guidelines 108, 109
foot baths 151
lavender baths after childbirth 219
beauty treatments 14
benefits of aromatherapy 16–17
benzoic acid 22
benzoin 42, 103, 233
bergamot 71, 233
expression of 44
bergaptene 23
bile 192
bitter orange 58, 68
black pepper 25, 96, 211, 233
bladder 194
blending essential oils 50–5, 59
carrier oils 52, 53
discovering notes 50
formulating a blend 52
Joanna Hoare method of 51–3
mixing a blend 54
sample blends 53
synergy 50
blood 175–6
blood flow through the heart 174–5
blood pressure 174
hypertension 178
in pregnancy 217
blood sugar levels 230
body systems 158–211
body temperature regulation 166
bone structure 206
Book of Healing (Avicenna) 12
borage (starflower) oil 49

Boswellia carteri (frankincense) 10, 63
bracts 25
brain 184–5
brain stem 185
Brazilian rosewood 62
breastfeeding 219
breasts 202, 216
bronchitis 16, 172
burns 12–13, 17
Bursera glabrifolia (linaloe) 62
Burseraceae plant family 60
business cards/leaflets 246
buttocks, massaging 127–8
buying carrier oils 46
buying essential oils 45

C

cabbage rose 12, 98, 99
calamine lotion 152
calendula oil 46, 47
camelina oil 49
camphor 41
Canaga odorata (ylang ylang) 21, 41, 64, 221, 233
cancellous bone 206
cancer 16, 121, 229, 231, 238–9
Canon of Medicine (Avicenna) 12, 112
capilliaries 176
capitate hairs (plants) 30
carbon 20, 21
carbon dioxide extraction 42–3
cardamom 215, 233
cardiac cycle 175
carminatives 193
carpal tunnel syndrome 188
carrier oils 46–9
for babies 221
blending with essential oils 52, 53
nut-based 53
for pregnant women 214
purchasing and storing 46
types of 46
carrot oil 46, 49

cartilaginous joints 208
caryophyllene 21
case notes, taking 119
cassia oil 45
castor oil 49
catabolism 161
Cayola, Dr Renato 13
cedarwood 21, 65, 233
Cedrus atlantica (Atlas
    cedarwood) 21, 65
cells (body systems)
    160–1
cells (plants) 24, 30
    distillation 40
centrioles 160
cerebellum 185
cerebral palsy 188
cerebrum 184–5
challenging behaviour
    227
chamomile
    German 87, 233
    Roman 66, 193, 211,
        218, 233
chemotherapy 121, 238,
    239
chemotypes 31
Chen Nang 10
cherry kernal oil 49
chest massage 140–1
childbirth 218–19
children and essential
    oils 108, 150
Chinese medicine 10,
    86, 134
chlorophyll 24, 26
cholagogues 193
chromosomes 161
Cinnamomum camphora
    (Howood leaf) 62
cinnamon 30
circulatory system
    174–9
    beneficial effects of
        massage 113
    blood 175–6
    cardiac cycle 175
    disorders 178–9
    essential oils 179
        bitter orange 68
        black pepper 96
        clary sage 101
        coriander 77
        cypress 78
        eucalyptus 81
        geranium 94
        German chamomile
            87
        ginger 107
        grapefruit 73
        juniper berry 84

lavender 85
lemon 72
lemon balm 90
lemongrass 79
lime 67
may chang 86
myrrh 76
neroli 69
patchouli 97
peppermint 91
pine 95
Roman chamomile
    66
rose 99
rosemary 100
sweet fennel 82
sweet marjoram 93
sweet orange 75
thyme 104
yarrow 61
ylang ylang 64
heart 174–5
    problems 121, 150
    and stress 231
citrus fruits, expression
    of 44
clary sage 101, 203, 211,
    233
    in childbirth 218
classical world 10
cleansers 152
clients
    consultation notes
        119–20
    evaluation and
        aftercare 148–9
    with existing medical
        conditions 121
    feedback 149
    focusing on 118
    with learning
        difficulties 226–8
    professional ethics
        248–9
    records of 248
    talking to 118
clinical studies 14
clinics
    setting up your own
        244–7
    working in therapy
        clinics 242
cocoa butter 49
coconut oil 48
cohabation 41
cold compresses 151
colds 150
collagen 165
comminution 40
Commiphora myrrha
    (myrrh) 76

compact bone 206
complementary
    medicine 14, 16–17
    and aromatherapy
        massage 121
    and cancer 238
compresses 151
Concerning Odours
    (Hippocrates) 10
concrete 42
condyloid joints 207
confidentiality 249
conifers 30
connective tissue 163
constipation 150
    in pregnancy 215
consultation notes
    119–20
continuing professional
    development (CPD)
    249
coriander 30, 77
corn oil 49
coughs 150
coumarins 23
covalent bonds (atoms)
    21
CPD (continuing
    professional
    development) 249
Culpepper, Nicholas 98
    Complete Herbal 12
Cupressaceae plant
    family 60
Cushings syndrome 198
Cymbopogon citrates
    (lemongrass) 22, 79
Cymbopogon martini
    (palmarosa) 80, 98
cypress 78
cystitis 16, 150
cytoplasm 30, 160, 161

D
Damask rose 41, 98, 99
De Materia Medica
    (Pedanius Dioscorides)
    10
degenerative nerve
    diseases 188
dementia 14, 235, 236
dendrites 185
depression 150, 188
    postnatal 219
depuratives 209
dermatitis 150
dermis 164, 165
detox 183
diabetes 198
    clients with 121
diastole cycle 175

diet 17, 204
digestive system 190–3
    accessory organs 192
    disorders 193
    essential oils
        basil 92
        bergamot 71
        bitter orange 68
        black pepper 96
        clary sage 101
        coriander 77
        German chamomile
            87
        ginger 107
        grapefruit 73
        lemon 72
        lemon balm 90
        lemongrass 79
        lime 67
        mandarin 74
        myrrh 76
        neroli 69
        palmarosa 80
        peppermint 91
        peppermint oil 14
        Roman chamomile
            66
        rose 99
        rosemary 100
        sandalwood 102
        sweet fennel 82
        sweet orange 75
        thyme 104
        yarrow 61
    in pregnancy 214
distillation 12, 21, 40–2
diterpenes 21
drugs
    medicinal 121
    recreational 121
dry skin 168
dysmenorrhoea 203

E
eczema 16, 49, 150, 168
effleurage (stroking)
    113, 114, 116
Egyptians 10, 11, 65
elastin 165
elderly people 234–7
electrons 20, 21
emmenagogue 203
emotional states, and
    essential oils 233
emphysema 172
endocrine system 196–9
    essential oils to
        benefit 83, 94, 99, 101
    pituitary gland 196
endometriosis 199, 203,
    204

endoplasmic reticulum
    160
enfleurage 44
enzymes 185
epidermis 34–5, 164, 165,
    167
epiglottis 170
epilepsy 16
    treating clients with
        121
epithelial tissue
    (epithelium) 162
equipment, setting up
    your own clinic 245
erythrocytes (red blood
    cells) 175
essential oils
    accidental swallowing
        of 109
    acne 169
    adding to bathwater
        35
    anorexia nervosa 188
    antibacterial 12, 14
    antiseptic 12, 14, 173
    antispasmodic 173,
        193, 203
    anxiety and tension
        headaches 189
    application to the skin
        17
    for babies 221
    back pain 208
    in baths 35, 108, 109,
        150
    blending 50–5, 59
    buying 45
    cancer patients 239
    chemical composition
        of 21
    in childbirth 218
    choosing and using
        36–53
    and complementary
        medicine 14
    detox 183
    dilutions 108
    directory of 56–109
        classification 58
        nature of 59
        distillation 12, 21,
            40–2
    eczema 168
    elderly people and
        236–7
    emphysema 172
    endometriosis 199,
        203, 204
    extraction 40–4
    for high stress levels
        179

home treatments
150–3
and homeopathic
remedies 14
hormonal imbalances
199
hypertension 178
irritable bowel
syndrome 193
learning difficulties
228
lymphatic system
183
massage
applying 122
dilutions of 108
measures of 54
record of 148
muscular pain 53, 211
pioneers of
aromatherapy 12–13
in pregnancy 108,
215–17
research studies of 14
retailing 249
safety guidelines
108–9
science of 18–35
seeds for
aromatherapy 25
sinusitis 173
skeletal disorders 209
solvent extraction 42
and stress relief 232,
233
undiluted 17
unsafe for general use
109
unsuitable for home
use 109
urinary system 195
see also carrier oils
esters 22–3
ethics, professional
248–9
eucalyptus 16, 22, 23, 81,
151
baby massage 221
eugenol 23
evening primrose oil
48
existing medical
conditions 121
expectorants 173
expression of citrus
fruits 44
extraction of essential
oils 40–4
extracts 42
eye irritation and
essential oils 109

F
face
facial steaming 152
massage 54, 136–9
Fallopian tubes 201
families of plants 27, 60
feet *see* foot massage
female reproductive
system 200, 201–4
fennel 30, 82
fevers 121
fibrocytes 163
fibroids 203
fibrous joints 208
fire safety 248
first aid 109, 248
fixed oils 46, 49
flaxseed (linseed) oil 49
floral waters 41
flowers
distillation 40
Lamiaceae family 27
reproduction 25
fluid retention 53, 150,
195
Foeniculum vulgare
(sweet fennel) 30, 82,
199
foot baths 151
foot massage 145–7
sanitizing 122
solar plexus point 133
fractional distillation 41
frankincense 10, 63, 168,
233
baby massage 221
in childbirth 218
fruits 25
distillation 40
fucocoumarins 23

G
Galen 10
gall bladder 192
ganglia (reflex points)
116
Garri, Dr Giovanni 13
Gattefossé,
René-Maurice 9, 12–13
genera (plants) 27
genital organs
female 201
male 205
genito-urinary system
essential oils
Atlas cedarwood 65
basil 92
bergamot 71
clary sage 101
cypress 78
geranium 94

German chamomile
87
juniper berry 84
myrrh 76
niaouli 89
pine 95
Roman chamomile
66
sandalwood 102
sweet fennel 82
sweet marjoram 93
yarrow 61
geranic acid 22
geranium 94, 98, 118,
168, 199, 233
Geriniaceae plant family
60
German chamomile 87,
233
Gesner, Conrad 12
ginger 107, 211, 215, 233
glandular cells 30
gliding joints 207
glucocorticoids 198
golgi body/apparatus
160
gomenol 89
gonadotrophic (sex)
hormones 196
granulocytes 175
grapefruit 73, 215, 233
grapeseed oil 46, 48, 214
Grasse Parfumerie
Museum 40
Graves disease 198
Greeks, ancient 10, 112
growth (somatotrophic)
hormone 196

H
haemorrhoids 219
hair
clary sage 101
glands 167
rosemary 100
yarrow 61
ylang ylang 64
hand massage 14, 142,
226
hand washing, and
massage 116, 122, 147,
228
hazelnut oil 48
head massage 124–5,
135
Indian 115
headaches 150
anxiety and tension
headaches 189
essential oils for
16

healing art,
aromatherapy as
16–17
health and safety *see*
safety
heart 174–5
heart disease 178
helium 20
hepatics 193
Hepatitis B 182
high blood pressure 150
Himalayan cedarwood
65
hinge joints 207
Hippocrates 10, 112
hips, massaging 127–7
history of aromatherapy
10–13
holistic medicine 14
home treatments 150–3
home visiting 243
home, working from 243
homeopathy 14
homeostasis 195
hormonal imbalances
199
hormones 196–9
pregnancy 214
and essential oils
217
hospital work 242–3
hot compresses 151
hot stone massage 115
Howood leaf 62
HRT (hormone
replacement therapy)
202
hyaline cartilage 163
hydro-massage 115
hydrocarbon extraction
43
hydrocotyle oil 49
hydrodiffusion 41
hydrogen 20, 21
hydrosols 41
hydrothermic massage
115
hypericum (St John's
wort) 49
hypersecretion 198
hypertension 178
hypertensives 179
hyperthermia 23
hyperthyroidism 121
hypotensives 179

I
immune response 182
immune system
essential oils 182–4
benzoin 103

bitter orange 68
Brazilian rosewood
62
juniper berry 84
lemon balm 90
niaouli 89
peppermint 91
pine 95
sweet orange 75
tea tree 88
immunization 121
immunostimulants 173
incense 10, 63
India 10
Indian head massage 115
indigestion 150
in pregnancy 215
Indus Valley civilization
13
inhalation of essential
oils 152
insect bites and stings
153
insect repellent 153
insomnia 150
in pregnancy 216
insulin 198
insurance 245
integral biology 16
intervertebral discs 208
intestines 190, 191
irritable bowel
syndrome 193
islets of Langerhans 198
isoprene units 21

J
jasmine 83, 233
in childbirth 218
solvent extraction 42
jet lag 121, 153
joints
essential oils to
benefit 234
clary sage 101
coriander 77
cypress 78
eucalyptus 81
German chamomile
87
ginger 107
juniper berry 84
lavender 85
lemongrass 79
myrrh 76
Roman chamomile
66
rosemary 100
sweet marjoram 93
yarrow 61
synovial 207, 208

ojoba oil 46, 48, 215
uniper berry 84
Juniperus (cedarwood)
  65

K
ketones 22, 23
kidney stones 195
kidneys 194
kukui nut oil 49

L
abour massage 219
actones 23
Lamiaceae (Labiatae)
  plant family 27, 30, 60
Langerhans, islets of
  198
arge intestine 190, 191
Lauraceae plant family
  60
avender 14, 27, 85, 233
  adulterated 45
  baby massage 221
  for burns 12–13, 17
  chemical composition
    21
  in childbirth 218
  memories attached to
    236
  sedative effect of 59
earning difficulties
  226–8
  dementia 14, 235, 236
eaves 24, 25
  distillation 40
egs, massaging 132–3,
  145–6
emon 72, 233
  in childbirth 218
  expression of 44
  for morning sickness
    215
emon balm (melissa) 90
emongrass 79
  aldehydes 22
igaments 208
imbic system 33
ime 49, 67, 233
inaloe (Bursera
  glabrifolia) 62
inden blossom 233
inseed (flaxseed) oil 49
Litsea cubeba (may
  chang) 86
the liver 191, 192
the Long Journey 141
ungs 170, 171
ymph 180
ymph ducts 181
ymph nodes 180–1

lymphatic capilliaries
  180
lymphatic drainage 116,
  140
  the Long Journey 141
lymphatic pressure
  points 114
lymphatic stimulation
  face 139
  feet and legs 146
lymphatic system
  180–1
lymphatic vessels 180
lymphocytes 175
lymphoid tissue 163

M
macadamia nut oil 49
macerated oils 46, 49
maceration 43–4
male reproductive
  system 200, 205
mandarin 74, 218, 221,
  233
manual lymphatic
  drainage (MLD) 115
marjoram, sweet 30, 93,
  211, 233
massage 16, 110–57
  acupressure 114
  ancient Egypt 10
  beneficial effects of
    113
  effleurage (stroking)
    113, 114, 116
  history of 112
  lymphatic pressure
    points 114
  need for 112
  oriental 115
  petrissage
    (compression) 114
  professional image
    117
  Swedish 113, 116
  western 115
  see also aromatherapy
    massage
Maury, Marguerite 13,
  17, 53, 117
may chang 86
meadowsweet oil 49
Medical Aromatherapy
  (Schnaubelt) 41
medicinal drugs 121
meditation 231
meiosis 161
Melaleuca alternifolia
  see tea tree
melanin 167
melatonin 199

melissa (Melissa
  officinalis) 89
membranes 163
memory problems 16,
  236
memory and scent 54
meningitis 16
menopause 16, 202, 204
menstrual cycle 202
menstrual problems 16,
  188, 203
menstrual regulation
  150
Mentha piperita
  (peppermint) 14, 16,
  45, 91
metabolic rate 161
Middle Ages 10–12
middle notes 50
mineralocorticoids 198
mitochondria 160, 161
mitosis 161
mixed neurons 185
moisturizers 152
molecules 21
monocytes 175
monoterpenes 21
morning sickness 215
motor neurons 185
MRSA superbug 14
MSH (melanocyte-
  stimulating hormone)
  196
mucous membranes 163
multiple schlerosis 113
muscoskeletal system
  206–9
muscular pain 53, 211
muscular system
  beneficial effects of
    massage 113
  essential oils
    black pepper 96
    blend for muscle
  pain 53, 211
    clary sage 101
    coriander 77
    cypress 78
    eucalyptus 81
    German chamomile
    87
    ginger 107
    juniper berry 84
    lavender 85
    lemongrass 79
    myrrh 76
    peppermint 91
    Roman chamomile
    66
    rose 99
    rosemary 100

sweet marjoram 93
  yarrow 61
muscle function 211
muscle structure
  210–11
music 245
myrrh 10, 76
Myrtaceae plant family
  27, 60
myrtle 221

N
nails 167
neck massage 124–5,
  130–1, 140–1
neroli 58, 69, 168, 215,
  233
nervine relaxants 189
nervine tonics 189
nervous reflexes 186
nervous system 184–9
  autonomic 186
  the brain 184–5
  clients with
    dysfunctions 121
  disorders 188–9
  essential oils
    Atlas cedarwood 65
    basil 92
    benzoin 103
    bitter orange 68
    black pepper 96
    Brazilian rosewood
    62
    clary sage 101
    coriander 77
    cypress 78
    eucalyptus 81
    frankincense 63
    geranium 94
    German chamomile
    87
    ginger 107
    grapefruit 73
    jasmine 83
    juniper berry 84
    lavender 85
    lemon 72
    lemon balm 90
    lemongrass 79
    lime 67
    mandarin 74
    may chang 86
    neroli 69
    palmarosa 80
    patchouli 97
    peppermint 91
    petitgrain 70
    pine 95
    Roman chamomile
    66

rose 99
rosemary 100
sandalwood 102
sweet marjoram 93
sweet orange 75
thyme 104
vetiver 105
yarrow 61
ylang ylang 64
nervous reflexes 186
neurons 185
peripheral 186
spinal chord 186
networking 246
neurological conditions
  188
neurons (nervous
  system) 185
neutrons 20
niaouli (Melaleuca
  viridiflora) 89
nose
  decongestion 138
  respiratory system
    170, 171
nucleus (atoms) 20, 21
nucleus (cells) 160, 161
nut allergies 53

O
Ocimum basilicum
  (basil) 23, 92, 189,
  233
oesophagus 190
oestoporosis 202
oestrogen 199, 202
oil canals 30
oil cells 30
oil, maceration in 43
oil reservoirs 31
oily skin 168
Oleaceae plant family
  60
olfaction 32–3
on-site (seated)
  massage 115, 154–7,
  243
orders of plants 27
organelles 24, 160
oriental massage 115
Origanum marjorana
  (sweet marjoram)
  30, 93
ossification 206
osteoarthritis 209, 234
osteomalacia 166
osteoporosis 209, 235
ovaries 201, 202
oxides 23
oxygen 20, 21
oxytocin 196

P

palm kernal oil 49
palmarosa 80, 98
palpitations 178
pancreas 192, 199
Paoli, Professor Rovesti 13
Parascelus 12
parathyroid glands 198
passion flower oil 49
patchouli 40, 97, 233
PCOS (polycystic ovary syndrome) 203
peach kernal oil 46
peanut oil 49
Pedanius Dioscorides 10
Pelargonium graveolens see geranium
peltate hairs (plants) 30
Pen Tsao 10
penis 200, 205
peppermint 16, 91, 233
    adulterated 45
    in childbirth 218
    digestive system 14, 193
perianth 25
periosteum 206
peripheral nervous system 186
peritoneum 190
perspiration 166
petitgrain 58, 70, 215
petrissage (compression) 114
pharnyx 190
phenols 23
photosynthesis 24, 26
phytonic process 43
Pinaceae plant family 60
pine 95, 233
pineal gland 199
Pinus sylvestris (pine) 95
pioneers of aromatherapy 12–13
piper nigrum (black pepper) 25, 96, 211
pituitary gland 196
pivot joints 207
plai 58, 106, 211
plants
    anatomy and metabolism 24–6
    classification 27–8
    families 27, 60
    macerated oils from 46
plasma 176

platelets (thrombocytes) 175–6
PMS (pre-menstrual syndrome) 203
Poaceae (*Graminae*) plant family 60
Pogostemon cablin (patchouli) 40, 97
polarity therapy 134
pollination 25
polycystic ovary syndrome 199
pomades 44
pomanders 12
post-operative massages 121
postnatal depression 219
The Practice of Aromatherapy (Valnet) 13
pregnancy 214–17
    and clary sage 203
    constipation 215
    female reproductive system 201, 202
    hormones 214
    indigestion/heartburn 215
    insomnia 216
    and massage 121, 154
    morning sickness 215
    skin rashes 216
    stretchmarks 216
    urinary tract infections 214, 216–17
    use of essential oils during 108, 215–17
preventive medicine 16
primary sense of smell 32
professional ethics 248–9
professional image 117
professional standards 248–9
progesterone 199, 202
promotion 246
prostate gland 205
protons 20
psoriasis 150
psychological disturbance 188
puberty 200, 201

Q

qualified aromatherapists going into practice 242–3

professional standards 248–9
setting up a clinic 244–7

R

radiotherapy 239
ravensara 30, 88, 211
receptionists 246
recreational drugs, and aromatherapy massage 121
red thyme oil 104
redistillation (rectification) 41
reflexology 115
Reiki 118
relaxation techniques 16
reproductive system 83, 200–4
    disorders 203
    female 200, 201–4
    male 200, 205
    puberty 200, 201
research studies 14
resin canals 30
resin cells 30
resinoids 42
respiratory system 170–1
    disorders 172–3
    essential oils
        Atlas cedarwood 65
        basil 92
        benzoin 103
        bergamot 71
        clary sage 101
        cypress 78
        eucalyptus 81
        frankincense 63
        ginger 107
        lavender 85
        lemon 72
        may chang 86
        myrrh 76
        niaouli 89
        peppermint 91
        pine 95
        plai 106
        rosemary 100
        sandalwood 102
        sweet fennel 82
        sweet marjoram 93
        tea tree 88
        thyme 104
    lungs 170, 171
    upper respiratory tract 170, 171
reticular fibres 165
rheumatism 150, 151
rheumatoid arthritis 209, 234

ribosomes 160, 161
rickets 166
Roman chamomile 66, 193, 211, 233
    baby massage 211
    in childbirth 218
Romans 10, 112
room fragrances 108
    sprays 153
    vaporizers and diffusers 153
root systems (plants) 24
Rosaceae plant family 60
rose 218, 233
    absolute (cabbage rose) 12, 98, 99
    otto (damask rose) 41, 98, 99
rosehip oil 49
rosemary 14, 30, 31, 100, 211, 233
    elderly people and 237
    and epilepsy 121
    identifying 51
    ketones 22,
rubifacients 179, 209
Rutaceae plant family 60

S

SAD (seasonal affective disorder) 199
saddle joints 207
safety
    client safety 249
    clients with challenging behaviour 227
    essential oils 108–9
        Atlas cedarwood 65
        basil 92
        benzoin 103
        bergamot 71
        bitter orange 68
        black pepper 96
        Brazilian rosewood 62
        clary sage 101
        coriander 77
        eucalyptus 81
        frankincense 63
        geranium 94
        German chamomile 87
        ginger 107
        grapefruit 73
        jasmine 83
        juniper berry 84
        lavender 85
        lemon 72
        lemon balm 90

lemongrass 79
        lime 67
        mandarin 74
        may chang 86
        myrrh 76
        neroli 69
        niaouli 89
        palmarosa 80
        patchouli 97
        peppermint 91
        petitgrain 70
        pine 95
        plai 106
        in pregnancy 217
        red thyme oil 104
        Roman chamomile 66
        rose 99
        rosemary 100
        sandalwood 102
        sweet fennel 82
        sweet marjoram 93
        sweet orange 75
        tea tree 88
        vetiver 105
        yarrow 61
        ylang ylang 64
    first aid 109
    health and safety 248
    personal safety 249
St John's wort (hypericum) oil 49
Salvia sclarea (clary sage) 101, 203, 211, 218, 233
sandalwood 102, 233
Santalaceae plant family 60
saunas 151
scalp massage 125, 135
Schnaubelt, Dr Kurt 41
sciatica 188
science of essential oils 18–35
    absorption through the skin 34–5
    chemistry basics 20–1
    functional groups 22–3
    oil-producing structures 30
    oil-storage structures 30–1
    plant anatomy and metabolism 24–5
    sense of smell 32–3
seated massage 115, 154–7
sebaceous glands 167
secondary sense of smell 32

The Secret of Life and
   Youth (Maury) 13, 17
seeds 25
selling essential oil
   blends 249
sensory nerve endings
   166
sequiterpenes 21
serous membrane 163
sex corticoids 198
sex glands 199
shampoos 151
shiastu 115
shingles 150
shock 150
shoot systems (plants)
   25
shoulders, massaging
   130–1
showering 151
sinus decongestion 139
sinusitis 172, 173
skeletal muscle 210
skeletal system 206–9
skin 164–7
   babies 220
   beneficial effects of
      massage 113
   dermis 164, 165
   epidermis 34–5, 164,
      165, 167
   and essential oils
      absorption of 34–5
      application of
         undiluted 108
   functions 166
   glands 167
   PH measurement 166
   in pregnancy 214, 216
   structure 164–5
   subcutaneous layer/
      hypodermis 165
skin conditions 16,
   168–9
   essential oils for
      Atlas cedarwood 65
      basil 92
      benzoin 103
      bergamot 71
      bitter orange 68
      black pepper 96
      Brazilian rosewood
         62
      clary sage 101
      cypress 78
      eucalyptus 81
      frankincense 63
      geranium 94
      German chamomile
         87
      grapefruit 73

      jasmine 83
      juniper berry 84
      lavender 85
      lemon 72
      lemon balm 90
      lemongrass 79
      lime 67
      mandarin 74
      may chang 86
      myrrh 76
      neroli 69
      niaouli 89
      palmarosa 80
      patchouli 97
      peppermint 91
      petitgrain 70
      Roman chamomile
         66
      rose 99
      rosemary 100
      sandalwood 102
      sweet marjoram 93
      sweet orange 75
      tea tree 88
      vetiver 105
      yarrow 61
      ylang ylang 64
   essential oils to avoid
      using 108
   treating clients with
      121
skin sensitivity, to
   essential oils 108, 109
sleep 17, 168, 229, 236–7
small intestine 190, 191
smell, sense of 32–3
smooth muscle 210
solar plexus point 133
Solomon, King 10
solvent extraction 42, 43
sore throats 53
specialist fixed oils 46
species (plants) 27
spinal chord 186
spinal curves 207
spine, massaging 126
spleen 182
sports massage 115
starflower (borage) oil
   49
steam distillation 21, 22,
   40–1
stems (plants) 25
stomach 190, 191
stomach ulcers 230
Stone, Dr Randolph 134
storing carrier oils 46
stress 16, 229–33
   alleviating 229
   aromatherapy
      massage for 231–2

   bodily effects of 230–1
   chemistry of 231
   elderly people 236
   essential oils for 179
   and illness 229, 231
   and massage 112
   and nervous system
      disorders 189
   in pregnancy 216
   reactions under
      229–30
   relief 150
   typical effects of 231
   and women 229, 231
stress therapy 115
stretchmarks 216
strokes 179
Styracaceae plant family
   60
Styrax benzoin (benzoin)
   42, 103
subcutaneous
   layer/hypodermis 165
subliminal promotion
   246
sunbed treatments 109
sunburn 121
sunlight 109
sweat glands 167
Swedish massage 113,
   116
sweet almond 30, 47,
   214
sweet fennel 30, 82, 199
sweet marjoram 30, 93,
   211, 233
sweet orange 75, 215,
   221
synergy 50
synovial joints 207, 208
systole cycle 175

T
tamanu oil 49
tea tree 14, 17, 88, 168
   baby massage 211
   hydrolat 122
   hydrosol 41
   inhalation 152
   terpenes 21
tendons 208
terpenes 21
terroir 31
testes 200, 205
Texas cedarwood 65
Thai massage 115
Theophrastus 10
thrombosis (DVT) 121
thuja 22
thujone 22
thyme 23, 104

thymol 23
thymus 182
thyroid gland 121, 198
tinctures 43
tissues (body cells)
   162–3
tissues (plant cells) 24
toners 152
tonics 179
tonsilitis 172
tonsils 182
top notes 50
towels 122
transpiration 26
travel sickness 153
trunks (plants) 25
TSH
   (thyroid-stimulating
      hormone) 196
tui na 115

U
umbellifers 30
urethra 194
urinary incontinence 195
urinary system 194–5
urinary tract infections
   195, 214
   in pregnancy 214,
      216–17
uterine tonics 203
uterus 201

V
vagina 201
Valnet, Dr Jean 13, 117
varicose veins 178
veins 176, 177
verbenone 22
vetiver 105, 233
Vitamin D production
   166
vulva 201

W
walnut oil 49
water distillation 40
water, drinking 183
western massage 115
wheatgerm oil 46, 49
white fibro-cartilage 163
white thyme oil 104
workplaces, on-site
   massage 115, 154–7,
   243
wormwood 22

Y
yarrow 58, 61, 233
yellow fibro-cartilage
   163

yin/yang and polarity
   therapy 134
ylang ylang 64, 233
   baby massage 221
   chemical composition
      21
   fractional distillation
      of 41

Z
zinc oxide cream 152
Zingiber cassumunar
   (plai) 106
Zingiber officinale
   (ginger) 107, 211, 215
Zingibercaceae plant
   family 60
zygotes 161

References and acknowledgements

References and further reading

Arcier, M., *Aromatherapy*, 1990, Hamlyn, London

Ball, J., M.D., *Understanding Disease*, 1990, C.W.Daniel, Saffron Walden

Battaglia, S., *The Complete Guide to Aromatherapy*, 1997, The Perfect Potion (Aust) Pty. Ltd

Botanical Information, Aromatherapy Quarterly, issue 48 – Spring 1996, Scottish Agricultural College

Bowles, E.J., *The Basic Chemistry of Aromatherapeutic Essential Oils*, 2000, E.Joy Bowles, Sydney Australia

Buckle, J., *Clinical Aromatherapy in Nursing*, 1997, Arnold (Hodder Headline Group) London

Davis, P., *Aromatherapy an A–Z*, 1995, C.W.Daniel, Saffron Walden

Fountain Centre, *Cancer Therapy Information*, St.Luke's Cancer Centre, The Royal Surrey County Hospital, Guildford

Gallant, A., *Body Treatments and Dietetics for the Beauty Therapist*, 1978, Stanley Thornes (Publishers) Ltd

Gattefossé, M., (edited by R. Tisserand), *Gattefossé's Aromatherapy*, 1992, C.W.Daniel, Saffron Walden

Johnson, C., *How to Be a Successful Therapist*, 2003, The Book Guild Ltd, Brighton

Lavabre, M., *Aromatherapy Workbook*, 1990, Healing Arts Press, Vermont

Lawless, J., *The Encyclopedia of Essential Oils*, 1992, Element, Shaftesbury

Maury, M., Ryman, D. and Maury, E.A., *Marguerite Maury's Guide to Aromatherapy: The Secret of Life & Youth*, 1990, C.W.Daniel, Saffron Walden

McGuiness, H., *Aromatherapy: Therapy Basics*, 2001, Hodder & Stoughton, London;
Anatomy & Physiology: Therapy Basics, 2002, Hodder & Stoughton, London

McNamara, P., *Massage for People with Cancer*, 1994, Wandsworth Cancer Support Centre, London

Pitman, V., *Aromatherapy: a Practical Approach*, 2004, Nelson Thornes Ltd, Cheltenham

Price, L., with Smith, I. and Price, S., *Carrier Oils for Aromatherapy & Massage*, 1999, Riverhead, Stratford-upon-Avon

Ross and Wilson, *Anatomy & Physiology in Health and Illness*, 1993, Churchill Livingstone, Oxford

Susskind, P., *Perfume: The Story of a Murderer*, 1986, Penguin, London

Tisserand and Balacs, *Essential Oil Safety*, 1995, Churchill Livingstone, London

Valnet, Dr J., *The Practice of Aromatherapy*, 1993, C.W.Daniel, Saffron Walden

Williams, D.G., *The Chemistry of Essential Oils*, 1996, Micelle Press, Weymouth

Worwood, V.A., *The Fragrant Mind*, 1995, Doubleday Transworld Publishers, London

The author would like to thank Sarah Wilson, Journalist, for help in putting together this book. Also thanks to Megan Joyce for computer and 'hands-on' help and for writing the section on helping those with learning difficulties, and to Pauline Allen of the IFA who encouraged me. Thanks to Sue Mousley for writing the Pregnancy and Childbirth section and to Charles and Jan Wells of Essentially Oils of Chipping Norton for allowing me to use their safety data statement. I am grateful to my friend Glenys Bennett, who taught me how to become a little more computer literate, and also for the support of all my good friends, particularly Anne Manning, Sarah Hutchings, Genie Allenby, Pauleen Dowsett and friends at The Fountain Centre, Guildford for their encouragement throughout this project. This book would not have been possible without the pioneers of Aromatherapy from Dr.Jean Valnet to Marguerite Maury but more recently the work of other professionals including my tutor and mentor, the late Micheline Arcier and of Patricia Davis, Julia Lawless, Robert Tisserand, Valerie Anne Worwood, Shirley and Len Price, Pierre Franchomme and Daniel Penoel amongst others

The publisher would like to thank Alternative Products Limited for supplying the Starlight massage table.

Special photography: © Octopus Publishing Group Limited/Ruth Jenkinson.

Other photography: Alamy Adam James 62; Chris Rout 46; flowerphotos 79, 88; Geoffrey Kidd 76; Image Source Black 115l; Interfoto 12; Jupiterimages/Pixland 173; MEPL 13; Natural History Museum 38; Natural Visions 64; Nature PL 69; niceartphoto 40, 44; Organics Image Library 77, 92 101; PhotoAlto 232; Pictopresto 166; RF Company 87; Rob Walls 96; Steffen Hauser 82; Zach Holmes 11. **Ancient Art & Architecture Collection** 11. **Biosphoto** Daniel Barthelemy 103. **Camera Press** Rebecca Lacey 238, Richard Stonehouse 209, Silke Wernet/Laif 183; **Corbis** Allana Wesley White 234; Douglas Peebles 102; Luca Tettoni 216, 226; zefa Value 113. **DK Images** Deni Bown 105. **FLPA** Roger Wilmshurst 78. **Gap Photos** Dianna Jazwinski 24; John Glover 83; Leigh Clapp 100; Mark Bolton 95; Pernilla Bergdahl 30; Rob Whitworth 91; Tim Gainey 59. **Garden Collection** Torie Chugg 104. **Garden World Images** Christopher Fairweather 65. **Getty Images** 200; Fabrice Lerouge 136; David Sieren 97; Kroeger/Gross 106; National Geographic 63; Shinya Sasaki/Neovision 51. **iStockphoto.com** Sondra Paulson 81. **John Glover** 75. **Jupiterimages** Cristina Cassinelli 28; Image Source 112; Nonstock 167; Roy McMahon/Corbis 169; Sally Peterson 236; Sang An 45. **Kenny Fung** 86. **Marianne Majerus Garden Images** Andrew Lawson 93. **Masterfile** 35, 115, 202. **Octopus Publishing Group Limited** 117 Russell Sadur 229; William Reavell 17. **Photolibrary** 27; Arthur 29; Brigitte Thomas 90; Carltons Carltons 68; Chassenet 107; Harley Seaway 89; Juliette Wade 99; Michele Lamontagne 98; Mick Rock/Cephas 31; Purestock 219. **Photoshot** Photos Horticultural 66, 71, 80. **Science Photo Library** Adrian Thomas 70; Crisitna Pedrazzini 15. **Shutterstock** Adam Borkowski 220; Artis Pusilds 84; Blaz Kure 67; Carme Balcells 235; Danilo Ascione 72; Fred Sgrosso 73; iofoto 94; Iryna Shpulak 179; Liv Friis-Larsen 231; Natalia Bratslavsky 85; Nicholas Rjabow 74; photosib com 47l, Sergey Chushkin 48 61; Stuart Taylor 47r.

Executive Editor Jessica Cowie
Senior Editor Lisa John
Executive Art Editor Darren Southern
Designer Geoff Borin
Illustrators Susan Tyler, Kate Nardoni and Sudden Impact Media Ltd
Picture Researcher Ciaran O'Reilly
Production Controller Marián Sumega